FACING ADDICTION IN AMERICA

The Surgeon General's Report on Alcohol, Drugs, and Health

2016
U.S. Department of Health & Human Services

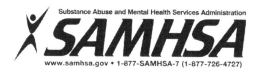

Suggested Citation

U.S. Department of Health and Human Services (HHS), Office of the Surgeon General, *Facing Addiction in America: The Surgeon General's Report on Alcohol, Drugs, and Health.* Washington, DC: HHS, November 2016.

For More Information

For more information about the Surgeon General's report or to download copies, visit Addiction.SurgeonGeneral.gov.

Use of trade names and specific programs are for identification only and do not constitute endorsement by the U.S. Department of Health and Human Services.

Non-discrimination

HHS complies with applicable federal civil rights laws and does not discriminate on the basis of race, color, national origin, age, disability, or sex. HHS does not exclude people or treat them differently because of race, color, national origin, age, disability, or sex.

HHS provides free aids and services to people with disabilities to communicate effectively with us, such as:
- Qualified sign language interpreters
- Written information in other formats (large print, audio, accessible electronic formats, other formats)

HHS provides free language services to people whose primary language is not English, such as:
- Qualified interpreters
- Information written in other languages

If you need these services, call 1-877-696-6775.

If you believe that HHS has failed to provide these services or discriminated in another way on the basis of race, color, national origin, age, disability, or sex, you can file a grievance with the U.S. Department of Health and Human Services, Office for Civil Rights, electronically through the Office for Civil Rights Complaint Portal, available at https://ocrportal.hhs.gov/ocr/portal/lobby.jsf, or by mail or phone at:

U.S. Department of Health and Human Services
200 Independence Avenue, SW
Room 509F, HHH Building
Washington, D.C. 20201
1-800-368-1019, 800-537-7697 (TDD)

Complaint forms are available at http://www.hhs.gov/ocr/office/file/index.html.

Español (Spanish) - ATENCIÓN: si habla español, tiene a su disposición servicios gratuitos de asistencia lingüística. Llame al 1-877-696-6775.

繁體中文 (Chinese) - 注意：如果您使用繁體中文，您可以免費獲得語言援助服務。請致電 1-877-696-6775.

Tiếng Việt (Vietnamese) - CHÚ Ý: Nếu bạn nói Tiếng Việt, có các dịch vụ hỗ trợ ngôn ngữ miễn phí dành cho bạn. Gọi số 1-877-696-6775.

한국어 (Korean) - 주의: 한국어를 사용하시는 경우, 언어 지원 서비스를 무료로 이용하실 수 있습니다. 1-877-696-6775 번으로 전화해 주십시오.

Tagalog - PAUNAWA: Kung nagsasalita ka ng Tagalog, maaari kang gumamit ng mga serbisyo ng tulong sa wika nang walang bayad. Tumawag sa 1-877-696-6775.

Русский (Russian) - ВНИМАНИЕ: Если вы говорите на русском языке, то вам доступны бесплатные услуги перевода. Звоните 1-877-696-6775.

العربية (Arabic) - ملحوظة: إذا كنت تتحدث اذكر اللغة، فإن خدمات المساعدة اللغوية تتوافر لك بالمجان. اتصل برقم 1-877-696-6775.

Kreyòl Ayisyen (Haitian Creole) - ATANSYON: Si w pale Kreyòl Ayisyen, gen sèvis èd pou lang ki disponib gratis pou ou. Rele 1-877-696-6775.

Français (French) - ATTENTION: Si vous parlez français, des services d'aide linguistique vous sont proposés gratuitement. Appelez le 1-877-696-6775.

Polski (Polish) - UWAGA: Jeżeli mówisz po polsku, możesz skorzystać z bezpłatnej pomocy językowej. Zadzwoń pod numer 1-877-696-6775.

Português (Portuguese) - ATENÇÃO: Se fala português, encontram-se disponíveis serviços linguísticos, grátis. Ligue para 1-877-696-6775.

Italiano (Italian) - ATTENZIONE: In caso la lingua parlata sia l'italiano, sono disponibili servizi di assistenza linguistica gratuiti. Chiamare il numero 1-877-696-6775.

Deutsch (German) - ACHTUNG: Wenn Sie Deutsch sprechen, stehen Ihnen kostenlos sprachliche Hilfsdienstleistungen zur Verfügung. Rufnummer: 1-877-696-6775.

日本語 (Japanese) - 注意事項：日本語を話される場合、無料の言語支援をご利用いただけます。1-877-696-6775 まで、お電話にてご連絡ください.

فارسی (Farsi) - توجه: اگر به زبان فارسی گفتگو می کنید، تسهیلات زبانی بصورت رایگان برای شما فراهم می باشد. با 1-877-696-6775 تماس بگیرید.

MESSAGE FROM THE SECRETARY, U.S. DEPARTMENT OF HEALTH AND HUMAN SERVICES

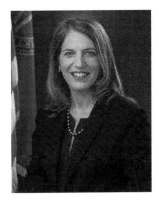

All across the United States, individuals, families, communities, and health care systems are struggling to cope with substance use, misuse, and substance use disorders. Substance misuse and substance use disorders have devastating effects, disrupt the future plans of too many young people, and all too often, end lives prematurely and tragically. Substance misuse is a major public health challenge and a priority for our nation to address.

Fortunately, we have made considerable progress in recent years. First, decades of scientific research and technological advances have given us a better understanding of the functioning and neurobiology of the brain and how substance use affects brain chemistry and our capacity for self-control. One of the important findings of this research is that addiction is a chronic neurological disorder and needs to be treated as other chronic conditions are. Second, this Administration and others before it, as well as the private sector, have invested in research, development, and evaluation of programs to prevent and treat substance misuse, as well as support recovery. We now have many of the tools we need to protect children, young people, and adults from the negative health consequences of substance misuse; provide individuals with substance use disorders the treatment they need to lead healthy and productive lives; and help people stay substance-free. Finally, the enactment of the Paul Wellstone and Pete Domenici Mental Health Parity and Addiction Equity Act of 2008 and the Affordable Care Act in 2010 are helping increase access to prevention and treatment services.

The effects of substance use are cumulative and costly for our society, placing burdens on workplaces, the health care system, families, states, and communities. *The Surgeon General's Report on Alcohol, Drugs, and Health* is another important step in our efforts to address the issue. This historic *Report* explains, in clear and understandable language, the effects on the brain of alcohol and drugs and how misuse can become a disorder. It describes the considerable evidence showing that prevention, treatment, and recovery policies and programs really do work. For example, minimum legal drinking age laws, funding for multi-sector community-based coalitions to plan and implement effective prevention interventions with fidelity, screening and brief intervention for alcohol use, needle/syringe exchange programs, behavioral counseling, pharmacologic interventions such as buprenorphine for opioid misuse, and mutual aid groups have all been shown effective in preventing, reducing, treating, and sustaining recovery from substance misuse and substance use disorders.

The *Report* discusses opportunities to bring substance use disorder treatment and mainstream health care systems into alignment so that they can address a person's overall health, rather than a substance misuse or a physical health condition alone or in isolation. It also provides suggestions and recommendations for action that everyone—individuals, families, community leaders, law enforcement, health care professionals, policymakers, and researchers—can take to prevent substance misuse and reduce its consequences.

MESSAGE FROM THE SECRETARY

Throughout, the *Report* provides examples of how individuals, organizations, and communities can partner to lessen and eliminate substance misuse. These efforts have to start now. Change takes time and long-term commitment, as well as collaboration among key stakeholders. As the Secretary of the Department of Health and Human Services, I encourage you to use the information and findings in this *Report* to take action so that we can improve the health of those we love and make our communities healthier and stronger.

Sylvia Mathews Burwell
Secretary
U.S. Department of Health and Human Services

FOREWORD FROM THE PRINCIPAL DEPUTY ADMINISTRATOR, SUBSTANCE ABUSE AND MENTAL HEALTH SERVICES ADMINISTRATION

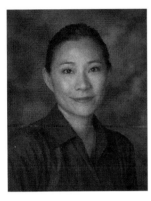

Substance misuse is one of the critical public health problems of our time. The most recent data on substance use, misuse, and substance use disorders reveal that the problem is deepening and the consequences are becoming more deadly than ever. There is an urgent need to raise awareness about the issue. At the same time, we need to spread the word that substance misuse and addiction are solvable problems. We can, and must, inspire and catalyze action on this crisis.

That's why I am so proud to support the Office of the Surgeon General in releasing this first report of its kind – *The Surgeon General's Report on Alcohol, Drugs, and Health.*

This *Report* takes a comprehensive look at the problem; covering topics including misuse of alcohol, prescription drugs, and other substances, and bringing together the best available science on the adverse health consequences of substance misuse. It also summarizes what we know about what works in prevention, treatment, and recovery. Our goal: to equip health care providers, communities, policymakers, law enforcement, and others with the evidence, the tools, and the information they need to take action to address this growing epidemic.

Now is the time for this *Report*. The substance misuse problem in America won't wait. Almost 22.5 million people reported use of an illegal drug in the prior year. Over 20 million people have substance use disorders, and 12.5 million Americans reported misusing prescription pain relievers in the past year. Seventy-eight people die every day in the United States from an opioid overdose, and those numbers have nearly quadrupled since 1999. Despite the fact that we have treatments we know are effective, only one in five people who currently need treatment for opioid use disorders is actually receiving it.

The addiction problem touches us all. We all need to play a part in solving it. *The Surgeon General's Report on Alcohol, Drugs, and Health* provides a roadmap for working together to move our efforts forward. I hope all who read it will be inspired to take action to stem the rising tide of this public health crisis and reduce the impact of substance misuse and addiction on individuals, communities, and our nation.

Kana Enomoto
Principal Deputy Administrator
Substance Abuse and Mental Health Services Administration
U.S. Department of Health and Human Services

PREFACE FROM THE SURGEON GENERAL, U.S. DEPARTMENT OF HEALTH AND HUMAN SERVICES

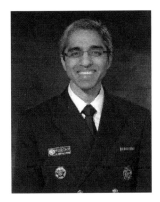

Before I assumed my position as U.S. Surgeon General, I stopped by the hospital where I had worked since my residency training to say goodbye to my colleagues. I wanted to thank them, especially the nurses, whose kindness and guidance had helped me on countless occasions. The nurses had one parting request for me. If you can only do one thing as Surgeon General, they said, please do something about the addiction crisis in America.

I have not forgotten their words. As I have traveled across our extraordinary nation, meeting people struggling with substance use disorders and their families, I have come to appreciate even more deeply something I recognized through my own experience in patient care: that substance use disorders represent one of the most pressing public health crises of our time.

Whether it is the rapid rise of prescription opioid addiction or the longstanding challenge of alcohol dependence, substance misuse and substance use disorders can—and do— prevent people from living healthy and productive lives. And, just as importantly, they have profound effects on families, friends, and entire communities.

I recognize there is no single solution. We need more policies and programs that increase access to proven treatment modalities. We need to invest more in expanding the scientific evidence base for prevention, treatment, and recovery. We also need a cultural shift in how we think about addiction. For far too long, too many in our country have viewed addiction as a moral failing. This unfortunate stigma has created an added burden of shame that has made people with substance use disorders less likely to come forward and seek help. It has also made it more challenging to marshal the necessary investments in prevention and treatment. We must help everyone see that addiction is not a character flaw – it is a chronic illness that we must approach with the same skill and compassion with which we approach heart disease, diabetes, and cancer.

I am proud to release *The Surgeon General's Report on Alcohol, Drugs, and Health.* As the first ever Surgeon General's Report on this important topic, this *Report* aims to shift the way our society thinks about substance misuse and substance use disorders while defining actions we can take to prevent and treat these conditions.

Over the past few decades, we have built a robust evidence base on this subject. We now know that there is a neurobiological basis for substance use disorders with potential for both recovery and recurrence. We have evidence-based interventions that prevent harmful substance use and related problems, particularly when started early. We also have proven interventions for treating substance use disorders, often involving a combination of medication, counseling, and social support. Additionally, we have

PREFACE

learned that recovery has many pathways that should be tailored to fit the unique cultural values and psychological and behavioral health needs of each individual.

As Surgeon General, I care deeply about the health and well-being of all who are affected by substance misuse and substance use disorders. This *Report* offers a way forward through a public health approach that is firmly grounded in the best available science. Recognizing that we all have a role to play, the *Report* contains suggested actions that are intended for parents, families, educators, health care professionals, public policy makers, researchers, and all community members.

Above all, we can never forget that the faces of substance use disorders are real people. They are a beloved family member, a friend, a colleague, and ourselves. Despite the significant work that remains ahead of us, there are reasons to be hopeful. I find hope in the people I have met in recovery all across America who are now helping others with substance use disorders find their way. I draw strength from the communities I have visited that are coming together to work on prevention initiatives and to connect more people to treatment. And I am inspired by the countless family members who have lost loved ones to addiction and who have transformed their pain into a passion for helping others. These individuals and communities are rays of hope. It is now our collective duty to bring such light to all corners of our country.

How we respond to this crisis is a moral test for America. Are we a nation willing to take on an epidemic that is causing great human suffering and economic loss? Are we able to live up to that most fundamental obligation we have as human beings: to care for one another?

Fifty years ago, the landmark Surgeon General's report on the dangers of smoking began a half century of work to end the tobacco epidemic and saved millions of lives. With *The Surgeon General's Report on Alcohol, Drugs, and Health*, I am issuing a new call to action to end the public health crisis of addiction. Please join me in taking the actions outlined in this *Report* and in helping ensure that all Americans can lead healthy and fulfilling lives.

> Vivek H. Murthy, M.D., M.B.A.
> Vice Admiral, U.S. Public Health Service
> Surgeon General

ACKNOWLEDGMENTS

This *Report* was prepared by the U.S. Department of Health and Human Services under the general direction of the Substance Abuse and Mental Health Services Administration.

Vice Admiral Vivek H. Murthy, M.D., M.B.A., Surgeon General, U.S. Public Health Service, Office of the Surgeon General, Office of the Assistant Secretary for Health, Office of the Secretary, U.S. Department of Health and Human Services, Washington, D.C.

Kana Enomoto, Principal Deputy Administrator, Substance Abuse and Mental Health Services Administration, Rockville, Maryland.

Science Editors

A. Thomas McLellan, Ph.D., Senior Scientific Editor, Chair of the Board and Co-Founder, Treatment Research Institute, Philadelphia, Pennsylvania.

Richard F. Catalano, Jr., Ph.D., M.A., Bartley Dobb Professor for the Study and Prevention of Violence; Co-Founder, Social Development Research Group, School of Social Work, University of Washington, Seattle, Washington.

H. Westley Clark, M.D., J.D., M.P.H., CAS, FASAM, Dean's Executive Professor of Public Health, Santa Clara University, Santa Clara, California.

Keith Humphreys, Ph.D., Professor, Department of Psychiatry and Behavioral Science, Stanford University, Stanford, California; Research Career Scientist, VA Palo Alto Health Care System, Palo Alto, California.

George F. Koob, Ph.D., Director, National Institute on Alcohol Abuse and Alcoholism, National Institutes of Health, Rockville, Maryland.

Nora D. Volkow, M.D., Director, National Institute on Drug Abuse, National Institutes of Health, Rockville, Maryland.

Constance M. Weisner, Dr.P.H., M.S.W., Associate Director, Behavioral Health, Aging, and Infectious Disease Section, Division of Research, Kaiser Permanente, Oakland, California; Professor of Psychiatry, Department of Psychiatry, Langley Porter Psychiatric Institute, University of California, San Francisco, California.

Managing Editors

Jinhee J. Lee, Pharm.D., Managing Editor, Senior Public Health Advisor, Division of Pharmacologic Therapies, Center for Substance Abuse Treatment, Substance Abuse and Mental Health Services Administration, Rockville, Maryland.

ACKNOWLEDGMENTS

Jorielle Brown Houston, Ph.D., Associate Managing Editor, Director, Division of Systems Development, Center for Substance Abuse Prevention, Substance Abuse and Mental Health Services Administration, Rockville, Maryland.

Richard Lucey, Jr., M.A., Associate Managing Editor, Special Assistant to the Director, Center for Substance Abuse Prevention, Substance Abuse and Mental Health Services Administration, Rockville, Maryland.

Contributing Editors

Nazleen H. Bharmal, M.D., Ph.D., M.P.P., Director of Science and Policy, Office of the Surgeon General, Office of the Assistant Secretary of Health, U.S. Department of Health and Human Services, Washington, D.C.

Christine A. Cichetti, Senior Behavioral Health Policy Advisor, Office of the Assistant Secretary for Health/Office of the Deputy Assistant Secretary for Health (Science and Medicine), Washington, D.C.

Tom Coderre, Chief of Staff, Substance Abuse and Mental Health Services Administration, Rockville, Maryland.

Tom Hill, M.S.W., Senior Advisor for Addiction and Recovery, Substance Abuse and Mental Health Services Administration, Rockville, Maryland.

Marion Cornelius Pierce, Public Health Analyst, Division of Systems Development, Center for Substance Abuse Prevention, Substance Abuse and Mental Health Services Administration, Rockville, Maryland.

Contributing Authors

Michael A. Arends, Senior Research Assistant in the Committee on the Neurobiology of Addictive Disorders, The Scripps Research Institute, La Jolla, California.

Maureen Boyle, Ph.D., Chief, Science Policy Branch, Office of Science Policy and Communications, National Institute on Drug Abuse, National Institutes of Health, Rockville, Maryland.

Felipe González Castro, Ph.D., M.S.W., Professor and Southwest Borderlands Scholar, Arizona State University, College of Nursing and Health Innovation, Phoenix, Arizona.

Mady Chalk, Ph.D., M.S.W., Managing Partner, The Chalk Group.

Laura J. Dunlap, Ph.D., Director, Behavioral Health Economics Program, RTI International, Research Triangle Park, North Carolina.

Vivian B. Faden, Ph.D., Director, Office of Science Policy and Communications and Associate Director of Behavioral Research, National Institute on Alcohol Abuse and Alcoholism, National Institutes of Health, Rockville, Maryland.

Abigail A. Fagan, Ph.D., Associate Professor of Criminology & Law, Department of Sociology and Criminology & Law, University of Florida, Gainesville, Florida.

Mark T. Greenberg, Ph.D., M.A., Edna Peterson Bennett Endowed Chair in Prevention Research, Professor of Human Development and Psychology, College of Health and Human Development, The Pennsylvania State University, State College, Pennsylvania.

Kevin P. Haggerty, Ph.D., M.S.W., Associate Professor; Director of Research; Director, Social Development Research Group; School of Social Work, University of Washington, Seattle, Washington.

Ralph W. Hingson, Sc.D., M.P.H., Director, Division of Epidemiology and Prevention Research, National Institute on Alcohol Abuse and Alcoholism, National Institutes of Health, Rockville, Maryland.

Jennifer A. Hobin, Ph.D., Senior Health Science Policy Analyst, Science Policy Branch, Office of Science Policy and Communications, National Institute on Alcohol Abuse and Alcoholism, National Institutes of Health, Rockville, Maryland.

John F. Kelly, Ph.D, Elizabeth R. Spallin Associate Professor of Psychiatry in the Field of Addiction Medicine, Harvard Medical School, Boston, Massachusetts; Director, Recovery Research Institute; Program Director, Addiction Recovery Management Service; Associate Director, Center for Addiction Medicine, Massachusetts General Hospital, Boston, Massachusetts.

Tami L. Mark, Ph.D., M.B.A., Vice President and Director, Center for Behavioral Health Services Research, Truven Health Analytics, Bethesda, Maryland.

Patrick O'Connor, M.D., M.P.H., F.A.C.P., Professor and Chief of General Internal Medicine, Yale University School of Medicine, New Haven, Connecticut.

Harold Pollack, Ph.D., M.P.P., Helen Ross Professor, School of Social Services Administration; Affiliate Professor, Biological Science Collegiate Divisions and the Department of Public Health Service; Co-Director, The University of Chicago Crime Lab, The University of Chicago, Chicago, Illinois.

Patricia A. Powell, Ph.D., Acting Deputy Director, Associate Director for Scientific Initiatives, National Institute on Alcohol Abuse and Alcoholism, National Institutes of Health, Rockville, Maryland.

Stacy A. Sterling, Dr.P.H., M.S.W., Practice Leader, Division of Research, Kaiser Permanente, Oakland, California.

Eric M. Wargo, Ph.D., Science Writer, Science Policy Branch, Office of Science Policy and Communications, National Institute on Drug Abuse, National Institutes of Health, Rockville, Maryland.

Deborah Klein Walker, Ed.D., Vice President & Senior Fellow, U.S. Health, Abt Associates, Cambridge, Massachusetts.

Bridget D. Williams-Simmons, Ph.D., Chief, Science Policy Branch, Office of Science Policy and Communications, National Institute on Alcohol Abuse and Alcoholism, National Institutes of Health, Rockville, Maryland.

Gary A. Zarkin, Ph.D., Vice President, Behavioral Health and Criminal Justice Research Division, RTI International, Research Triangle Park, North Carolina.

ACKNOWLEDGMENTS

Science Writer

Anne B. Rodgers, Science Writer, Falls Church, Virginia.

Reviewers

Hortensia Amaro, Ph.D., Dean's Professor, School of Social Work; Professor, Department of Preventive Medicine, Keck School of Medicine; and Associate Vice Provost, Community Research Initiatives, University of Southern California, Los Angeles, California.

Trina Menden Anglin, M.D., Ph.D., Chief, Adolescent Health Branch, Maternal and Child Health Bureau, Health Resources and Services Administration, Rockville, Maryland.

Bethany Applebaum, M.P.H., M.A., Public Health Analyst, Office of Women's Health, Health Resources and Services Administration, Rockville, Maryland.

Marsha L. Baker, LCSW, Public Health Advisor, Center for Substance Abuse Treatment, Substance Abuse and Mental Health Services Administration, Rockville, Maryland.

David S. Barry, Psy.D., Public Health Advisor, Substance Abuse and Mental Health Services Administration, Rockville, Maryland.

Mirtha R. Beadle, Director, Office of Tribal Affairs and Policy, Office of Policy, Planning, and Innovation, Substance Abuse and Mental Health Services Administration, Rockville, Maryland.

David J. Beckstead, Ph.D., A.P.B.B., Clinical Director, Desert Visions Youth Wellness Center, Indian Health Services, Sacaton, Arizona.

B. Steven Bentsen, M.D., D.F.A.P.A., Regional Chief Medical Officer, Beacon Health Options, Morrisville, North Carolina.

Mitchell Berger, Public Health Advisor, Office of Policy, Planning, and Innovation, Substance Abuse and Mental Health Services Administration, Rockville, Maryland.

Jonaki Bose, Branch Chief, Populations Survey Branch, Center for Behavioral Health Statistics and Quality, Substance Abuse and Mental Health Services Administration, Rockville, Maryland.

Cheryl A. Boyce, Ph.D., Division of Clinical Neuroscience and Behavioral Research, National Institute on Drug Abuse, National Institutes of Health, Rockville, Maryland.

Katharine A. Bradley, M.D., M.P.H., Senior Investigator and Internal Medicine Physician, Group Health Research Institute, Seattle, Washington.

Robert D. Brewer, M.D., M.S.P.H., Epidemiologist - Lead, Alcohol Program, Division of Population Health, National Center for Chronic Disease Prevention and Health Promotion, Centers for Disease Control and Prevention, Atlanta, Georgia.

Jeffrey A. Buck, Ph.D., Centers for Medicare & Medicaid Services, Washington, D.C.

ACKNOWLEDGMENTS

A. Kathleen Burlew, Ph.D., M.A., McMicken Professor, McMicken College of Arts and Sciences, University of Cincinnati, Cincinnati, Ohio.

John Campbell, M.A., Chief, Performance Partnership Grant Branch, Division of State and Community Assistance, Chief Medical Officer, Office of the Director, Center for Substance Abuse Treatment, Substance Abuse and Mental Health Services Administration, Rockville, Maryland.

Melinda Campopiano, M.D., Chief Medical Officer, Office of the Director, Center for Substance Abuse Treatment, Substance Abuse and Mental Health Services Administration, Rockville, Maryland.

Christopher D. Carroll, M.Sc., Director of Health Care Financing and Systems Integration, Substance Abuse and Mental Health Services Administration, Rockville, Maryland.

Walter B. Castle, M.S.S.W., Senior Public Health Advisor, Division of Behavioral Health, Indian Health Service, Rockville, Maryland.

Nancy Cheal, M.S., Ph.D., Health Scientist, Division of Congenital and Developmental Disorders, National Center on Birth Defects and Developmental Disabilities, Centers for Disease Control and Prevention, Atlanta, Georgia.

Laura W. Cheever, M.D., Sc.M., Associate Administrator, HIV/AIDS Bureau, Health Resources and Services Administration, Rockville, Maryland.

Dominic Chiapperino, Ph.D., Regulatory and Liaison Team Lead, Controlled Substance Staff, Center for Drug Evaluation and Research, U.S. Food and Drug Administration, Silver Spring, Maryland.

Wilson M. Compton, M.D., M.P.E., Deputy Director, National Institute on Drug Abuse, National Institutes of Health, Rockville, Maryland.

Jessica H. Cotto, Health Scientist Administrator, Science Policy Branch, National Institute on Drug Abuse, National Institutes of Health, Rockville, Maryland.

Don L. Coyhis, Mohican Nation, President and Founder, White Bison, Inc., Colorado Springs, Colorado.

Steven Dettwyler, Ph.D., Public Health Advisor, State Grants Western Branch, Division of State and Community Systems Development, Center for Mental Health Services, Substance Abuse and Mental Health Services Administration, Rockville, Maryland.

Lori Ducharme, Ph.D., Program Director for Health Services Research, Division of Treatment and Recovery Research, National Institute on Alcohol Abuse and Alcoholism, National Institutes of Health, Rockville, Maryland.

Marissa Esser, M.P.H., Ph.D., Heath Scientist, Division of Population Health, National Center for Chronic Disease Prevention and Health Promotion, Centers for Disease Control and Prevention, Atlanta, Georgia.

Monica Feit, Ph.D., Director of the Office of Policy, Planning, and Innovation, Substance Abuse and Mental Health Services Administration, Rockville, Maryland.

Corinne Ferdon, Ph.D., Deputy Associate Director for Science, Division of Violence Prevention, National Center for Injury Prevention and Control, Centers for Disease Control and Prevention, Atlanta, Georgia.

ACKNOWLEDGMENTS

David A. Fiellin, M.D., Professor of Medicine (General Medicine) and Public Health (Health Policy), Institute for Social and Policy Studies; Director, Community Research and Implementation Core, Center for Interdisciplinary Research on AIDS, Yale School of Medicine, New Haven, Connecticut.

Pennie Foster-Fishman, Ph.D., Professor, Department of Psychology; Senior Outreach Fellow, University Outreach and Engagement, Michigan State University. East Lansing, Michigan.

Henry L. Francis, M.D., Director for Data Mining and Informatics Evaluation and Research, Office of Translational Sciences, Center for Drug Evaluation and Research, U.S. Food and Drug Administration, Silver Spring, Maryland.

Rebecca Freeman, Ph.D., R.N., P.M.P., Chief Nursing Officer, Office of the National Coordinator for Health IT, U.S. Department of Health and Human Services, Washington, D.C.

Peter Gaumond, Chief, Recovery Branch, Office of National Drug Control Policy, Executive Office of the President, Washington, D.C.

Udi E. Ghitza, Ph.D., Health Scientist Administrator, Program Officer, Center for the Clinical Trials Network, National Institute on Drug Abuse, National Institutes of Health, Rockville, Maryland.

Gregory Goldstein, M.S.H.S., Deputy Director, Center for Substance Abuse Prevention, Substance Abuse and Mental Health Services Administration, Rockville, Maryland.

Althea M. Grant, M.P.H., Ph.D., Chief, Epidemiology and Surveillance Branch, Division of Blood Disorders, National Center on Birth Defects and Developmental Disabilities, Office of Noncommunicable Diseases, Injury and Environmental Health, Centers for Disease Control and Prevention, Atlanta, Georgia.

Stephen J. Gumbley, M.A., Independent Consultant; Former Director, New England Addiction Technology Transfer Center, Providence, Rhode Island.

Susan Marsiglia Gray, M.P.H., Senior Public Health Advisor, Center for Substance Abuse Prevention, Substance Abuse and Mental Health Services Administration, Rockville, Maryland.

Frances M. Harding, Director, Center for Substance Abuse Prevention, Substance Abuse and Mental Health Services Administration, Rockville, Maryland.

R. Adron Harris, Ph.D., M. June & J. Virgil Waggoner Chair in Molecular Biology; Director, Waggoner Center for Alcohol and Addiction Research, University of Texas at Austin, Austin, Texas.

Marla Hendriksson, M.P.M., Director, Office of Communications, Substance Abuse and Mental Health Services Administration, Rockville, Maryland.

Anne M. Herron, M.S., Director, Division of Regional and National Policy Liaison, and Agency Lead, SAMHSA Workforce Development Strategic Initiative, Substance Abuse and Mental Health Services Administration, Rockville, Maryland.

Sharon Hertz, M.D., Director, Division of Anesthesia, Analgesia, and Addiction Products, Center for Drug Evaluation and Research, U.S. Food and Drug Administration, Silver Spring, Maryland.

Kevin C. Heslin, Ph.D., Staff Research Fellow, Agency for Healthcare Research and Quality, U.S. Department of Health and Human Services, Rockville, Maryland.

Donna Hillman, M.A., Lead Public Health Advisor, Center for Substance Abuse Treatment, Substance Abuse and Mental Health Services Administration, Rockville, Maryland.

Margaret (Peggy) Honein, Ph.D., M.P.H., Chief, Birth Defects Branch, National Center on Birth Defects and Developmental Disabilities, Centers for Disease Control and Prevention, Atlanta, Georgia.

Alexis G. Horan, M.P.P., Expert Consultant, Addiction Policy, Office of the Assistant Secretary for Planning and Evaluation, U.S. Department of Health and Human Services, Washington, D.C.

Constance M. Horgan, M.A., Sc.D., Professor; Director, Institute for Behavioral Health, The Heller School for Social Policy and Management, Brandeis University, Waltham, Massachusetts.

Larke N. Huang, Ph.D., Director, Office of Behavioral Health Equity, Office of Policy, Planning, and Innovation, Substance Abuse and Mental Health Services Administration, Rockville, Maryland.

Robert B. Huebner, Ph.D., Acting Director, Division of Treatment and Recovery Research, National Institute on Alcohol Abuse and Alcoholism, National Institutes of Health, Rockville, Maryland.

Kristen V. Huntley Ph.D., Health Science Administrator, Center for the Clinical Trials Network, National Institute on Drug Abuse, National Institutes of Health, Rockville, Maryland.

Corinne G. Husten, M.D., M.P.H., Senior Medical Advisor, Office of the Center Director, Center for Tobacco Products, U.S. Food and Drug Administration, Silver Spring, Maryland.

Linda Hutchings, M.S.J., Special Assistant to the Director, Center for Substance Abuse Treatment, Substance Abuse and Mental Health Services Administration, Rockville, Maryland.

Pamela S. Hyde, J.D., Former Administrator, Substance Abuse and Mental Health Services Administration, Rockville, Maryland.

Carrie L. Jeffries, A.N.P.-B.C., M.S., M.P.H., R.N., A.A.C.R.N., Chief Nursing Officer, HIV/AIDS Bureau, Health Resources and Services Administration, Rockville, Maryland.

Amelia (Amy) Jewett, M.P.H., Epidemiologist, Transportation Safety Team, Division of Unintentional Injury Prevention, National Center for Injury Prevention and Control, Centers for Disease Control and Prevention, Atlanta, Georgia.

Kimberly A. Johnson, Ph.D., Director, Center for Substance Abuse Treatment, Substance Abuse and Mental Health Services Administration, Rockville, Maryland.

Wanda K. Jones, Dr.P.H., M.P.H., Principal Deputy Assistant Secretary for Health, U.S. Department of Health and Human Services, Washington, D.C.

Elliot Kennedy, J.D., Special Expert, LGBT Affairs, Substance Abuse and Mental Health Services Administration, Rockville, Maryland.

ACKNOWLEDGMENTS

Paul J. Kenny, Ph.D., Ward-Coleman Professor; Chair, Dorothy H. and Lewis Rosentiel Department of Pharmacology and Systems Therapeutics; Director, Experimental Therapeutics Institute, Mount Sinai Hospital, New York, New York.

Thomas Kresina, Ph.D., Senior Public Health Advisor, Center for Substance Abuse Treatment, Substance Abuse and Mental Health Services Administration, Rockville, Maryland.

Alexandre B. Laudet, Ph.D., Director, Center for the Study of Addictions and Recovery, National Development and Research Institutes, Inc. (NDRI), New York, New York.

Jennifer LeClercq, M.P.H., C.H.E.S., Public Health Analyst, Division of Population Health, National Center for Chronic Disease Prevention and Health Promotion, Centers for Disease Control and Prevention, Atlanta, Georgia.

Raye Z. Litten, Ph.D., Acting Director, Division of Medications Development, National Institute on Alcohol Abuse and Alcoholism, National Institutes of Health, Rockville, Maryland.

Xiang Sharon Liu, Statistician, Treatment Service Branch, Center for Behavioral Health Statistics and Quality, Substance Abuse and Mental Health Services Administration, Rockville, Maryland.

Jacqueline J. Lloyd, Ph.D., M.S.W., Deputy Branch Chief and Health Scientist Administrator, Prevention Research Branch, Division of Epidemiology, Services, and Prevention Research, National Institute on Drug Abuse, National Institutes of Health, Rockville, Maryland.

Joshua Lloyd, M.D., Lead Medical Officer, Division of Anesthesia, Analgesia, and Addiction Products, Center for Drug Evaluation and Research, U.S. Food and Drug Administration, Silver Spring, Maryland.

Peter G. Lurie, M.D., M.P.H., Associate Commissioner for Public Health Strategy and Analysis, U.S. Food and Drug Administration, Silver Spring, Maryland.

Robert Lyerla, Ph.D., Research Officer, Center for Behavioral Health Statistics and Quality, Substance Abuse and Mental Health Services Administration, Rockville, Maryland.

Spero M. Manson, Ph.D., Distinguished Professor of Public Health and Psychiatry; Director, Centers for American Indian and Alaska Native Health; The Colorado Trust Chair in American Indian Health; Associate Dean of Research, Colorado School of Public Health, Aurora, Colorado.

Tim McAfee, Director, Medical Officer, Office on Smoking and Health, National Center for Chronic Disease Prevention and Health Promotion, Centers for Disease Control and Prevention, Atlanta, Georgia.

Dennis McCarty, Ph.D., M.A., Professor; Division Head, Health Services Research; OHSU-PSU School of Public Health, Oregon Health & Science University, Portland, Oregon.

David K. Mineta, M.S.W., President and CEO, Momentum for Mental Health, San Jose, California.

Ivan D. Montoya, M.D., M.P.H., Deputy Director, Division of Therapeutics and Medical Consequences, National Institute on Drug Abuse, National Institutes of Health, Rockville, Maryland.

Michele LaTour Monroe, Senior Communications Specialist, Office of Communications, Substance Abuse and Mental Health Services Administration, Rockville, Maryland.

Jon Morgenstern, Ph.D., Director of Addiction Services, Northwell Health, Great Neck, New York.

Charlotte A. Mullican, M.P.H., Senior Advisor for Mental Health Research, Center for Evidence and Practice Improvement, Agency for Healthcare Research and Quality, Rockville, Maryland.

Lisa M. Najavits, Ph.D., Professor, Department of Psychiatry, Boston University School of Medicine, Boston, Massachusetts; Director, Treatment Innovations, Newton Centre, Massachusetts.

Jon P. Nelson, Ph.D., Professor Emeritus of Economics, The Pennsylvania State University, State College, Pennsylvania.

Phyllis Holditch Niolon, Ph.D., Behavioral Scientist, Division of Violence Prevention, National Center for Injury Prevention and Control, Centers for Disease Control and Prevention, Atlanta, Georgia.

Antonio Noronha, Ph.D., Director, Division of Neuroscience and Behavior, National Institute on Alcohol Abuse and Alcoholism, National Institutes of Health, Rockville, Maryland.

Thomas E. Novotny, M.D., M.P.H., Deputy Assistant Secretary for Health (Science and Medicine), U.S. Department of Health and Human Services, Washington, D.C.

John P. O'Brien, Senior Policy Advisor, Disabled and Elderly Health Programs Group, Centers for Medicare & Medicaid Services, Baltimore, Maryland.

David L. Olds, Ph.D., Professor of Pediatrics; Director, Prevention Research Center for Family and Child Health; Department of Pediatrics, University of Colorado, Aurora, Colorado.

Dee S. Owens, M.P.A., Special Assistant to the Director, Center for Behavioral Health Statistics and Quality, Substance Abuse and Mental Health Services Administration, Rockville, Maryland.

Derek W. Patton, M.S., M.B.A., Division Director, Integrated Behavioral Health, Office of Health Programs, Indian Health Service, Phoenix, Arizona.

Len Paulozzi, M.D., Medical Officer, Division of Unintentional Injury Prevention, National Center for Injury Prevention and Control, Centers for Disease Control and Prevention, Atlanta, Georgia.

Adolf Pfefferbaum, M.D., Senior Program Director and Distinguished Scientist, Center for Health Sciences, SRI International, Menlo Park, California.

Kathryn Piscopo, Ph.D., Survey Statistician, Populations Survey Branch, Center for Behavioral Health Statistics and Quality, Substance Abuse and Mental Health Services Administration, Rockville, Maryland.

Jean O. Plascke, M.S.W., Youth Programs Officer, Office of Indian Alcohol and Substance Abuse, Center for Substance Abuse Prevention, Substance Abuse and Mental Health Services Administration, Rockville, Maryland.

Richard A. Rawson, Ph.D., Research Professor, Department of Psychiatry, University of Vermont, Burlington, Vermont; Professor Emeritus Department of Psychiatry; Geffen School of Medicine, University of California, Los Angeles, California.

ACKNOWLEDGMENTS

Kenneth W. Robertson, Lead Public Health Advisor, Criminal Justice Grants, Targeted Populations Branch, Division of Systems Improvement, Center for Substance Abuse Treatment, Substance Abuse and Mental Health Services Administration, Rockville, Maryland.

Susan Robilotto, D.O., Clinical Advisor/Medical Officer, HIV/AIDS Bureau, Health Resources and Services Administration, Rockville, Maryland.

Letitia B. Robinson, Ph.D., R.N., Senior Advisor, HIV/AIDS Bureau, Health Resources and Services Administration, Rockville, Maryland.

Alexander F. Ross, Sc.D., Senior Behavioral Health Advisor, Office of Planning, Evaluation, and Analysis, Health Resources and Services Administration, Rockville, Maryland.

Tyler Sadwith, Health Insurance Specialist, Center for Medicaid and CHIP Services, Centers for Medicare & Medicaid Services, San Francisco, California.

Onaje M. Salim, M.A., Ed.D., Director, Division of State and Community Assistance, Center for Substance Abuse Treatment, Substance Abuse and Mental Health Services Administration, Rockville, Maryland.

David R. Shillcutt, J.D., Disabled and Elderly Health Programs Group, Center for Medicaid and CHIP Services, Centers for Medicare & Medicaid Services, Baltimore, Maryland.

Ruth Shults, Ph.D., M.P.H., Senior Epidemiologist, Division of Unintentional Injury Prevention, National Center for Injury Prevention and Control, Centers for Disease Control and Prevention, Atlanta, Georgia.

Belinda Sims, Ph.D., Health Scientist Administrator, Prevention Research Branch, Division of Epidemiology, Services and Prevention Research, National Institute on Drug Abuse, National Institutes of Health, Rockville, Maryland.

Geetha A. Subramaniam, M.D., Deputy Director, Center for Clinical Trials Network, National Institute on Drug Abuse, National Institutes of Health, Rockville, Maryland.

Tison Thomas, M.S.W., Chief, State Grants Eastern Branch, Division of State and Community Systems Development, Center for Mental Health Services, Substance Abuse and Mental Health Services Administration, Rockville, Maryland.

Christine Timko, Ph.D., Research Career Scientist, Health Services Research and Development, U.S. Department of Veterans Affairs, Menlo Park, California.

Traci L. Toomey, Ph.D., Professor, Division of Epidemiology and Community Health, School of Public Health, University of Minnesota, Minneapolis, Minnesota.

Paolo del Vecchio, M.S.W., Director, Center for Mental Health Services, Substance Abuse and Mental Health Services Administration, Rockville, Maryland.

Mary Kate Weber, M.P.H, Behavioral Scientist, Division of Congenital and Developmental Disorders, National Center on Birth Defects and Developmental Disabilities, Centers for Disease Control and Prevention, Atlanta, Georgia.

Aaron White, Ph.D., Senior Advisor to the Director, National Institute on Alcohol Abuse and Alcoholism, National Institutes of Health, Rockville, Maryland.

William L. White, M.A., Emeritus Senior Research Consultant, Chestnut Health Systems, Bloomington, Illinois.

Gary B. Wilcox, M.A., Ph.D., John A. Beck Centennial Professor in Communication, Moody College of Communication, Stan Richards School of Advertising and Public Relations, The University of Texas at Austin, Austin, Texas.

David Wilson, Public Affairs Specialist, Center for Substance Abuse Prevention, Substance Abuse and Mental Health Services Administration, Rockville, Maryland.

Ellen Witt, Ph.D., (retired) Deputy Director, Division of Neuroscience and Behavior, National Institute on Alcohol Abuse and Alcoholism, National Institutes of Health, Rockville, Maryland.

Amy Funk Wolkin, Dr.P.H., M.S.P.H., Chief, Health Studies Branch, Division of Environmental Hazards and Health Effects, National Center for Environmental Health, Centers for Disease Control and Prevention, Atlanta, Georgia.

Albert M Woodward, Ph.D., Chief, Analysis and Services Research Branch, Division of Evaluation, Analysis and Quality, Center for Behavioral Health Statistics and Quality, Substance Abuse and Mental Health Services Administration, Rockville, Maryland.

Marie Zeimetz, Ph.D., Writer-Editor, Office of the Director, Center for Substance Abuse Treatment, Substance Abuse and Mental Health Services Administration, Rockville, Maryland.

Terry S. Zobeck, Ph.D., Associate Director, Office of Research/Data Analysis, Office of National Drug Control Policy, Executive Office of the President, Washington, D.C.

Other contributors were

Deepa Avula, M.P.H., Director, Office of Financial Resources, Substance Abuse and Mental Health Services Administration, Rockville, Maryland.

Amy Berninger, M.P.H., Senior Analyst, Abt Associates, Cambridge, Massachusetts.

Margaret K. Gwaltney, M.B.A., Principal Associate, Abt Associates, Bethesda, Maryland.

Kevin Hennessy, Ph.D., Former Deputy Director, Center for Behavioral Health Statistics and Quality, Substance Abuse and Mental Health Services Administration, Rockville, Maryland.

Janet Hightower, Digital Artist, Encinitas, California.

Mariel J. McLeod, Research Assistant, Abt Associates, Bethesda, Maryland.

Cori K. Sheedy, Ph.D., Senior Associate, Abt Associates, Cambridge, Massachusetts.

Daniel J. Smith, Senior Graphic Designer, Abt Associates, Bethesda, Maryland.

Alicia C. Sparks, Ph.D., Senior Analyst, Abt Associates, Bethesda, Maryland.

Melanie Whitter, Principal Associate, Abt Associates, Bethesda, Maryland.

TABLE OF CONTENTS

CHAPTER 1 - INTRODUCTION AND OVERVIEW OF THE REPORT		
	Chapter 1 Preview	1-1
	Substances Discussed in this Report	1-4
	Prevalence of Substance Use, Misuse Problems, and Disorders	1-7
	Costs and Impact of Substance Misuse	1-12
	Vulnerability to Substance Misuse Problems and Disorders	1-15
	Diagnosing a Substance Use Disorder	1-16
	The Separation of Substance Use Treatment and General Health Care	1-19
	Recent Changes in Health Care Policy and Law	1-20
	Marijuana: A Changing Legal and Research Environment	1-21
	Purpose, Focus, and Format of the *Report*	1-22
	References	1-26

CHAPTER 2 - THE NEUROBIOLOGY OF SUBSTANCE USE, MISUSE, AND ADDICTION		
	Chapter 2 Preview	2-1
	Conducting Research on the Neurobiology of Substance Use, Misuse, and Addiction	2-3
	The Primary Brain Regions Involved in Substance Use Disorders	2-5
	The Addiction Cycle	2-6
	Binge/Intoxication Stage: Basal Ganglia	2-8
	Withdrawal/Negative Affect Stage: Extended Amygdala	2-12
	Factors that Increase Risk for Substance Use, Misuse, and Addiction	2-21
	Use of Multiple Substances and Co-occurring Mental Health Conditions	2-22
	Biological Factors Contributing to Population-based Differences in Substance Misuse and Substance Use Disorders	2-23
	Recommendations for Research	2-24
	References	2-27

TABLE OF CONTENTS

CHAPTER 3 - PREVENTION PROGRAMS AND POLICIES		
	Chapter 3 Preview	3-1
	Why We Should Care About Prevention	3-3
	Risk and Protective Factors	3-4
	Types of Prevention Interventions	3-7
	Evidence-Based Prevention Programs	3-8
	Evidence-based Community Coalition-based Prevention Models	3-14
	Evidence-Based Prevention Policies	3-17
	Prevention Interventions for Specific Populations	3-27
	Improving the Dissemination and Implementation of Evidence-based Programs	3-32
	Recommendations for Research	3-35
	References	3-37

CHAPTER 4 - EARLY INTERVENTION, TREATMENT, AND MANAGEMENT OF SUBSTANCE USE DISORDERS		
	Chapter 4 Preview	4-1
	Continuum of Treatment Services	4-3
	Early Intervention: Identifying and Engaging Individuals At Risk for Substance Misuse and Substance Use Disorders	4-5
	Treatment Engagement: Reaching and Reducing Harm Among Those Who Need Treatment	4-8
	Principles of Effective Treatment and Treatment Planning	4-13
	Evidence-based Treatment: Components of Care	4-19
	Emerging Treatment Technologies	4-32
	Considerations for Specific Populations	4-36
	Recommendations for Research	4-40
	References	4-43

TABLE OF CONTENTS

CHAPTER 5 - RECOVERY: THE MANY PATHS TO WELLNESS	Chapter 5 Preview	5-1
	Definitions, Pathways, and Prevalence of Recovery	5-2
	Perspectives of Those in Recovery	5-4
	Estimating the Number of People "In Recovery"	5-5
	Recovery-oriented Systems of Care	5-6
	Recovery Supports	5-7
	Social and Recreational Recovery Infrastructures and Social Media	5-16
	Specific Populations and Recovery	5-16
	Recommendations for Research	5-17
	References	5-18
CHAPTER 6 - HEALTH CARE SYSTEMS AND SUBSTANCE USE DISORDERS	Chapter 6 Preview	6-1
	Key Components of Health Care Systems	6-3
	Substance Use Disorder Services Have Traditionally Been Separate From Mental Health and General Health Care	6-5
	A Growing Impetus for Integration	6-6
	Financing Systems for Substance Use Disorder Services	6-23
	Challenges Facing the Integration of Substance Use Services and Health Care	6-27
	Promising Innovations That Improve Access to Substance Use Disorder Treatment	6-34
	Recommendations for Research	6-43
	References	6-45
CHAPTER 7 - VISION FOR THE FUTURE: A PUBLIC HEALTH APPROACH	Time for a Change	7-2
	Specific Suggestions for Key Stakeholders	7-7
	Conclusion	7-16
	References	7-18

TABLE OF CONTENTS

GLOSSARY OF TERMS	1
LIST OF ABBREVIATIONS	7
LIST OF TABLES AND FIGURES	11
APPENDIX A - REVIEW PROCESS FOR PREVENTION PROGRAMS	15
APPENDIX B - EVIDENCE-BASED PREVENTION PROGRAMS AND POLICIES	17
APPENDIX C - RESOURCE GUIDE	41
APPENDIX D - IMPORTANT FACTS ABOUT ALCOHOL AND DRUGS	53

CHAPTER 1.
INTRODUCTION AND OVERVIEW OF THE REPORT

Chapter 1 Preview

The United States has a serious substance misuse problem. Substance misuse is the use of alcohol or drugs in a manner, situation, amount, or frequency that could cause harm to the user or to those around them. Alcohol and drug misuse and related substance use disorders affect millions of Americans and impose enormous costs on our society. In 2015, 66.7 million people in the United States reported binge drinking in the past month and 27.1 million people were current users of illicit drugs or misused prescription drugs.[3] The accumulated costs to the individual, the family, and the community are staggering and arise as a consequence of many direct and indirect effects, including compromised physical and mental health, increased spread of infectious disease, loss of productivity, reduced quality of life, increased crime and violence, increased motor vehicle crashes, abuse and neglect of children, and health care costs.

The most devastating consequences are seen in the tens of thousands of lives that are lost each year as a result of substance misuse. Alcohol misuse contributes to 88,000 deaths in the United States each year; 1 in 10 deaths among working adults are due to alcohol misuse.[6] In addition, in 2014 there were 47,055 drug overdose deaths including 28,647 people who died from a drug overdose involving some type of opioid, including prescription pain relievers and heroin—more than in any previous year on record.[7]

Even though the United States spends more than any other country on health care, it ranks 27th in life expectancy, which has plateaued or decreased for some segments of the population at a time when life expectancy continues to increase in other developed countries—and the difference is largely due to substance misuse and associated physical and mental health problems. For example, recent research has shown an unprecedented increase in mortality among middle-aged White Americans between 1999 and 2014 that was largely driven by alcohol and drug misuse and suicides, although this trend was not seen within other racial and ethnic populations such as Blacks and Hispanics.[8] An analysis from the Centers for Disease Control and Prevention (CDC) demonstrated that alcohol and drug misuse accounted for a roughly 4-month decline in life expectancy among White Americans; no other cause of death had a larger negative impact in this population.[9]

INTRODUCTION

Substance misuse and substance use disorders also have serious economic consequences, costing more than $400 billion annually in crime, health, and lost productivity.[10,11] These costs are of a similar order of magnitude to those associated with other serious health problems such as diabetes, which is estimated to cost the United States $245 billion each year.[12] Alcohol misuse and alcohol use disorders alone costs the United States approximately $249 billion in lost productivity, health care expenses, law enforcement, and other criminal justice costs.[10] The costs associated with drug use disorders and use of illegal drugs and non-prescribed medications were estimated to be more than $193 billion in 2007.[11]

Despite decades of expense and effort focused on a criminal justice–based model for addressing substance use-related problems, substance misuse remains a national public health crisis that continues to rob the United States of its most valuable asset: its people. In fact, high annual rates of past-month illicit drug use and binge drinking among people aged 12 years and older from 2002 through 2014 (**Figure 1.1**) emphasize the importance of implementing evidence-based public-health-focused strategies to prevent and treat alcohol and drug problems in the United States.[13] A public health approach seeks to improve the health and safety of the population by addressing underlying social, environmental, and economic determinants of substance misuse and its consequences, to improve the health, safety, and well-being of the entire population.

Figure 1.1: Past Month Rates of Substance Use Among People Aged 12 or Older: Percentages, 2002-2014, 2014 National Survey on Drug Use and Health (NSDUH)

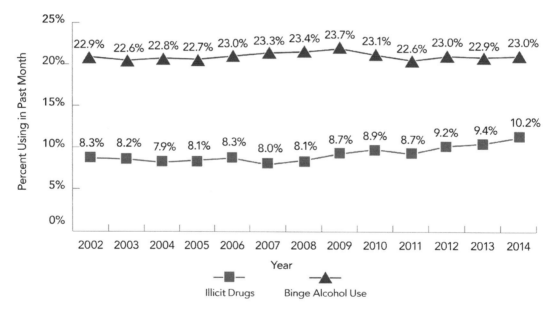

Notes: *The National Survey on Drug Use and Health* (NSDUH) obtains information on nine categories of illicit drugs: marijuana (including hashish), cocaine (including crack), heroin, hallucinogens, and inhalants, as well as the nonmedical use of prescription-type pain relievers, tranquilizers, stimulants, and sedatives; see the section on nonmedical use of psychotherapeutic drugs for the definition of nonmedical use. Estimates of "illicit drug use" reported from NSDUH reflect the use of these nine drug categories. Difference between the Illicit Drug Use estimate for 2002-2013 and the 2014 estimate is statistically significant at the .05 level for all years against 2014. Binge drinking for NSDUH data collected in 2014 is defined as five or more drinks on the same occasion on at least one day in the past 30 days. There was no significant difference between 2002-2013 against 2014. In 2015, changes were made to the NSDUH questionnaire and data collection procedures that do not allow comparisons between 2015 and previous years for a number of outcomes.

Source: Center for Behavioral Health Statistics and Quality, (2015).[13]

This *Surgeon General's Report* has been created because of the important health and social problems associated with alcohol and drug misuse in America. As described in this *Report*, a comprehensive approach is needed to address substance use problems in the United States that includes several key components:

- Enhanced public education to improve awareness about substance use problems and demand for more effective policies and practices to address them;
- Widespread implementation of evidence-based prevention policies and programs to prevent substance misuse and related harms;
- Improved access to evidence-based treatment services, integrated with mainstream health care, for those at risk for or affected by substance use disorders;
- Recovery support services (RSS) to assist individuals in maintaining remission and preventing relapse; and
- Research-informed public policies and financing strategies to ensure that substance misuse and use disorder services are accessible, compassionate, efficient, and sustainable.

> **KEY TERMS**
>
> **The Public Health System.** The Public Health System is defined as "all public, private, and voluntary entities that contribute to the delivery of essential public health services within a jurisdiction" and includes state and local public health agencies, public safety agencies, health care providers, human service and charity organizations, recreation and arts-related organizations, economic and philanthropic organizations, and education and youth development organizations.[2]
>
> **The Health Care System.** The World Health Organization defines a health care system as (1) all the activities whose primary purpose is to promote, restore, and/or maintain health, and (2) the people, institutions, and resources, arranged together in accordance with established policies, to improve the health of the population they serve. The health care system is made up of diverse health care organizations ranging from primary care, specialty substance use disorder treatment (including residential and outpatient settings), mental health care, infectious disease clinics, school clinics, community health centers, hospitals, emergency departments, and others.[5]

Recognizing these needs, the *Report* explains the neurobiological basis for substance use disorders and provides the biological, psychological, and social frameworks for improving diagnosis, prevention, and treatment of alcohol and drug misuse. It also describes evidence-based prevention strategies, such as public policies that can reduce substance misuse problems (e.g., driving under the influence [DUI]); effective treatment strategies, including medications and behavioral therapies for treating substance use disorders; and RSS for people who have completed treatment. Additionally, the *Report* describes recent changes in health care financing, including changes in health insurance regulations, which support the integration of clinical prevention and treatment services for substance use disorders into mainstream health care practice, and defines a research agenda for addressing alcohol and drug misuse as medical conditions.

Thus, this first *Surgeon General's Report on Alcohol, Drugs, and Health* is not issued simply because of the prevalence of substance misuse or even the related devastating harms and costs, but also to help inform policymakers, health care professionals, and the general public about effective, practical, and sustainable strategies to address these problems. These strategies have the potential to substantially reduce substance misuse and related problems; promote early intervention for substance misuse and substance use disorders; and improve the availability of high-quality treatment and RSS for persons with substance use disorders.

A Public Health Model for Addressing Substance Misuse and Related Consequences

A public health systems approach to substance misuse and its consequences, including substance use disorders, aims to:

- Define the problem through the systematic collection of data on the scope, characteristics, and consequences of substance misuse;
- Identify the risk and protective factors that increase or decrease the risk for substance misuse and its consequences, and the factors that could be modified through interventions;
- Work across the public and private sector to develop and test interventions that address social, environmental, or economic determinants of substance misuse and related health consequences;
- Support broad implementation of effective prevention and treatment interventions and recovery supports in a wide range of settings; and
- Monitor the impact of these interventions on substance misuse and related problems as well as on risk and protective factors.

A healthy community is one with not just a strong health care system but also a strong public health educational system, safe streets, effective public transportation and affordable, high quality food and housing – where all individuals have opportunities to thrive. Thus, community leaders should work together to mobilize the capacities of health care organizations, social service organizations, educational systems, community-based organizations, government health agencies, religious institutions, law enforcement, local businesses, researchers, and other public, private, and voluntary entities that can contribute to the above aims. Everyone has a role to play in addressing substance misuse and its consequences and thereby improving the public health.

Substances Discussed in this Report

This *Report* defines a **substance** as a psychoactive compound with the potential to cause health and social problems, including substance use disorders (and their most severe manifestation, addiction). These substances can be divided into three major categories: Alcohol, Illicit Drugs (a category that includes prescription drugs used nonmedically), and Over-the-Counter Drugs. Some specific examples of the substances included in each of these categories are included in Table 1.1. Over-the-Counter Drugs are not discussed in this *Report*, but are included in Appendix D – Important Facts about Alcohol and Drugs.

Although different in many respects, the substances discussed in this *Report* share three features that make them important to public health and safety. *First, many people use and misuse these substances:* 66.7 million individuals in the United States aged 12 or older admitted to binge drinking in the past month and 27.1 million people aged 12 or older used an illicit drug in the past month.[3]

Table 1.1: Categories and Examples of Substances

Substance Category	Representative Examples
Alcohol	<ul><li>Beer</li><li>Wine</li><li>Malt liquor</li><li>Distilled spirits</li></ul>
Illicit Drugs	<ul><li>Cocaine, including crack</li><li>Heroin</li><li>Hallucinogens, including LSD, PCP, ecstasy, peyote, mescaline, psilocybin</li><li>Methamphetamines, including crystal meth</li><li>Marijuana, including hashish*</li><li>Synthetic drugs, including K2, Spice, and "bath salts"**</li><li>Prescription-type medications that are used for nonmedical purposes<ul><li>Pain Relievers - Synthetic, semi-synthetic, and non-synthetic opioid medications, including fentanyl, codeine, oxycodone, hydrocodone, and tramadol products</li><li>Tranquilizers, including benzodiazepines, meprobamate products, and muscle relaxants</li><li>Stimulants and Methamphetamine, including amphetamine, dextroamphetamine, and phentermine products; mazindol products; and methylphenidate or dexmethylphenidate products</li><li>Sedatives, including temazepam, flurazepam, or triazolam and any barbiturates</li></ul></li></ul>
Over-the-Counter Drugs and Other Substances	<ul><li>Cough and cold medicines**</li><li>Inhalants, including amyl nitrite, cleaning fluids, gasoline and lighter gases, anesthetics, solvents, spray paint, nitrous oxide</li></ul>

Notes: The *Report* discusses the substances known to have a significant public health impact. These substances are also included in NSDUH. Additionally, NSDUH includes tobacco products (cigarettes, smokeless tobacco, cigars, and pipe tobacco); however, tobacco products are not discussed in this *Report* at length because they have been covered extensively in other Surgeon General's Reports.[14-17]

* As of June 2016, 25 states and the District of Columbia have legalized medical marijuana use, four states have legalized retail marijuana sales, and the District of Columbia has legalized personal use and home cultivation (both medical and recreational). It should be noted that none of the permitted uses under state laws alter the status of marijuana and its constituent compounds as illicit drugs under Schedule I of the federal Controlled Substances Act. See the section on Marijuana: A Changing Legal and Research Environment later in this chapter for more detail on this issue.

** These substances are not included in NSDUH and are not discussed in this *Report*. However, important facts about these drugs are included in Appendix D - Important Facts about Alcohol and Drugs.

Second, individuals can use these substances in a manner that causes harm to the user or those around them. This is called **substance misuse** and often results in health or social problems, referred to in this *Report* as **substance misuse problems.** Misuse can be of low severity and temporary, but it can also result in serious, enduring, and costly consequences due to motor vehicle crashes,[18,19] intimate partner and sexual violence,[20] child abuse and neglect,[21] suicide attempts and fatalities,[22] overdose deaths,[23] various forms of cancer[24] (e.g., breast cancer in women),[25] heart and liver diseases,[26] HIV/AIDS,[27] and problems related to drinking or using drugs during pregnancy, such as fetal alcohol spectrum disorders (FASDs) or neonatal abstinence syndrome (NAS).[28]

*Third, prolonged, repeated misuse of any of these substances can produce changes to the brain that can lead to a **substance use disorder**, an independent illness that significantly impairs health and function and may require specialty treatment.* Disorders can range from mild to severe. Severe and chronic substance use disorders are commonly referred to as **addictions.**

> **FOR MORE ON THIS TOPIC**
>
> See the section on *Diagnosing a Substance Use Disorder* later in this chapter.

Key Terms Used in the Report

Addiction: The most severe form of substance use disorder, associated with compulsive or uncontrolled use of one or more substances. Addiction is a chronic brain disease that has the potential for both recurrence (relapse) and recovery.

Substance: A psychoactive compound with the potential to cause health and social problems, including substance use disorders (and their most severe manifestation, addiction). For a list of substance categories included in this *Report* see <u>Table 1.1.</u> Note: Cigarettes and other tobacco products are only briefly discussed here due to extensive coverage in prior Surgeon General's Reports.[14-17]

Substance Use: The use—even one time—of any of the substances in this *Report*.

Substance Misuse: The use of any substance in a manner, situation, amount, or frequency that can cause harm to users or to those around them. For some substances or individuals, any use would constitute misuse (e.g., underage drinking, injection drug use).

Binge Drinking: Binge drinking for men is drinking 5 or more standard alcoholic drinks, and for women, 4 or more standard alcoholic drinks on the same occasion on at least 1 day in the past 30 days.

Heavy Drinking: Defined by the CDC as consuming 8 or more drinks per week for women, and 15 or more drinks per week for men, and by the Substance Abuse and Mental Health Services Administration (SAMHSA), for research purposes, as binge drinking on 5 or more days in the past 30 days.

Standard Drink: Based on the *2015-2020 Dietary Guidelines for Americans*, a standard drink is defined as shown in the graphic below. All of these drinks contain 14 grams (0.6 ounces) of pure alcohol.

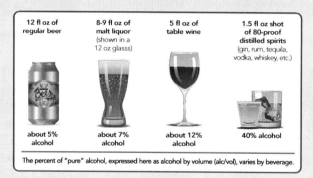

Source: U.S. Department of Health and Human Services and U.S. Department of Agriculture, (2015).[29]

Substance Misuse Problems or Consequences: Any health or social problem that results from substance misuse. Substance misuse problems or consequences may affect the substance user or those around them, and they may be acute (e.g., an argument or fight, a motor vehicle crash, an overdose) or chronic (e.g., a long-term substance-related medical, family, or employment problem, or chronic medical condition, such as various cancers, heart disease, and liver disease). These problems may occur at any age and are more likely to occur with greater frequency of substance misuse.

Substance Use Disorder: A medical illness caused by repeated misuse of a substance or substances. According to the Fifth Edition of the *Diagnostic and Statistical Manual of Mental Disorders* (DSM-5),[30] substance use disorders are characterized by clinically significant impairments in health, social function, and impaired control over substance use and are diagnosed through assessing cognitive, behavioral, and psychological symptoms. Substance use disorders range from mild to severe and from temporary to chronic. They typically develop gradually over time with repeated misuse, leading to changes in brain circuits governing incentive salience (the

> ability of substance-associated cues to trigger substance seeking), reward, stress, and executive functions like decision making and self-control. Multiple factors influence whether and how rapidly a person will develop a substance use disorder. These factors include the substance itself; the genetic vulnerability of the user; and the amount, frequency, and duration of the misuse. Note: A severe substance use disorder is commonly called an addiction.
>
> **Relapse:** The return to drug use after a significant period of abstinence.
>
> **Recovery:** A process of change through which individuals improve their health and wellness, live a self-directed life, and strive to reach their full potential. Even individuals with severe and chronic substance use disorders can, with help, overcome their substance use disorder and regain health and social function. This is called remission. When those positive changes and values become part of a voluntarily adopted lifestyle, that is called "being in recovery." Although abstinence from all substance misuse is a cardinal feature of a recovery lifestyle, it is not the only healthy, pro-social feature.

Prevalence of Substance Use, Misuse Problems, and Disorders

How widespread are substance use, misuse, and substance use disorders in the United States? The annual *National Survey on Drug Use and Health* (NSDUH) gathers data on the scope and prevalence of substance use, misuse, and related disorders, as well as utilization of substance use disorder treatment, among Americans aged 12 and older, representing more than 265 million people. Table 1.2 provides selected findings from the 2015 NSDUH. The table provides only general statistics for the United States as a whole; readers are urged to consult NSDUH's detailed tables[3] for subpopulation estimates.

Over 175 million persons aged 12 and older (65.7 percent of this population) reported alcohol use in the past year, with over 66 million (24.9 percent) reporting binge drinking in the past month (Table 1.2). More than 36 million (13.5 percent) reported using marijuana in the past year, 12.5 million reported misusing prescription pain relievers, and over 300,000 reported using heroin in the past year. Almost 8 percent of the population met diagnostic criteria for a substance use disorder for alcohol or illicit drugs, and another 1 percent met diagnostic criteria for both an alcohol and illicit drug use disorder. Although 20.8 million people (7.8 percent of the population) met the diagnostic criteria for a substance use disorder in 2015, only 2.2 million individuals (10.4 percent) received any type of treatment. Of those treated, 63.7 percent received treatment in specialty substance use disorder treatment programs.[3]

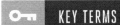

KEY TERMS

Prevalence. The proportion of a population who have (or had) a specific characteristic—for example, an illness, condition, behavior, or risk factor— in a given time period.

Several specific findings shown in Table 1.2 bear emphasis. Past year misuse of prescription psychotherapeutic drugs was reported by 18.9 million individuals in 2015 (7.1 percent of the population).[3] Within this category, prescribed opioid pain relievers (e.g., OxyContin®, Vicodin®, Lortab®) accounted for 12.5 million people, followed by tranquilizers, such as Xanax®, reported by 6.1 million people; stimulants, such as Adderall® or Ritalin®, reported by 5.3 million people; and sedatives, such as Valium®, reported by 1.5 million people.[3]

> ## Substance Use Disorder Treatment Programs
>
> Historically, treatment services were designed for people with severe substance use disorders (addictions), and programs were generally referred to as "specialty addiction treatment programs." Today, individuals with mild to severe substance use disorders may receive treatment. These treatments are delivered by specialty programs, as well as by more generalist providers (e.g., primary care and general mental health providers). Not everyone with a substance use disorder will need ongoing treatment; many will require only a brief intervention and monitoring. Because treatments vary substantially in level of specialization, content, duration, and setting, and because those receiving services may differ substantially in the severity, duration, and complexity of their substance use disorder, this *Report* uses the phrase "substance use disorder treatment" as the generic term to capture the broad spectrum of advice, therapies, services, and monitoring provided to the group of individuals with mild to severe substance use disorders. The programs and services that provide specialty treatment are referred to as "substance use disorder treatment programs or services."

The prevalence of past 30-day use of "any illicit drugs" (a broad category including marijuana/hashish, cocaine/crack, heroin, hallucinogens, inhalants, and prescription psychotherapeutic medications used nonmedically) rose from 9.4 percent in 2013 to 10.2 percent in 2014 among persons aged 12 and older (**Figure 1.2**). This 2014 prevalence rate for illicit drugs is significantly higher than it was in any year from 2002 to 2013. However, no significant changes were observed that year specifically in the use of prescription psychotherapeutic drugs, cocaine, or hallucinogens, suggesting that the observed increase was primarily related to increased use of marijuana. Marijuana was the most frequently used illicit drug (35.1 million past year users).[31] The rate for past month marijuana use in 2014 was significantly higher than it was in any year from 2002 to 2013, with the prevalence of past 30-day marijuana use rising from 7.5 percent in 2013 to 8.4 percent in 2014.[13] (Note: In 2015, changes were made to the NSDUH questionnaire and data collection procedures that do not allow for the presentation of trend data beyond 2014. For more information, see *Summary of the Effects of the 2015 NSDUH Questionnaire Redesign: Implications for Data Users.*[32])

Demographics of Substance Use

Table 1.3 and Table 1.4 show substance use by demographic characteristics. Prevalence of substance misuse and substance use disorders differs by race and ethnicity and gender, and these factors can also influence access to health care and substance use disorder treatment. Past year alcohol use for men was 68.6 percent and for women it was 62.9 percent. Past month binge alcohol use was 29.6 percent for men and 20.5 percent for women. The prevalence of past month binge alcohol use was 24.1 percent for American Indians or Alaska Natives, 25.7 percent for Hispanics or Latinos, and 26.0 for Whites. Prevalence of an alcohol use disorder was 7.8 percent for men and 4.1 percent for women. The prevalence of an illicit drug use disorder was 3.8 percent for men and 2.0 percent for women.

Table 1.2: Past Year Substance Use, Past Year Initiation of Substance Use, and Met Diagnostic Criteria for a Substance Use Disorder in the Past Year Among Persons Aged 12 Years or Older for Specific Substances: Numbers in Millions and Percentages, 2015 National Survey on Drug Use and Health (NSDUH)

Substance	Past Year Use or Misuse[v]		Past Year Initiation Among Total Population[vi]		Met Diagnostic Criteria for a Substance Use Disorder[vi,vii]	
	#	%	#	%	#	%
Alcohol	175.8	65.7	4.8	1.8	15.7	5.9
Drinking Pattern						
Binge Drinking[i]	66.7	24.9	da	da	da	da
Heavy Drinking[i]	17.3	6.5	da	da	da	da
Any Illicit Drug[ii]	47.7	17.8	nr	nr	7.7	2.9
Cocaine/Crack	36.0	1.8	1.0	0.4	0.9	0.3
Heroin	0.8	0.3	0.1	0.1	0.6	0.2
Hallucinogens	4.7	1.8	1.2	0.4	0.3	0.1
Marijuana[iii]	36.0	13.5	2.6	1.0	4.0	1.5
Inhalants	1.8	0.7	0.6	0.2	0.1	0.0
Misuse of Psychotherapeutics[iv]	18.9	7.1	nr	nr	2.7	1.0
Pain Relievers	12.5	4.7	2.1	0.8	2.0	0.8
Tranquilizers	6.1	2.3	1.4	0.5	0.7	0.3
Stimulants	5.3	2.0	1.3	0.5	0.4	0.2
Sedatives	1.5	0.6	0.4	0.2	0.2	0.1
Alcohol or Any Illicit Drugs[ii]	182.3	68.1	nr	nr	20.8	7.8
Alcohol and Any Illicit Drugs[ii]	41.3	15.4	nr	nr	2.7	1.0

Notes: Past year initiates are defined as persons who used the substance(s) for the first time in the 12 months before the date of interview. The "nr = not reported due to measurement issues" notation indicates that the estimate could be calculated based on available data but is not calculated due to potential measurement issues. The "da" indication means does not apply.

i. Binge and heavy drinking, as defined by SAMHSA, are reported only for the period of 30 days before the interview date. SAMHSA defines binge use of alcohol for males and females as "drinking five (males)/four (females) or more drinks on the same occasion (i.e., at the same time or within a couple of hours of each other) on at least 1 day in the past 30 days" and heavy use of alcohol for both males and females as "binge drinking on each of 5 or more days in the past 30 days."

ii. Illicit drug use includes the misuse of prescription psychotherapeutics or the use of marijuana, cocaine (including crack), heroin, hallucinogens, inhalants, or methamphetamine.

iii. As of June 2016, 25 states and the District of Columbia have legalized medical marijuana use. Four states have legalized retail marijuana sales; the District of Columbia has legalized personal use and home cultivation (both medical and recreational). It should be noted that none of the permitted uses under state laws alter the status of marijuana and its constituent compounds as illicit drugs under Schedule I of the federal Controlled Substances Act.

iv. Misuse of prescription-type psychotherapeutics includes the nonmedical use of pain relievers, tranquilizers, stimulants, or sedatives and does not include over-the-counter drugs.

v. Estimates of misuse of psychotherapeutics and stimulants include data from new methamphetamine items added in 2005 and 2006 and are not comparable with estimates presented in NSDUH reports before 2007. See Section B.4.8 in Appendix B of the Results from the 2008 NSDUH.

vi. Estimates of misuse of psychotherapeutics and stimulants do not include data from new methamphetamine items added in 2005 and 2006.

vii. Diagnostic criteria for a substance use disorder is based on definitions found in the Fourth Edition of the *Diagnostic and Statistical Manual of Mental Disorders* (DSM-IV).

Source: Center for Behavioral Health Statistics and Quality, (2016).[3]

Figure 1.2: Trends in Binge Drinking and Past 30-Day Use of Illicit Drugs among Persons Aged 12 Years or Older, 2014 National Survey on Drug Use and Health (NSDUH)

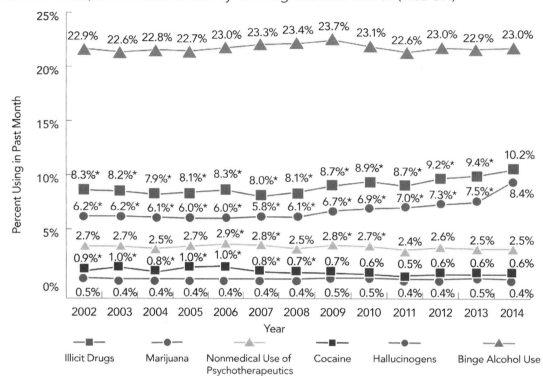

Notes: *Difference between this estimate and the 2014 estimate is statistically significant at the .05 level. Illicit drugs include marijuana/hashish, cocaine (including crack), heroin, hallucinogens, inhalants, or prescription psychotherapeutics used non-medically. Nonmedical use of prescription psychotherapeutics includes the nonmedical use of pain relievers, tranquilizers, stimulants, or sedatives. In 2015, changes were made to the NSDUH questionnaire and data collection procedures that do not allow comparisons between 2015 and previous years for a number of outcomes.

Source: Center for Behavioral Health Statistics and Quality, (2015).[13]

Relevance of Substance Use and Misuse

It is sometimes thought that concern over substance use and misuse should be secondary to the *real* issue of substance use disorders and especially their severest manifestation, addiction, which has captured media headlines and has been linked to many health and social problems. This is an important misconception. Individuals with substance use disorders have elevated rates of substance misuse–related health and social problems and costs, but as shown in the last columns of Table 1.2, Table 1.3, and Table 1.4, many people who misuse substances do not meet the diagnostic criteria for a substance use disorder. For example, binge drinking at least once during the past month was self-reported by over 66 million individuals. By definition, those episodes have the potential for producing harm to the user and/or to those around them, through increases in motor vehicle crashes, violence, and alcohol-poisonings.[33] Similarly, in 2015, 12.5 million individuals misused a pain reliever in the past year—setting the stage for a potential overdose—but only 2.9 million met diagnostic criteria for a prescription medication disorder.[3]

Table 1.3: Past Year Alcohol Use, Past Month Binge Alcohol Use, and Met Diagnostic Criteria for a Substance Use Disorder in the Past Year Among Persons Aged 12 Years or Older: Numbers in Millions and Percentages, 2015 National Survey on Drug Use and Health (NSDUH)

Demographic Group	Past Year Alcohol Use		Past Month Binge Alcohol Use[ii]		Met Diagnostic Criteria for a Substance Use Disorder in Past Year[i]	
	#	%	#	%	#	%
Alcohol						
Male	89.0	68.6	38.4	29.6	10.1	7.8
Female	86.9	62.9	28.3	20.5	5.6	4.1
White	119.9	70.3	44.4	26.0	10.4	6.1
Black or African American	18.6	58.0	7.5	23.4	1.6	4.9
American Indian or Alaska Native	0.7	51.4	0.3	24.1	0.1	9.7
Native Hawaiian or Other Pacific Islander	0.4	51.1	0.1	17.8	0.04	5.4
Asian	7.8	53.1	2.1	14.0	0.5	3.2
Two or More Races	2.7	57.0	1.1	22.9	0.3	6.2
Hispanic or Latino	25.7	59.0	11.2	25.7	2.8	6.4

Table 1.4: Past Year Substance Use, Past 30-Day Illicit Drug Use, and Met Diagnostic Criteria for a Substance Use Disorder in the Past Year Among Persons Aged 12 Years or Older: Numbers in Millions and Percentages, 2015 National Survey on Drug Use and Health (NSDUH)

Demographic Group	Past Year Use		Past 30-Day Illicit Drug Use		Met Diagnostic Criteria for a Substance Use Disorder in Past Year[i]	
	#	%	#	%	#	%
Any Illicit Drug[iii]						
Male	26.6	20.5	16.2	12.5	5.0	3.8
Female	21.2	15.3	10.9	7.9	2.8	2.0
White	30.5	17.9	17.4	10.2	4.8	2.8
Black or African American	6.6	20.7	4.0	12.5	1.1	3.5
American Indian or Alaska Native	0.3	22.9	0.2	14.2	0.06	4.1
Native Hawaiian or Other Pacific Islander	0.1	20.5	0.07	9.8	0.03	4.5
Asian	1.4	9.2	0.6	4.0	0.2	1.2
Two or More Races	1.3	27.1	0.8	17.2	0.2	4.9
Hispanic or Latino	7.4	17.2	4.0	9.2	1.3	3.0

i. Diagnostic criteria for a substance use disorder is based on definitions found in the Fourth Edition of the *Diagnostic and Statistical Manual of Mental Disorders* (DSM-IV).

ii. Binge drinking, as defined by SAMHSA, are reported only for the period of 30 days before the interview date. SAMHSA defines binge use of alcohol for males and females as "drinking five (males)/four (females) or more drinks on the same occasion (i.e., at the same time or within a couple of hours of each other) on at least 1 day in the past 30 days.

iii. Illicit drugs include marijuana/hashish, cocaine (including crack), heroin, hallucinogens, inhalants, or misuse of prescription-type psychotherapeutics, including data from original methamphetamine questions but not including new methamphetamine items added in 2005 and 2006.

Source: Center for Behavioral Health Statistics and Quality, (2016).[3]

The clear implications of these data are that a comprehensive approach to reducing the misuse of alcohol and drugs—one that includes the implementation of effective prevention programs and policy strategies as well as high-quality treatment services—is needed to reduce the problems and costs of substance misuse in the United States. In fact, greater impact is likely to be achieved by reducing substance misuse in the general population—that is, among people who are *not* addicted—than among those with severe substance use problems. Of course, efforts to reduce general population rates of substance use and misuse are also likely to reduce rates of substance use disorders, because substance use disorders typically develop over time following repeated episodes of misuse (often at escalating rates) that result in the progressive changes to brain circuitry that underlie addiction.

> **FOR MORE ON THIS TOPIC**
>
> See Chapter 2 - *The Neurobiology of Substance Use, Misuse, and Addiction.*

Costs and Impact of Substance Use and Misuse

Alcohol misuse, illicit drug use, misuse of medications, and substance use disorders are estimated to cost the United States more than $400 billion in lost workplace productivity (in part, due to premature mortality), health care expenses, law enforcement and other criminal justice costs (e.g., drug-related crimes), and losses from motor vehicle crashes.[10,11] Furthermore, about three quarters of the costs associated with alcohol use were due to binge drinking, and about 40 percent of those costs were paid by government, emphasizing the huge cost of alcohol misuse to taxpayers.[34]

These costs are not unique to the United States. A 2010 study examined the global burden of disability attributable to substance misuse problems and disorders, focusing particularly on lost ability to work and years of life lost to premature mortality. Costs were calculated for 20 age groups and both sexes in 187 countries.[35] Mental and substance use disorders were the leading causes of years lived with disability worldwide, largely because these problems strike individuals early in their lives and can continue—especially if untreated—for long periods.

In addition to the costs to society, substance misuse can have many direct and indirect health and personal consequences for individuals. The direct effects on the user depend on the specific substances used, how much and how often they are used, how they are taken (e.g., orally vs. injected), and other factors. Acute effects can range from changes in mood and basic body functions, such as heart rate or blood pressure, to overdose and death. Alcohol misuse and drug use can also have long-term effects on physical and mental health and can lead to substance use disorders. For example, drug use is associated with chronic pain conditions and cardiovascular and cardiopulmonary diseases.[36,37] Alcohol misuse is associated with liver and pancreatic diseases, hypertension, reproductive system disorders, trauma, stroke, FASD, and cancers of the oral cavity, esophagus, larynx, pharynx, liver, colon, and rectum.[26,28] For breast cancer, studies have shown that even moderate drinking may increase the risk.[25] Although alcohol consumption is associated with adverse health effects as noted above, the *2015-2020 Dietary Guidelines for*

Americans indicate that moderate alcohol use can be part of a healthy diet, but only when used by adults of legal drinking age.[i]

In addition, alcohol and drug use by pregnant women can have profound effects on the developing fetus. Alcohol use during pregnancy can lead to a wide range of disabilities in children, the most severe of which is FASD, characterized by intellectual disabilities, speech and language delays, poor social skills, and sometimes facial deformities. Use of drugs, such as opioids during pregnancy, can result in NAS, a drug-withdrawal syndrome requiring medical intervention and extended hospital stay for newborns. Use of some drugs, such as cocaine, during pregnancy may also lead to premature birth or miscarriage. In addition, substance use during pregnancy may interfere with a child's brain development and result in later consequences for mental functioning and behavior.

Substance misuse also can affect a user's nutrition and sleep, as well as increase the risk for trauma, violence, injury, and contraction of communicable diseases, such as HIV/AIDS and Hepatitis C. These consequences can all contribute to the spectrum of public health consequences of substance misuse and need to be considered both independently and collectively when developing and implementing clinical and public health interventions.

Substance misuse problems can also result in other serious and sometimes fatal health problems and extraordinary costs; they may also lead to unexpected death from other causes. Three examples of these serious, sometimes lethal, problems related to substance misuse are highlighted below.

Driving Under the Influence

In 2014, 9,967 people were killed in motor vehicle crashes while driving under the influence of alcohol, representing nearly one third (31 percent) of all traffic-related fatalities in the United States.[38] DUI continues to be among the most frequent causes for arrests every year.[39] But at approximately 1.3 million per year, these arrests represent only about 1 percent of the actual alcohol-impaired driving incidents reported in national surveys, suggesting that there are many more people who drive while impaired that have not been arrested, putting themselves and others at high risk of being harmed.[18,40] In addition to the deaths that result from DUI, the National Highway Traffic Safety Administration (NHTSA) estimates that DUI costs the United States more than $44 billion each year in prosecution, higher insurance rates, higher taxes, medical claims, and property damage.[41]

As important as they are, these statistics account for only alcohol-related driving impairment and fail to measure other impairing substances. A study by NHTSA tested oral fluid and blood specimens from a random sample of drivers at the roadside (during daytime on Friday or nighttime Friday to Sunday) and

---

i   Moderate alcohol use is defined by the *2015-2020 Dietary Guidelines for Americans* as up to 1 drink per day for women and up to 2 drinks per day for men—and only by adults of legal drinking age. Many individuals should not consume alcohol, including individuals who are taking certain over-the-counter or prescription medications or who have certain medical conditions, those who are recovering from an alcohol use disorder or are unable to control the amount they drink, and anyone younger than age 21 years. In addition, drinking during pregnancy may result in negative behavioral or neurological consequences in the offspring.

found 12 to 15 percent had used one or more illegal substances.[42] Drivers tested positive for drugs in approximately 16 percent of all motor vehicle crashes.[43]

Overdose Deaths

Overdose deaths are typically caused by consuming substances at high intensity and/or by consuming combinations of substances such as alcohol, sedatives, tranquilizers, and opioid pain relievers to the point where critical areas in the brain that control breathing, heart rate, and body temperature stop functioning.

Alcohol Overdose (Alcohol Poisoning)

The CDC reports more than 2,200 alcohol overdose deaths in the United States each year—an average of six deaths every day.[44] More than three quarters (76 percent) of alcohol overdose deaths occur among adults between ages 35 and 64, and 76 percent of those who die from alcohol overdose are men.

Drug Overdose (Illicit and Prescription Drugs)

Opioid analgesic pain relievers are now the most prescribed class of medications in the United States, with more than 289 million prescriptions written each year.[45,46] The increase in prescriptions of opioid pain relievers has been accompanied by dramatic increases in misuse (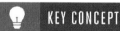) and by a more than 200 percent increase in the number of emergency department visits from 2005 to 2011.[47] In 2014, 47,055 drug overdose deaths occurred in the United States, and 61 percent of these deaths were the result of opioid use, including prescription opioids and heroin.[7] Heroin overdoses have more than tripled from 2010 to 2014.[7] Heroin overdoses were more than five times higher in 2014 (10,574) then ten years before in 2004 (1,878). Additionally, rates of cocaine overdose were higher in 2014 than in the previous six years (5,415 deaths from cocaine overdose). In 2014, there were 17,465 overdoses from illicit drugs and 25,760 overdoses from prescription drugs.[48] Drug overdose deaths also occur as a result of the illicit manufacturing and distribution of synthetic opioids, such as fentanyl, and the illegal diversion of prescription opioids. Illicit fentanyl, for example, is often combined with heroin or counterfeit prescription drugs or sold as heroin, and may be contributing to recent increases in drug overdose deaths.[7,49]

> **KEY CONCEPT**
>
> **The Opioid Crisis.** Over-prescription of powerful opioid pain relievers beginning in the 1990s led to a rapid escalation of use and misuse of these substances by a broad demographic of men and women across the country.[1] This led to a resurgence of heroin use, as some users transitioned to using this cheaper street cousin of expensive prescription opioids. As a result, the number of people dying from opioid overdoses soared—increasing nearly four-fold between 1999 and 2014.[4]

Intimate Partner Violence, Sexual Assault, and Rape

Intimate partner violence, sexual assault, and rape are crimes with long-lasting effects on victims and great cost to society.[50,51] These crimes happen to both women and men and are often associated with substance use. A recent national survey found that 22 percent of women and 14 percent of men reported experiencing severe physical violence from an intimate partner in their lifetimes.[52] In this survey, 19.3 percent of women and 1.7 percent of men reported being raped in their lifetimes, while 43.9 percent of women and 23.4 percent of men reported some other form of sexual violence in their lifetimes.[52] Substance misuse is often related to these crimes.

Numerous studies have found a high correlation between substance use and intimate partner violence,[53-56] although this does not mean that substance use causes intimate partner violence. In addition to evidence from the criminal justice arena, recent systematic reviews have found that substance use is both a risk factor for and a consequence of intimate partner violence.[57-59]

A recent survey of sexual assault and sexual misconduct on college campuses found that use of alcohol and drugs are important risk factors for nonconsensual sexual contact among undergraduate, graduate, and professional students.[20] It is clear that substance use and intimate partner violence and sexual assault are closely linked; however, more research is needed on the nature of the relationship between substance use and these forms of violence to determine how substance use contributes to the perpetration of violence and victimization and how violence contributes to subsequent substance use among both perpetrators and victims.

Vulnerability to Substance Misuse Problems and Disorders

Risk and Protective Factors: Keys to Vulnerability

Substance misuse problems and substance use disorders are not inevitable. An individual's vulnerability may be partly predicted by assessing the nature and number of their community, caregiver/family, and individual-level risk and protective factors.

Significant community-level risk factors for substance misuse and use disorders include easy access to inexpensive alcohol and other substances. Caregiver/family-level risk factors include low parental monitoring, a family history of substance use or mental disorders, and high levels of family conflict or violence. At the individual level, major risk factors include current mental disorders, low involvement in school, a history of abuse and neglect, and a history of substance use during adolescence, among others.[60]

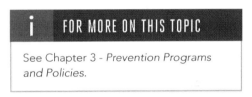

FOR MORE ON THIS TOPIC

See Chapter 3 - *Prevention Programs and Policies*.

Community-level protective factors include higher cost for alcohol and other drugs (often achieved by increasing taxes on these products); regulating the number and concentration of retailers selling various substances (e.g., density of alcohol outlets or marijuana dispensaries); preventing illegal alcohol and other drug sales by enforcing existing laws and holding retailers accountable for harms caused by illegal sales (e.g., commercial host [dram shop] liability); availability of healthy recreational and social activities; and other population-level policies and their enforcement.[61] Caregiver/family-level protective factors include support and regular monitoring by parents.[60] Some important individual-level protective factors include involvement in school, engagement in healthy recreational and social activities, and good coping skills.[60]

Three important points about vulnerability should be highlighted. First, no single individual or community-level factor determines whether an individual will develop a substance misuse problem or disorder. Second, most risk and protective factors can be modified through preventive programs and policies to reduce vulnerability. Third, although substance misuse problems and disorders may occur at any age, adolescence and young adulthood are particularly critical at-risk periods. Research now indicates that the majority of those who meet criteria for a substance use disorder in their lifetime

> **FOR MORE ON THIS TOPIC**
>
> See Chapter 2 - *The Neurobiology of Substance Use, Misuse, and Addiction.*

started using substances during adolescence and met the criteria by age 20 to 25.[62-64] One likely reason for this vulnerability in adolescence and young adulthood is that alcohol and other substances have particularly potent effects on developing brain circuits, and recent scientific findings indicate that brain development is not complete until approximately age 21 to 23 in women and 23 to 25 in men.[65-67] Among the last brain regions to reach maturity is the prefrontal cortex, the brain region primarily responsible for "adult" abilities, such as delay of reward, extended reasoning, and impulse control. This area of the brain is one of the most affected regions in a substance use disorder.

Substance misuse can begin at any age. Therefore, it is important to focus on prevention of substance misuse across the lifespan as well as the prevention of substance use disorders.

Diagnosing a Substance Use Disorder

Changes in Understanding and Diagnosis of Substance Use Disorders

Repeated, regular misuse of any of the substances listed in <u>Figure 1.2</u> may lead to the development of a substance use disorder. Severe substance use disorders are characterized by compulsive use of substance(s) and impaired control of substance use. Substance use disorder diagnoses are based on criteria specified in the American Psychiatric Association's *Diagnostic and Statistical Manual of Mental Disorders* (DSM). Much of the substance use disorder data included in this *Report* is based on definitions included in the DSM-IV, which described two distinct disorders: substance abuse and substance dependence, with specific diagnostic criteria for each. Anyone meeting one or more of the abuse criteria—which focused largely on the negative consequences associated with substance misuse, such as being unable to fulfill family or work obligations, experiencing legal trouble, or engaging in hazardous behavior as a result of drug use—would receive the "abuse" diagnosis. Anyone with three or more of the dependence criteria, which included symptoms of drug tolerance, withdrawal, escalating and uncontrolled substance use, and the use of the substance to the exclusion of other activities, would receive the "dependence" diagnosis. Notably, addiction is not listed as a formal diagnosis in the DSM. However, substance

> **KEY CONCEPT**
>
> **Misuse versus Abuse.** This *Report* uses the term substance misuse, a term that is roughly equivalent to substance *abuse*. Substance abuse, an older diagnostic term, was defined as use that is unsafe (e.g., drunk or drugged driving), use that leads a person to fail to fulfill responsibilities or gets them in legal trouble, or use that continues despite causing persistent interpersonal problems like fights with a spouse.
>
> However, "substance abuse" is increasingly avoided by professionals because it can be shaming. Instead, substance misuse is now the preferred term. Although misuse is not a diagnostic term, it generally suggests use in a manner that could cause harm to the user or those around them.

dependence was often used interchangeably with addiction, and tolerance and withdrawal were considered, by many, cardinal features of addiction.

The DSM-5, which is the fifth and current version of the DSM, integrates the two DSM-IV disorders, substance abuse and substance dependence, into a single disorder called *substance use disorder* with *mild*, *moderate*, and *severe* sub-classifications. Individuals are evaluated for a substance use disorder based on 10 or 11 (depending on the substance) equally weighted diagnostic criteria (Table 1.5). Most of these overlap with those used to diagnose DSM-IV dependence and abuse. Individuals exhibiting fewer than two of the symptoms are not considered to have a substance use disorder. Those exhibiting two or three symptoms are considered to have a "mild" disorder, four or five symptoms constitutes a "moderate" disorder, and six or more symptoms is considered a "severe" substance use disorder.[30] In this *Report*, addiction is used to refer to substance use disorders at the severe end of the spectrum and are characterized by compulsive substance use and impaired control over use.

> **KEY TERMS**
>
> **Tolerance.** Alteration of the body's responsiveness to alcohol or a drug such that higher doses are required to produce the same effect achieved during initial use.
>
> **Withdrawal.** A set of symptoms that are experienced when discontinuing use of a substance to which a person has become dependent or addicted, which can include negative emotions such as stress, anxiety, or depression, as well as physical effects such as nausea, vomiting, muscle aches, and cramping, among others. Withdrawal symptoms often lead a person to use the substance again.

Table 1.5: Criteria for Diagnosing Substance Use Disorders

Diagnostic Criteria for Substance Use Disorders
Using in larger amounts or for longer than intended
Wanting to cut down or stop using, but not managing to
Spending a lot of time to get, use, or recover from use
Craving
Inability to manage commitments due to use
Continuing to use, even when it causes problems in relationships
Giving up important activities because of use
Continuing to use, even when it puts you in danger
Continuing to use, even when physical or psychological problems may be made worse by use
Increasing tolerance
Withdrawal symptoms

Notes: Fewer than 2 symptoms = no disorder; 2-3 = mild disorder; 4-5 = moderate disorder; 6 or more = severe disorder.

Source: American Psychiatric Association, (2013).[30]

Implications of the New Diagnostic Criteria

The new diagnostic criteria are likely to reduce the "all or nothing" thinking that has characterized the substance use field. Tolerance and withdrawal remain major clinical symptoms, but they are no longer the deciding factor in whether an individual "has an addiction." Substance use disorders, including addiction, can occur with *all* substances listed in Table 1.1, *not* just those that are able to produce

What is an Intervention?

Intervention here and throughout this *Report* means a professionally delivered program, service, or policy designed to prevent substance misuse or treat an individual's substance use disorder. It does not refer to an arranged meeting or confrontation intended to persuade a friend or loved one to quit their substance misuse or enter treatment—the type of "intervention" sometimes depicted on television. Planned surprise confrontations of the latter variety—a model developed in the 1960s, sometimes called the "Johnson Intervention"—have not been demonstrated to be an effective way to engage people in treatment.[68] Confrontational approaches in general, though once the norm even in many behavioral treatment settings, have not been found effective and may backfire by heightening resistance and diminishing self-esteem on the part of the targeted individual.[69]

tolerance and withdrawal. It is also important to understand that substance use disorders do not occur immediately but over time, with repeated misuse and development of more symptoms. This means that it is both possible and highly advisable to identify emerging substance use disorders, and to use evidence-based early interventions to stop the addiction process before the disorder becomes more chronic, complex, and difficult to treat.

This type of proactive clinical monitoring and management is already done within general health care settings to address other potentially progressive illnesses that are brought about by unhealthy behaviors.[70] For example, patients with high blood pressure may be told to adjust their activity and stress in order to reduce the progression of hypertension. Typically, these individuals are also clinically monitored for key symptoms to ensure that symptoms do not worsen.

> **FOR MORE ON THIS TOPIC**
>
> See Chapter 6 - *Health Care Systems and Substance Use Disorders*.

There are compelling reasons to apply similar procedures in emerging cases of substance misuse. Routine screening for alcohol and other substance use should be conducted in primary care settings to identify early symptoms of a substance use disorder (especially among those with known risk and few protective factors). This should be followed by informed clinical guidance on reducing the frequency and amount of substance use, family education to support lifestyle changes, and regular monitoring.

Research has shown that substance use disorders are similar in course, management, and outcome to other chronic illnesses, such as hypertension, diabetes, and asthma.[71] Unfortunately, substance use disorders have not been treated, monitored, or managed like other chronic illnesses, nor has care for these conditions been covered by insurance to the same degree. Nonetheless, it is possible to adopt the same type of chronic care management approach to the treatment of substance use disorders as is now used to manage most other chronic illnesses.[70-72] Evidence-based behavioral interventions, medications, social support services, clinical monitoring, and RSS make this type of chronic care management possible, often by the same health care teams that currently treat other chronic illnesses.

> **FOR MORE ON THIS TOPIC**
>
> See Chapter 4 - *Early Intervention, Treatment, and Management of Substance Use Disorders* and Chapter 6 - *Health Care Systems and Substance Use Disorders*.

Evidence also shows that such an approach will improve the effectiveness of treatments for substance use disorders. Remission of substance use and even full recovery can now be achieved if evidence-based care is provided for adequate periods of time, by properly trained health care professionals, and augmented by supportive monitoring, RSS, and social services. This fact is supported by a national survey showing that there are more than 25 million individuals who once had a problem with alcohol or drugs who no longer do.[73]

The Separation of Substance Use Treatment and General Health Care

Until quite recently, substance misuse problems and substance use disorders were viewed as social problems, best managed at the individual and family levels, and sometimes through the existing social infrastructure—such as schools and places of worship, and, when necessary, through civil and criminal justice interventions.[74] In the 1970s, when rates of substance misuse increased, including by college students and Vietnam War veterans, most families and traditional social services were not prepared to handle this problem.[75] Despite a compelling national need for treatment, the existing health care system was neither trained to care for nor especially eager to accept patients with substance use disorders.

For these reasons, a new system of substance use disorder treatment programs was created, but with administration, regulation, and financing placed outside mainstream health care.[74,75] This meant that with the exception of detoxification in hospital-based settings, virtually all treatment was delivered by programs that were geographically, financially, culturally, and organizationally separate from mainstream health care. Of equal historical importance was the decision to focus treatment only on addiction. This left few provisions for detecting or intervening clinically with the far more prevalent cases of early-onset, mild, or moderate substance use disorders.

Creating this system of substance use disorder treatment programs was a critical element in addressing the burgeoning substance use disorder problems in our nation. However, that separation also created unintended and enduring impediments to the quality and range of care options. For example, separate systems for substance use disorder treatment and other health care needs may have exacerbated the negative public attitudes toward people with substance use disorders. Additionally, the pharmaceutical industry was hesitant to invest in the development of new medications for individuals with substance use disorders, because they were not convinced that a market for these medications existed. Consequently, until the 1990s, few U.S. Food and Drug Administration (FDA) approved medications were available to treat addictions.[76,77]

Meanwhile, despite numerous research studies documenting high prevalence rates of substance use disorders among patients in emergency departments, hospitals, and general medical care settings, mainstream health care generally failed to recognize or address substance use disorders.[78] In fact, a recent study by the CDC found that in 2011, only 1 in 6 United States adults and 1 in 4 binge drinkers had *ever* been asked by a health professional about their drinking behavior.[79] Furthermore, the percent of adult binge drinkers who had been asked about their drinking had not changed since 1997, reflecting the challenges involved in fostering implementation of screening and counseling services for alcohol misuse in clinical settings. This has been a costly mistake, with often deadly consequences. A recent study showed that the presence of a substance use disorder often doubles the odds for the subsequent development of chronic and expensive medical illnesses, such as arthritis, chronic pain, heart disease, stroke, hypertension, diabetes, and asthma.[80]

In this regard, fatal medication errors due to unforeseen interactions between a prescribed medication for a diagnosed medical condition and unscreened, unaddressed patient substance use increased tenfold over the past 20 years.[81] To address this problem, researchers suggested "…(1) screening patients for use…of alcohol and/or street drugs; (2) taking extra precautions when prescribing medicines with known dangerous interactions with alcohol and/or street drugs; and (3) teaching the patient the risks of mixing medicines with alcohol and/or street drugs."[81] Similar recommendations focusing on prescribed opioids have been issued by the CDC to curb the rise in opioid overdose deaths.[82] Again, screening for substance use and substance use disorders before and during the course of opioid prescribing, combined with patient education, are recommended.[82]

Yet despite these and other indications of extreme threats to health care quality, safety, effectiveness, and cost containment, as of this writing, few general health care organizations screen for, or offer services for, the early identification and treatment of substance use disorders. Moreover, few medical, nursing, dental, or pharmacy schools teach their students about substance use disorders;[83-86] and, until recently, few insurers offered adequate reimbursement for treatment of substance use disorders.[87,88]

Recent Changes in Health Care Policy and Law

The longstanding separation of substance use disorders from the rest of health care began to change with enactment of the Paul Wellstone and Pete Domenici Mental Health Parity and Addiction Equity Act of 2008 (MHPAEA) and the Affordable Care Act in 2010.[89,90] MHPAEA requires that the financial requirements and treatment limitations imposed by health plans and insurers for substance use disorders be no more restrictive than the financial requirements and treatment limitations they impose for medical and surgical conditions. The Affordable Care Act requires the majority of United States health plans and insurers to offer prevention, screening, brief interventions, and other forms of treatment for substance use disorders.[89]

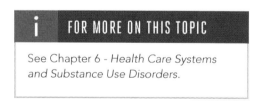

FOR MORE ON THIS TOPIC

See Chapter 6 - *Health Care Systems and Substance Use Disorders.*

It is difficult to overstate the importance of these two Acts for creating a public health-oriented approach to reducing substance misuse and related disorders. These laws and related changes in health care financing are creating incentives for health care organizations to integrate substance use disorder treatment with general health care. Many questions remain, but those questions are no longer *whether* but *how* this much-needed integration will occur. These changes combine to create a new, challenging but exceptionally promising era for the prevention and treatment of substance use disorders and set the context for this *Report.*

Marijuana: A Changing Legal and Research Environment

Although this *Report* does not examine the issue of marijuana legalization, its continually evolving legal status is worth mentioning because of implications for both research and policy. As mentioned elsewhere, marijuana is the most commonly used illicit drug in the United States, with 22.2 million people aged 12 or older using it in the past month.[3] In recent years marijuana use has become more socially acceptable among both adults and youth, while perceptions of risk among adolescents of the drug's harms have been declining over the past 13 years.[91]

As use of marijuana and its constituent components and derivatives becomes more widely accepted, it is critical to strengthen understanding of the effects and consequences for individual users and for public health and safety. Conducting such research can be complex as laws and policies vary significantly from state to state. For example, some states use a decriminalization model, which means production and sale of marijuana are still illegal and no legal marijuana farms, distributors, companies, stores, or advertising are permitted. Through ballot initiatives, other states have "legalized" marijuana use, which means they allow the production and sales of marijuana for personal use. Additionally, some states have legalized marijuana for medical purposes, and this group includes a wide variety of different models dictating how therapeutic marijuana is dispensed. The impacts of state laws regarding therapeutic and recreational marijuana are still being evaluated, although the differences make comparisons between states challenging.[92]

As of June 2016, 25 states and the District of Columbia have legalized medical marijuana use. Four states have legalized retail sales; the District of Columbia has legalized personal use and home cultivation (both medical and recreational), with more states expecting to do so. None of the permitted uses under state laws alters the status of marijuana and its constituent compounds as illicit drugs under Schedule I of the federal Controlled Substances Act.[93] It should also be noted that use for recreational purposes has not been legalized by any jurisdiction for people under age 21, and few jurisdictions have legalized medical marijuana for young people. While laws are changing, so too is the drug itself with average potency more than doubling over the past decade (1998 to 2008).[94] The ways marijuana is used are also changing – in addition to smoking, consuming edible forms like baked goods and candies, using vaporizing devices, and using high-potency extracts and oils (e.g., "dabbing") are becoming increasingly common.[95] Because these products and methods are unregulated even in states that have legalized marijuana use, users may not have accurate information about dosage or potency, which can lead and has led to serious consequences such as hospitalizations for psychosis and other overdose-related symptoms.[95] Marijuana use can also impair driving skills and, while estimates vary, is linked to a roughly two-fold increase in accident risk.[96-98] The risk is compounded when marijuana is used with alcohol.[96,99]

There is a growing body of research suggesting the potential therapeutic value of marijuana's constituent cannabinoid chemicals in numerous health conditions including pain, nausea, epilepsy, obesity, wasting disease, addiction, autoimmune disorders, and other conditions. Given the possibilities around therapeutic use, it is necessary to continue to explore ways of easing existing barriers to research. Marijuana has more than 100 constituent cannabinoid compounds, with cannabidiol (CBD) and tetrahydrocannabinol (THC, the chemical responsible for most of marijuana's intoxicating effects) being the most well-studied. Evidence collected so far in clinical investigations of the marijuana plant is still insufficient to meet

FDA standards for a finding of safety and efficacy for any therapeutic indications. However, the FDA has approved three medications containing synthetically derived cannabinoids: Marinol capsules and Syndros oral solution (both containing dronabinol, which is identical in chemical structure to THC), and Cesamet capsules (containing nabilone, which is similar in structure to THC) for severe nausea and wasting in certain circumstances, for instance in AIDS patients. Recognizing the potential therapeutic importance of compounds found in marijuana, the FDA has granted Fast Track designation to four development programs of products that contain marijuana constituents or their synthetic equivalents. The therapeutic areas in which products are being developed granted Fast Track by FDA include the treatment of pain in patients with advanced cancer; treatment of Dravet syndrome (two programs), a rare and catastrophic treatment-resistant form of childhood epilepsy; and treatment of neonatal hypoxic ischemic encephalopathy, brain injury resulting from oxygen deprivation during birth.

Additionally, there are clinical investigations for the treatment of refractory seizure syndromes, including Lennox Gastaut Syndrome, and for treatment of post-traumatic stress disorder (PTSD). However, further exploration of these issues always requires consideration of the serious health and safety risks associated with marijuana use. Research shows that risks can include respiratory illnesses, dependence, mental health-related problems, and other issues affecting public health such as impaired driving. Within this context of changing marijuana policies at the state level, research is needed on the impact of different models of legalization and how to minimize harm based on what has been learned from legal substances subject to misuse, such as alcohol and tobacco. Continued assessment of barriers to research and surveillance will help build the best scientific foundation to support good public policy while also protecting the public health.

Purpose, Focus, and Format of the *Report*

The Audience

This *Report* is intended for individuals, families, community members, educators, health care professionals, public health practitioners, advocates, public policymakers, and researchers who are looking for effective, sustainable solutions to the problems created by alcohol and other substances. To meet those needs, the *Report* reviews and synthesizes the most important and reliable scientific findings in key topic areas and distills those findings into recommendations for:

- Improving public awareness of substance misuse and related problems;
- Reducing negative attitudes related to substance use disorders;
- Closing the gap between what is known to reduce substance misuse at the population level and within specific subgroups, and the implementation of these effective programs, policies, and environmental strategies at the federal, state, and community levels;
- Understanding the need for and effectiveness of programs for high-risk populations;
- Expanding the capacity of health care systems to deliver evidence-based substance use disorder treatment;
- Integrating financing and health care system models to facilitate access and affordability of care for substance use disorders;

- Continuing to build the science base of effective prevention, treatment, and recovery practices and policies; and
- Engaging stakeholders in reducing substance use and misuse problems and protecting the health of all individuals across the lifespan.

Because of the broad audience, the *Report* is purposely written in accessible language without excessive scientific jargon. The *Report* also focuses on current issues and practical questions that trouble so many people:

- What are the health and social impacts of alcohol and drug use and misuse in the United States? What key factors influence these behaviors?
- What are the major substance misuse problems facing the United States?
- What causes substance use disorders and why do they change people so dramatically?
- Can substance misuse problems and disorders be prevented? How?
- What constitutes effective treatment?
- Can addicted individuals recover? What will it take to manage their disorders and sustain recovery?

Topics Covered in the *Report*

Individual chapters in the *Report* review the science associated with the major substance use, misuse, and disorder issues for specific topics. Tobacco, also an addictive substance, is mentioned only briefly, because problems associated with tobacco use and nicotine addiction have been covered extensively in other Surgeon General's Reports.[14-16,100-103]

Because of the broad audience and the practical emphasis, the *Report* is intentionally selective rather than exhaustive, emphasizing findings that have the potential for the greatest public health impact and the greatest potential for action. For readers wanting greater scientific detail or more specific information, detailed research reports, as well as supplemental resource materials, are supplied in references, in the Appendices, and in special emphasis boxes throughout the *Report*.

Scientific Standards Used to Develop the *Report*

Findings cited in all of the chapters came from electronic database searches of research articles published in English. Within those searches, priority was given to systematic literature reviews and to findings that were replicated by multiple controlled trials. However, many important issues in prevention, treatment, recovery, and health care systems have not yet been examined in rigorous controlled trials, or are not appropriate for such research designs. In these cases, the best available evidence was cited and labeled according to the reporting conventions published by the CDC:[104]

- *Well-supported*: Evidence derived from multiple controlled trials or large-scale population studies.
- *Supported*: Evidence derived from rigorous but fewer or smaller trials or restricted samples.
- *Promising*: Findings that do not derive from rigorously controlled studies but that nonetheless make practical or clinical sense and are widely practiced.

In cases in which evidence was based on findings of neurobiological research, the CDC standards were adapted.

A summary of the key findings appears at the beginning of each chapter. The key findings highlight what is currently known from available research about the chapter topic, as well as the strength of the evidence. As with the rest of the *Report*, the key findings are not intended to be exhaustive, but are instead considered the important "take-aways" from each chapter. Readers interested in a fuller discussion of the topics are encouraged to read the chapters in their entirety.

Addressing Substance Use in Specific Populations

As indicated, the chapters are designed to prioritize best available research findings that apply most broadly across different substances and across various subgroups, while also identifying program and policy interventions that have strong evidence for particular substances (e.g., alcohol), when available. The rationale for this decision is that the available research suggests that the genetic, neurobiological, and environmental processes underlying substance use, misuse, and disorders are largely similar across most known substances and unrelated to the age, sex, race and ethnicity, gender identity, or culture of the individual. The available research also clearly indicates that many of the interventions, including population-level policies, focused programs, behavioral therapies, medications, and social services shown to be effective in one subgroup are *generally* effective for other subgroups. Put differently, it is reasonable to assume that the findings presented in this *Report* are relevant for many substance use types and patterns; for most age, gender, racial and ethnic, and cultural subgroups; and for many special needs subgroups (e.g., those with co-occurring mental or physical illnesses; those involved with the criminal justice system).

However, this general statement has some important caveats. First, the statement depends heavily on the phrase "available research." There is insufficient research examining subgroup differences in the neurobiology of substance use disorders and in interventions aimed at preventing, treating, and promoting recovery from substance use disorders. Additional research designed to examine these differences and to test interventions in specific populations is needed.

A second caveat is that individual variability in response to standard prevention, treatment, and recovery support interventions is common throughout health care. Individuals with the same disease often react quite differently to the same medicine or behavioral intervention. Accordingly, general health care has moved toward "personalized medicine," an individualized treatment regimen derived from specific information about the individual's genetics and stage of illness, as well as lifestyle, language, culture, and personal preferences. Personalized care is not common in the substance use disorder field because many prevention, treatment, and recovery regimens were created as standardized "programs" rather than individualized protocols.

The third caveat to the statement on general research findings is that even if research has shown that certain medications, therapies, or recovery support services are likely to be *effective*, this does not mean that they will be *adequate*, especially for groups with specific needs. For example, a medication that is effective in blocking the rewarding effects of opioid use will not fully address the multiple, complex problems of those with opioid use disorders, nor address any co-occurring health conditions such as depression or HIV/AIDS.

Recognizing these limitations to the generalizability of research findings, each chapter has a dedicated section on Specific Populations that focuses particularly on age, racial and ethnic subgroups, and individuals with co-occurring mental and physical illnesses. Findings relevant to other important groups (e.g., military veterans; lesbian, gay, bisexual, and transgender [LGBT] populations; those with criminal justice involvement; those in rural areas) are referred to throughout the *Report* when available.

The Organization of the Report

This *Report* is divided into Chapters, highlighting the key issues and most important research findings in those topics. The final chapter concludes with recommendations for key stakeholders, including implications for practice and policy.

This **Chapter 1 - Introduction and Overview** describes the overall rationale for the *Report*, defines key terms used throughout the *Report*, introduces the major issues covered in the topical chapters, and describes the organization, format, and the scientific standards that dictated content and emphasis within the *Report*.

Chapter 2 - The Neurobiology of Substance Use, Misuse, and Addiction reviews brain research on the neurobiological processes that turn casual substance use into a compulsive disorder.

Chapter 3 - Prevention Program and Policies reviews the scientific evidence on preventing substance misuse, substance use-related problems, and substance use disorders.

Chapter 4 - Early Intervention, Treatment, and Management of Substance Use Disorders describes the goals, settings, and stages of treatment, and reviews the effectiveness of the major components of early intervention and treatment approaches, including behavioral therapies, medications, and social services.

Chapter 5 - Recovery: The Many Paths to Wellness discusses perspectives on remission and recovery from substance use disorders and reviews the types and effectiveness of RSS.

Chapter 6 - Health Care Systems and Substance Use Disorders reviews ongoing changes in organization, delivery, and financing of care for substance use disorders in both specialty treatment programs and in mainstream health care settings.

Chapter 7 - Vision for the Future: A Public Health Approach presents a realistic vision for a comprehensive, effective, and humane public health approach to addressing substance misuse and substance use disorders in our country, including actionable recommendations for parents, families, communities, health care organizations, educators, researchers, and policymakers.

The **Appendices** provide additional detail about the topics covered in this *Report*. **Appendix A - Review Process for Prevention Programs** details the review process for the prevention programs included in Chapter 3 and the evidence on these programs; **Appendix B - Evidence-Based Prevention Programs and Policies** provides detail on scientific evidence grounding the programs and policies discussed in Chapter 3; **Appendix C - Resource Guide** provides resources specific to those seeking information on preventing and treating substance misuse or substance use disorders; and **Appendix D - Important Facts about Alcohol and Drugs** contains facts about alcohol and specific drugs, including descriptions, uses and possible health effects, treatment options, and statistics as of 2015.

References

1. Kolodny, A., Courtwright, D. T., Hwang, C. S., Kreiner, P., Eadie, J. L., Clark, T. W., & Alexander, G. C. (2015). The prescription opioid and heroin crisis: A public health approach to an epidemic of addiction. *Annual Review of Public Health, 36*, 559-574.

2. Centers for Disease Control and Prevention. (2014). The public health system and the 10 essential public health services. Retrieved from http://www.cdc.gov/nphpsp/essentialservices.html. Accessed on August 16, 2016.

3. Center for Behavioral Health Statistics and Quality. (2016). *Results from the 2015 National Survey on Drug Use and Health: Detailed tables.* Rockville, MD: Substance Abuse and Mental Health Services Administration.

4. Volkow, N. D. (2014). *America's addiction to opioids: Heroin and prescription drug abuse.* Senate Caucus on International Narcotics Control: National Institute on Drug Abuse. Retrieved from https://www.drugabuse.gov/about-nida/legislative-activities/testimony-to-congress/2015/americas-addiction-to-opioids-heroin-prescription-drug-abuse. Accessed on February 16, 2016.

5. World Health Organization. (2015). Health systems strengthening glossary, G-H. *Health Systems.* Retrieved from http://www.who.int/healthsystems/hss_glossary/en/index5.html. Accessed on August 16, 2016.

6. Stahre, M., Roeber, J., Kanny, D., Brewer, R. D., & Zhang, X. (2014). Contribution of excessive alcohol consumption to deaths and years of potential life lost in the United States. *Preventing Chronic Disease, 11*(E109).

7. Rudd, R. A., Aleshire, N., Zibbel, J. E., & Gladden, R. M. (2016). Increases in drug and opioid overdose deaths — United States, 2000–2014. *MMWR, 64*(50), 1378-1382.

8. Case, A., & Deaton, A. (2015). Rising morbidity and mortality in midlife among white non-Hispanic Americans in the 21st century. *Proceedings of the National Academy of Sciences, 112*(49), 15078-15083.

9. Kochanek, K. D., Arias, E., & Bastian, B. A. (2016). *The effect of changes in selected age-specific causes of death on non-Hispanic white life expectancy between 2000 and 2014.* (NCHS Data Brief No. 250). Atlanta, GA: Centers for Disease Control and Prevention.

10. Sacks, J. J., Gonzales, K. R., Bouchery, E. E., Tomedi, L. E., & Brewer, R. D. (2015). 2010 national and state costs of excessive alcohol consumption. *American Journal of Preventive Medicine, 49*(5), e73-e79.

11. National Drug Intelligence Center. (2011). *National drug threat assessment.* Washington, DC: U.S. Department of Justice.

12. Centers for Disease Control and Prevention. (2014). *National Diabetes Statistics Report: Estimates of diabetes and its burden in the United States, 2014.* Atlanta, GA: U.S. Department of Health and Human Services.

13. Center for Behavioral Health Statistics and Quality. (2015). *Behavioral health trends in the United States: Results from the 2014 National Survey on Drug Use and Health.* (HHS Publication No. SMA 15-4927 NSDUH Series H-50). Rockville, MD: Substance Abuse and Mental Health Services Administration.

14. U.S. Department of Health and Human Services. (2000). *Reducing tobacco use: A report of the Surgeon General.* Atlanta, GA: U.S. Department of Health and Human Services, Centers for Disease Control and Prevention, National Center for Chronic Disease Prevention and Health Promotion, Office on Smoking and Health.

15. U.S. Department of Health and Human Services. (2004). *The health consequences of smoking: A report of the Surgeon General.* Atlanta, GA: U.S. Department of Health and Human Services, Centers for Disease Control and Prevention, National Center for Chronic Disease Prevention and Health Promotion, Office on Smoking and Health.

16. U.S. Department of Health and Human Services. (2014). *The health consequences of smoking: 50 years of progress. A Report of the Surgeon General.* Atlanta, GA: U.S. Department of Health and Human Services, Centers for Disease Control and Prevention, National Center for Chronic Disease Prevention and Health Promotion, Office on Smoking and Health.

17. U.S. Department of Health and Human Services. (2012). *Preventing tobacco use among youth and young adults: A report of the Surgeon General.* Atlanta, GA: Centers for Disease Control and Prevention, National Center for Chronic Disease Prevention and Health Promotion, Office on Smoking and Health.

18. Jewett, A., Shults, R. A., Banerjee, T., & Bergen, G. (2015). Alcohol-impaired driving among adults—United States, 2012. *MMWR, 64*(30), 814-817.

19. McMillan, G. P., & Lapham, S. (2006). Effectiveness of bans and laws in reducing traffic deaths: Legalized Sunday packaged alcohol sales and alcohol-related traffic crashes and crash fatalities in New Mexico. *American Journal of Public Health, 96*(11), 1944-1948.

20. Cantor, D., Fisher, B., Chibnall, S., Townsend, R., Lee, H., Bruce, C., & Thomas, C. (2015). *Report on the AAU campus climate survey on sexual assault and sexual misconduct assault and sexual misconduct.* Rockville, MD: The Association of American Universities.

21. Runyan, D., Wattam, C., Ikeda, R., Hassan, F., & Ramiro, L. (2002). Child abuse and neglect by parents and other caregivers. In E. Krug, L. L. Dahlberg, J. A. Mercy, A. B. Zwi, & R. Lozano (Eds.), *World report on violence and health.* (pp. 59-86). Geneva, Switzerland: World Health Organization.

22. U.S. Department of Health and Human Services, Office of the Surgeon General, & National Action Alliance for Suicide Prevention. (2012). *2012 National strategy for suicide prevention: Goals and objectives for action.* Washington, DC: U.S. Department of Health and Human Services.

23. Paulozzi, L. J., Kilbourne, E. M., & Desai, H. A. (2011). Prescription drug monitoring programs and death rates from drug overdose. *Pain Medicine, 12*(5), 747-754.

24. Bagnardi, V., Rota, M., Botteri, E., Tramacere, I., Islami, F., Fedirko, V., . . . Pasquali, E. (2015). Alcohol consumption and site-specific cancer risk: A comprehensive dose–response meta-analysis. *British Journal of Cancer, 112*(3), 580-593.

25. Jung, S., Wang, M., Anderson, K., Baglietto, L., Bergkvist, L., Bernstein, L., . . . Eliassen, A. H. (2015). Alcohol consumption and breast cancer risk by estrogen receptor status: In a pooled analysis of 20 studies. *International Journal of Epidemiology.*

26. Rehm, J., Mathers, C., Popova, S., Thavorncharoensap, M., Teerawattananon, Y., & Patra, J. (2009). Global burden of disease and injury and economic cost attributable to alcohol use and alcohol-use disorders. *The Lancet, 373*(9682), 2223-2233.

27. Baliunas, D., Rehm, J., Irving, H., & Shuper, P. (2010). Alcohol consumption and risk of incident human immunodeficiency virus infection: A meta-analysis. *International Journal of Public Health, 55*(3), 159-166.

28. Sokol, R. J., Delaney-Black, V., & Nordstrom, B. (2003). Fetal alcohol spectrum disorder. *JAMA, 290*(22), 2996-2999.

29. U.S. Department of Health and Human Services, & U.S. Department of Agriculture. (2015). 2015–2020 Dietary Guidelines for Americans: Appendix 9. Alcohol. *Dietary guidelines for Americans, 2015-2020.* (8th ed.).

30. American Psychiatric Association. (2013). *Diagnostic and statistical manual of mental disorders (DSM-5)* (5th ed.). Arlington, VA: American Psychiatric Publishing.

31. Center for Behavioral Health Statistics and Quality. (2015). *Results from the 2014 National Survey on Drug Use and Health: Detailed tables.* Rockville, MD: Substance Abuse and Mental Health Services Administration.

32. Center for Behavioral Health Statistics and Quality. (2016). *Summary of the effects of the 2015 NSDUH questionnaire redesign: Implications for data users.* Rockville, MD: Substance Abuse and Mental Health Services Administration.

33. Centers for Disease Control and Prevention. (n.d.). Alcohol and public health: Alcohol-related disease impact (ARDI). Retrieved from https://nccd.cdc.gov/DPH_ARDI/Default/Default.aspx. Accessed on July 9, 2016.

34. Centers for Disease Control and Prevention. (2016). Excessive drinking is draining the U.S. economy. Retrieved from http://www.cdc.gov/features/costsofdrinking/. Accessed on July 5, 2016.

35. Whiteford, H. A., Degenhardt, L., Rehm, J., Baxter, A. J., Ferrari, A. J., Erskine, H. E., . . . Vos, T. (2013). Global burden of disease attributable to mental and substance use disorders: Findings from the Global Burden of Disease Study 2010. *The Lancet, 382*(9904), 1575-1586.

36. Lange, R. A., & Hillis, L. D. (2001). Cardiovascular complications of cocaine use. *New England Journal of Medicine, 345*(5), 351-358.

37. Degenhardt, L., & Hall, W. (2012). Extent of illicit drug use and dependence, and their contribution to the global burden of disease. *The Lancet, 379,* 55-70.

38. National Highway Traffic Safety Administration. (2015). *Traffic safety facts 2014 data: Alcohol-impaired driving.* (DOT HS 812 231). Washington, DC: U.S. Department of Transportation.

39. National Highway Traffic Safety Administration (NHTSA). (2014). *Traffic safety facts 2013 data: Alcohol-impaired driving.* (DOT HS 812 102). Washington, DC: U.S. Department of Transportation.

40. Federal Bureau of Investigation (FBI). (2012). Estimated number of arrests: United States, 2012 *Crime in the United States 2012: Uniform crime reports.* Retrieved from https://www.fbi.gov/about-us/cjis/ucr/crime-in-the-u.s/2012/crime-in-the-u.s.-2012/tables/29tabledatadecpdf. Accessed on April 11, 2016.

41. Blincoe, L., Miller, T. R., Zaloshnja, E., & Lawrence, B. A. (2015). *The economic and societal impact of motor vehicle crashes, 2010 (Revised).* (DOT HS 812 013). Washington, DC: National Highway Traffic Safety Administration.

42. Berning, A., Compton, R., & Wochinger, K. (2015). *Results of the 2013–2014 National Roadside Survey of Alcohol and Drug Use by drivers.* (DOT HS 812 118). Washington, DC: National Highway Traffic Safety Administration.

43. Compton, R. P., & Berning, A. (2015). *Drug and alcohol crash risk.* (DOT HS 812 117). Washington, DC: National Highway Traffic Safety Administration.

44. Centers for Disease Control and Prevention. (2015). Alcohol poisoning deaths. Vital signs: Alcohol poisoning kills six people each day. Retrieved from http://www.cdc.gov/media/dpk/2015/dpk-vs-alcohol-poisoning.html. Accessed on April 6, 2016.

45. Levy, B., Paulozzi, L., Mack, K. A., & Jones, C. M. (2015). Trends in opioid analgesic–prescribing rates by specialty, US, 2007–2012. *American Journal of Preventive Medicine, 49*(3), 409-413.

46. Volkow, N. D., McLellan, T. A., Cotto, J. H., Karithanom, M., & Weiss, S. R. B. (2011). Characteristics of opioid prescriptions in 2009. *JAMA, 305*(13), 1299-1301.

47. Crane, E. H. (2013). *The CBHSQ Report: Emergency department visits involving narcotic pain relievers.* Rockville, MD: Substance Abuse and Mental Health Services Administration, Center for Behavioral Health Statistics and Quality.

48. Centers for Disease Control and Prevention. (2016). CDC Wonder: Multiple cause of death 1999 - 2014. Retrieved from http://wonder.cdc.gov/wonder/help/mcd.html. Accessed on May 17, 2016.

49. Drug Enforcement Administration. (2016). DEA Report: Counterfeit pills fueling U.S. fentanyl and opioid crisis: Problems resulting from abuse of opioid drugs continue to grow. Retrieved from https://www.dea.gov/divisions/hq/2016/hq072216.shtml. Accessed on August 16, 2016.

50. McCollister, K. E., French, M. T., & Fang, H. (2010). The cost of crime to society: New crime-specific estimates for policy and program evaluation. *Drug and Alcohol Dependence, 108*(1-2), 98-109.

51. National Center for Injury Prevention and Control. (2003). *Costs of intimate partner violence against women in the United States.* Atlanta, GA: Centers for Disease Control and Prevention.

52. Breiding, M. J. (2014). Prevalence and characteristics of sexual violence, stalking, and intimate partner violence victimization—National Intimate Partner and Sexual Violence Survey, United States, 2011. *MMWR, 63*(8), 1-18.

53. Klein, A. R. (2009). *Practical implications of current domestic violence research: For law enforcement, prosecutors and judges.* (NCJ 225722). Washington, DC: U.S. Department of Justice, Office of Justice Programs.

54. Friday, P. C., Lord, V. B., Exum, M. L., & Hartman, J. L. (2006). *Evaluating the impact of a specialized domestic violence police unit. Final report for National Institute of Justice.* (215916). Washington, DC: U.S. Department of Justice, National Institute of Justice.

55. Brookoff, D. (1997). *Drugs, alcohol, and domestic violence in Memphis.* Washington, DC: U.S. Department of Justice, National Institute of Justice.

56. Smith, P. H., Homish, G. G., Leonard, K. E., & Cornelius, J. R. (2012). Intimate partner violence and specific substance use disorders: Findings from the National Epidemiologic Survey on Alcohol and Related Conditions. *Psychology of Addictive Behaviors, 26*(2), 236-245.

57. Vagi, K. J., Rothman, E. F., Latzman, N. E., Tharp, A. T., Hall, D. M., & Breiding, M. J. (2013). Beyond correlates: A review of risk and protective factors for adolescent dating violence perpetration. *Journal of Youth and Adolescence, 42*(4), 633-649.

58. Stith, S. M., Smith, D. B., Penn, C. E., Ward, D. B., & Tritt, D. (2004). Intimate partner physical abuse perpetration and victimization risk factors: A meta-analytic review. *Aggression and Violent Behavior, 10*(1), 65-98.

59. Exner-Cortens, D., Eckenrode, J., & Rothman, E. (2013). Longitudinal associations between teen dating violence victimization and adverse health outcomes. *Pediatrics, 131*(1), 71-78.

60. Stone, A. L., Becker, L. G., Huber, A. M., & Catalano, R. F. (2012). Review of risk and protective factors of substance use and problem use in emerging adulthood. *Addictive Behaviors, 37*(7), 747-775.

61. Elder, R. W., Lawrence, B., Ferguson, A., Naimi, T. S., Brewer, R. D., Chattopadhyay, S. K., . . . Task Force on Community Preventive Services. (2010). The effectiveness of tax policy interventions for reducing excessive alcohol consumption and related harms. *American Journal of Preventive Medicine, 38*(2), 217-229.

62. Kessler, R. C., Berglund, P., Demler, O., Jin, R., Merikangas, K. R., & Walters, E. E. (2005). Lifetime prevalence and age-of-onset distributions of DSM-IV disorders in the National Comorbidity Survey Replication. *Archives of General Psychiatry, 62*(6), 593-602.

63. Compton, W. M., Thomas, Y. F., Stinson, F. S., & Grant, B. F. (2007). Prevalence, correlates, disability, and comorbidity of DSM-IV drug abuse and dependence in the United States: Results from the national epidemiologic survey on alcohol and related conditions. *Archives of General Psychiatry, 64*(5), 566-576.

64. Hasin, D. S., Stinson, F. S., Ogburn, E., & Grant, B. F. (2007). Prevalence, correlates, disability, and comorbidity of DSM-IV alcohol abuse and dependence in the United States: Results from the National Epidemiologic Survey on Alcohol and Related Conditions. *Archives of General Psychiatry, 64*(7), 830-842.

65. Hanson, K. L., Medina, K. L., Padula, C. B., Tapert, S. F., & Brown, S. A. (2011). Impact of adolescent alcohol and drug use on neuropsychological functioning in young adulthood: 10-year outcomes. *Journal of Child and Adolescent Substance Abuse, 20*(2), 135-154.

66. Giedd, J. N., Blumenthal, J., Jeffries, N. O., Castellanos, F. X., Liu, H., Zijdenbos, A., . . . Rapoport, J. L. (1999). Brain development during childhood and adolescence: A longitudinal MRI study. *Nature Neuroscience, 2*(10), 861-863.

67. Squeglia, L. M., Tapert, S. F., Sullivan, E. V., Jacobus, J., Meloy, M. J., Rolfing, T., & Pfefferbaum, A. (2015). Brain development in heavy-drinking adolescents. *American Journal of Psychiatry, 172*(6), 532-542.

68. Miller, W. R., Meyers, R. J., & Tonigan, J. S. (1999). Engaging the unmotivated in treatment for alcohol problems: A comparison of three strategies for intervention through family members. *Journal of Consulting and Clinical Psychology, 67*(5), 688-697.

69. White, W. L., & Miller, W. R. (2007). The use of confrontation in addiction treatment: History, science and time for change. *Counselor, 8*(4), 12-30.

70. Bodenheimer, T., Wagner, E. H., & Grumbach, K. (2002). Improving primary care for patients with chronic illness: The chronic care model, Part 2. *JAMA, 288*(15), 1909-1914.

71. McLellan, A. T., Lewis, D. C., O'Brien, C. P., & Kleber, H. D. (2000). Drug dependence, a chronic medical illness: Implications for treatment, insurance, and outcomes evaluation. *JAMA, 284*(13), 1689-1695.

72. McLellan, A. T., Starrels, J. L., Tai, B., Gordon, A. J., Brown, R., Ghitza, U., . . . Horton, T. (2014). Can substance use disorders be managed using the chronic care model? Review and recommendations from a NIDA Consensus Group. *Public Health Reviews, 35*(2), 1-14.

73. Feliz, J. (2012). Survey: Ten percent of American adults report being in recovery from substance abuse or addiction. Retrieved from http://www.drugfree.org/newsroom/survey-ten-percent-of-american-adults-report-being-in-recovery-from-substance-abuse-or-addiction/. Accessed on April 12, 2016.

74. White, W. (2014). *Slaying the dragon: The history of addiction treatment and recovery in America* (2nd Ed.). Bloomington, IL: Chestnut Health Systems.

75. Musto, D. F. (1987). *The American disease: Origins of narcotic control* (Expanded ed.). New York, NY: Oxford University Press.

76. Rettig, R. A., Yarmolinsky, A., & Institute of Medicine (US) Committee on Federal Regulation of Methadone Treatment (Eds.). (1995). *Federal regulation of methadone treatment*. Washington, DC: National Academies Press.

77. Ries, R. K., Fielen, D. A., Miller, S. C., & Saltz, R. (Eds.). (2014). *The ASAM principles of addiction medicine* (5th ed.): Wolters Kluwer.

78. Institute of Medicine, & Committee on Crossing the Quality Chasm. (2006). *Improving the quality of health care for mental and substance-use conditions*. Washington, DC: National Academies Press.

79. McKnight-Eily, L. R., Liu, Y., Brewer, R. D., Kanny, D., Lu, H., Denny, C. H., . . . Centers for Disease Control and Prevention. (2014). Vital signs: Communication between health professionals and their patients about alcohol use - 44 states and the District of Columbia, 2011. *MMWR, 63*(1), 16-22.

80. Scott, K. M., Lim, C., Al-Hamzawi, A., Alonso, J., Bruffaerts, R., Caldas-de-Almeida, J. M., . . . de Jonge, P. (2016). Association of mental disorders with subsequent chronic physical conditions: World mental health surveys from 17 countries. *JAMA Psychiatry, 73*(2), 150-158.

81. Phillips, D. P., Barker, G. E., & Eguchi, M. M. (2008). A steep increase in domestic fatal medication errors with use of alcohol and/or street drugs. *Archives of Internal Medicine, 168*(14), 1561-1566.

82. Dowell, D., Haegerich, T. M., & R., C. (2016). CDC guideline for prescribing opioids for chronic pain - United States. *MMWR, 65*(1), 1-49.

83. Parish, C. L., Pereyra, M. R., Pollack, H. A., Cardenas, G., Castellon, P. C., Abel, S. N., . . . Metsch, L. R. (2015). Screening for substance misuse in the dental care setting: Findings from a nationally representative survey of dentists. *Addiction, 110*(9), 1516-1523.

84. Denisco, R. C., Kenna, G. A., O'Neil, M. G., Kulich, R. J., Moore, P. A., Kane, W. T., . . . Katz, N. P. (2011). Prevention of prescription opioid abuse: The role of the dentist. *The Journal of the American Dental Association, 142*(7), 800-810.

85. Krause, M., Vainio, L., Zwetchkenbaum, S., & Inglehart, M. R. (2010). Dental education about patients with special needs: A survey of US and Canadian dental schools. *Journal of Dental Education, 74*(11), 1179-1189.

86. Tommasello, A. C. (2004). Substance abuse and pharmacy practice: What the community pharmacist needs to know about drug abuse and dependence. *Harm Reduction Journal, 1*(3), 1-15.

87. Barry, C. L., & Huskamp, H. A. (2011). Moving beyond parity—mental health and addiction care under the ACA. *New England Journal of Medicine, 365*(11), 973-975.

88. McLellan, A. T., & Meyers, K. (2004). Contemporary addiction treatment: A review of systems problems for adults and adolescents. *Biological Psychiatry, 56*(10), 764-770.

89. Patient Protection and Affordable Care Act, 42 U.S.C. § 18001, H.R. 3590, Public Law No. 111–148, 124 Stat. 119 Stat. (2010).

90. Paul Wellstone and Pete Domenici Mental Health Parity and Addiction Equity Act of 2008, H.R. 6983 (2008).

91. Miech, R. A., Johnston, L. D., O'Malley, P. M., Bachman, J. G., & Schulenberg, J. E. (2016). *Monitoring the Future national survey results on drug use, 1975-2015: Volume I, secondary school students.* Ann Arbor, MI: Institute for Social Research, The University of Michigan.

92. Pacula, R. L., Powell, D., Heaton, P., & Sevigny, E. L. (2015). Assessing the effects of medical marijuana laws on marijuana use: The devil is in the details. *Journal of Policy Analysis and Management, 34*(1), 7-31.

93. Office of National Drug Control Policy. (n.d.). Answers to frequently asked questions about marijuana. Retrieved from https://www.whitehouse.gov/ondcp/frequently-asked-questions-and-facts-about-marijuana. Accessed on June 27, 2016.

94. Mehmedic, Z., Chandra, S., Slade, D., Denham, H., Foster, S., Patel, A. S., . . . ElSohly, M. A. (2010). Potency trends of 9-THC and other cannabinoids in confiscated cannabis preparations from 1993 to 2008. *Journal of Forensic Sciences, 55*(5), 1209-1217.

95. National Institute on Drug Abuse. (2016). DrugFacts: Marijuana. Retrieved from https://www.drugabuse.gov/publications/drugfacts/marijuana. Accessed on June 20, 2016.

96. Ramaekers, J. G., Berghaus, G., van Laar, M., & Drummer, O. H. (2004). Dose related risk of motor vehicle crashes after cannabis use. *Drug and Alcohol Dependence, 73*(2), 109-119.

97. Li, M.-C., Brady, J. E., DiMaggio, C. J., Lusardi, A. R., Tzong, K. Y., & Li, G. (2012). Marijuana use and motor vehicle crashes. *Epidemiologic Reviews, 34*(1), 65-72.

98. Asbridge, M., Hayden, J. A., & Cartwright, J. L. (2012). Acute cannabis consumption and motor vehicle collision risk: Systematic review of observational studies and meta-analysis. *BMJ, 344*, e536.

99. Hartman, R. L., & Huestis, M. A. (2013). Cannabis effects on driving skills. *Clinical Chemistry, 59*(3), 478-492.

100. U.S. Department of Health, Education, and Welfare. (1964). *Smoking and health: Report of the advisory committee to the Surgeon General of the Public Health Service.* Washington, DC: U.S. Public Health Service, Office of the Surgeon General.

101. U.S. Department of Health and Human Services. (1986). *The health consequences of using smokeless tobacco: A report of the Advisory Committee to the Surgeon General.* Washington, DC: U.S. Department of Health and Human Services.

102. U.S. Department of Health and Human Services. (1994). *Preventing tobacco use among young people: A report of the Surgeon General.* Atlanta, GA: U.S. Department of Health and Human Services, Centers for Disease Control and Prevention, National Center for Chronic Disease Prevention and Health Promotion, Office on Smoking and Health.

103. U.S. Department of Health and Human Services. (2010). *How tobacco smoke causes disease: The biology and behavioral basis for smoking-attributable disease: A report of the Surgeon General.* Atlanta, GA: U.S. Department of Health and Human Services, Centers for Disease Control and Prevention, National Center for Chronic Disease Prevention and Health Promotion, Office on Smoking and Health.

104. Puddy, R. W., & Wilkins, N. (2011). *Understanding evidence Part 1: Best available research evidence. A guide to the continuum of evidence of effectiveness.* Atlanta, GA: Centers for Disease Control and Prevention.

CHAPTER 2.
THE NEUROBIOLOGY OF SUBSTANCE USE, MISUSE, AND ADDICTION

Chapter 2 Preview

A substantial body of research has accumulated over several decades and transformed our understanding of substance use and its effects on the brain. This knowledge has opened the door to new ways of thinking about prevention and treatment of substance use disorders.

This chapter describes the neurobiological framework underlying substance use and why some people transition from using or misusing alcohol or drugs to a substance use disorder—including its most severe form, addiction. The chapter explains how these substances produce changes in brain structure and function that promote and sustain addiction and contribute to relapse. The chapter also addresses similarities and differences in how the various classes of addictive substances affect the brain and behavior and provides a brief overview of key factors that influence risk for substance use disorders.

An Evolving Understanding of Substance Use Disorders

Scientific breakthroughs have revolutionized the understanding of substance use disorders. For example, severe substance use disorders, commonly called *addictions*, were once viewed largely as a moral failing or character flaw, but are now understood to be chronic illnesses characterized by clinically significant impairments in health, social function, and voluntary control over substance use.[3] Although the mechanisms may be different, addiction has many features in common with disorders such as diabetes, asthma, and hypertension. All of these disorders are chronic, subject to relapse, and influenced by genetic, developmental, behavioral, social, and environmental factors. In all of these disorders, affected individuals may have difficulty in complying with the prescribed treatment.[4]

This evolving understanding of substance use disorders as medical conditions has had important implications for prevention and treatment. Research demonstrating that addiction is driven by changes in the brain has helped to reduce the negative attitudes associated with substance use disorders and provided support for integrating treatment for substance use disorders into mainstream health care. Moreover, research on the basic neurobiology of addiction has already resulted in several effective

NEUROBIOLOGY

> **KEY FINDINGS***
>
> - Well-supported scientific evidence shows that addiction to alcohol or drugs is a chronic brain disease that has potential for recurrence and recovery.
> - Well-supported evidence suggests that the addiction process involves a three-stage cycle: binge/intoxication, withdrawal/negative affect, and preoccupation/anticipation. This cycle becomes more severe as a person continues substance use and as it produces dramatic changes in brain function that reduce a person's ability to control his or her substance use.
> - Well-supported scientific evidence shows that disruptions in three areas of the brain are particularly important in the onset, development, and maintenance of substance use disorders: the basal ganglia, the extended amygdala, and the prefrontal cortex. These disruptions: (1) enable substance-associated cues to trigger substance seeking (i.e., they increase incentive salience); (2) reduce sensitivity of brain systems involved in the experience of pleasure or reward, and heighten activation of brain stress systems; and (3) reduce functioning of brain executive control systems, which are involved in the ability to make decisions and regulate one's actions, emotions, and impulses.
> - Supported scientific evidence shows that these changes in the brain persist long after substance use stops. It is not yet known how much these changes may be reversed or how long that process may take.
> - Well-supported scientific evidence shows that adolescence is a critical "at-risk period" for substance use and addiction. All addictive drugs, including alcohol and marijuana, have especially harmful effects on the adolescent brain, which is still undergoing significant development.
>
> * Well-supported: when evidence is derived from multiple rigorous human and nonhuman studies; Supported: when evidence is derived from rigorous but fewer human and nonhuman studies.

medications for the treatment of alcohol, opioid, and nicotine use disorders, and clinical trials are ongoing to test other potential new treatments.[5]

All addictive substances have powerful effects on the brain. These effects account for the euphoric or intensely pleasurable feelings that people experience during their initial use of alcohol or other substances, and these feelings motivate people to use those substances again and again, despite the risks for significant harms.

> **FOR MORE ON THIS TOPIC**
>
> See the section on "Factors that Increase Risk for Substance Use, Misuse, and Addiction" later in this chapter.

As individuals continue to misuse alcohol or other substances, progressive changes, called *neuroadaptations*, occur in the structure and function of the brain. These neuroadaptations compromise brain function and also drive the transition from controlled, occasional substance use to chronic misuse, which can be difficult to control. Moreover, these brain changes endure long after an individual stops using substances. They may produce continued, periodic craving for the substance that can lead to relapse: More than 60 percent of people treated for a substance use disorder experience relapse within the first year after they are discharged from treatment,[4,6] and a person can remain at increased risk of relapse for many years.[7,8]

However, addiction is not an inevitable consequence of substance use. Whether an individual ever uses alcohol or another substance, and whether that initial use progresses to a substance use disorder of any severity, depends on a number of factors. These include: a person's genetic makeup and other individual biological factors; the age when use begins; psychological factors related to a person's unique history and personality; and environmental factors, such as the availability of drugs, family and peer dynamics, financial resources, cultural norms, exposure to stress, and access to social support.[9] Some of these factors increase risk for substance use, misuse, and use disorders, whereas other factors provide buffers against those risks. Nonetheless, specific combinations of factors can drive the emergence and continuation of substance misuse and the progression to a disorder or an addiction.

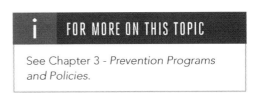

FOR MORE ON THIS TOPIC

See Chapter 3 - *Prevention Programs and Policies.*

Conducting Research on the Neurobiology of Substance Use, Misuse, and Addiction

Until recently, much of our knowledge about the neurobiology of substance use, misuse, and addiction came from the study of laboratory animals. Although no animal model fully reflects the human experience, animal studies let researchers investigate addiction under highly controlled conditions that may not be possible or ethical to replicate in humans. These types of studies have greatly helped to answer questions about how particular genes, developmental processes, and environmental factors, such as stressors, affect substance-taking behavior.

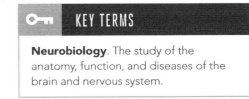

KEY TERMS

Neurobiology. The study of the anatomy, function, and diseases of the brain and nervous system.

Neurobiology studies in animals have historically focused on what happens in the brain right after taking an addictive substance (this is called the acute impact), but research has shifted to the study of how ongoing, long-term (or chronic) substance use changes the brain. One of the main goals of this research is to understand at the most basic level the mechanisms through which substance use alters brain structure and function and drives the transition from occasional use to misuse, addiction, and relapse.[10]

A growing body of substance use research conducted with humans is complementing the work in animals. For example, human studies have benefited greatly from the use of brain-imaging technologies, such as magnetic resonance imaging (MRI) and positron emission tomography (PET) scans. These technologies allow researchers to "see" inside the living human brain so that they can investigate and characterize the biochemical, functional, and structural changes in the brain that result from alcohol and drug use. The technologies also allow them to understand how differences in brain structure and function may contribute to substance use, misuse, and addiction.

Animal and human studies build on and inform each other, and in combination provide a more complete picture of the neurobiology of addiction. The rest of this chapter weaves together the most compelling data from both types of studies to describe a neurobiological framework for addiction.

A Basic Primer on the Human Brain

To understand how addictive substances affect the brain, it is important to first understand the basic biology of healthy brain function. The brain is an amazingly complex organ that is constantly at work. Within the brain, a mix of chemical and electrical processes controls the body's most basic functions, like breathing and digestion. These processes also control how people react to the multitudes of sounds, smells, and other sensory stimuli around them, and they organize and direct individuals' highest thinking and emotive powers so that they can interact with other people, carry out daily activities, and make complex decisions.

The brain is made of an estimated 86 billion nerve cells—called neurons—as well as other cell types. Each neuron has a cell body, an axon, and dendrites (Figure 2.1). The cell body and its nucleus control the neuron's activities. The axon extends out from the cell body and transmits messages to other neurons. Dendrites branch out from the cell body and receive messages from the axons of other neurons.

Neurons communicate with one another through chemical messengers called neurotransmitters. The neurotransmitters cross a tiny gap, or synapse, between neurons and attach to receptors on the receiving neuron. Some neurotransmitters are inhibitory—they make it less likely that the receiving neuron will carry out some action. Others are excitatory, meaning that they stimulate neuronal function, priming it to send signals to other neurons.

Neurons are organized in clusters that perform specific functions (described as networks or circuits). For example, some networks are involved with thinking, learning, emotions, and memory. Other networks communicate with muscles, stimulating them into action. Still others receive and interpret stimuli from the sensory organs, such as the eyes and ears, or the skin. The addiction cycle disrupts the normal functions of some of these neuronal networks.

Figure 2.1: A Neuron and its Parts

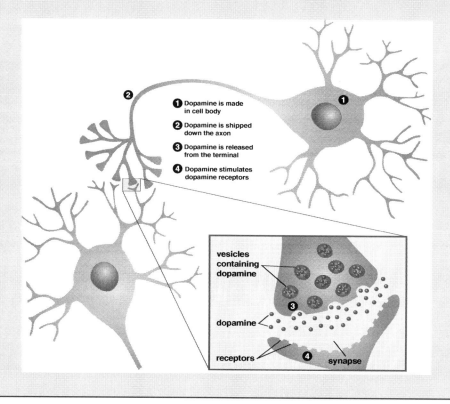

The Primary Brain Regions Involved in Substance Use Disorders

The brain has many regions that are interconnected with one another, forming dynamic networks that are responsible for specific functions, such as attention, self-regulation, perception, language, reward, emotion, and movement, along with many other functions. This chapter focuses on three regions that are the key components of networks that are intimately involved in the development and persistence of substance use disorders: the **basal ganglia**, the **extended amygdala**, and the **prefrontal cortex** ([Figure 2.2](#)). The basal ganglia control the rewarding, or pleasurable, effects of substance use and are also responsible for the formation of habitual substance taking. The extended amygdala is involved in stress and the feelings of unease, anxiety, and irritability that typically accompany substance withdrawal. The prefrontal cortex is involved in executive function (i.e., the ability to organize thoughts and activities, prioritize tasks, manage time, and make decisions), including exerting control over substance taking.

These brain areas and their associated networks are not solely involved in substance use disorders. Indeed, these systems are broadly integrated and serve many critical roles in helping humans and other animals survive. For example, when people engage in certain activities, such as consuming food or having sex, chemicals within the basal ganglia produce feelings of pleasure. This reward motivates individuals to continue to engage in these activities, thereby ensuring the survival of the species. Likewise, in the face of danger, activation of the brain's stress systems within the extended amygdala drives "fight or flight" responses. These responses, too, are critical for survival. As described in more detail below, these and other survival systems are "hijacked" by addictive substances.

Figure 2.2: Areas of the Human Brain that Are Especially Important in Addiction

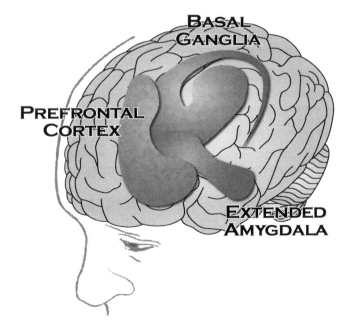

The Basal Ganglia

The basal ganglia are a group of structures located deep within the brain that play an important role in keeping body movements smooth and coordinated. They are also involved in learning routine behaviors and forming habits. Two sub-regions of the basal ganglia are particularly important in substance use disorders:

- The nucleus accumbens, which is involved in motivation and the experience of reward, and
- The dorsal striatum, which is involved in forming habits and other routine behaviors.[11]

The Extended Amygdala

The extended amygdala and its sub-regions, located beneath the basal ganglia, regulate the brain's reactions to stress-including behavioral responses like "fight or flight" and negative emotions like unease, anxiety, and irritability. This region also interacts with the hypothalamus, an area of the brain that controls activity of multiple hormone-producing glands, such as the pituitary gland at the base of the brain and the adrenal glands at the top of each kidney. These glands, in turn, control reactions to stress and regulate many other bodily processes.[12]

The Prefrontal Cortex

The prefrontal cortex is located at the very front of the brain, over the eyes, and is responsible for complex cognitive processes described as "executive function." Executive function is the ability to organize thoughts and activities, prioritize tasks, manage time, make decisions, and regulate one's actions, emotions, and impulses.[13]

The Addiction Cycle

Addiction can be described as a repeating cycle with three stages. Each stage is particularly associated with one of the brain regions described above—basal ganglia, extended amygdala, and prefrontal cortex (Figure 2.3).[10] This three-stage model draws on decades of human and animal research and provides a useful way to understand the symptoms of addiction, how it can be prevented and treated, and how people can recover from it.[14] The three stages of addiction are:

- **Binge/Intoxication**, the stage at which an individual consumes an intoxicating substance and experiences its rewarding or pleasurable effects;
- **Withdrawal/Negative Affect**, the stage at which an individual experiences a negative emotional state in the absence of the substance; and
- **Preoccupation/Anticipation**, the stage at which one seeks substances again after a period of abstinence.

Figure 2.3: The Three Stages of the Addiction Cycle and the Brain Regions Associated with Them

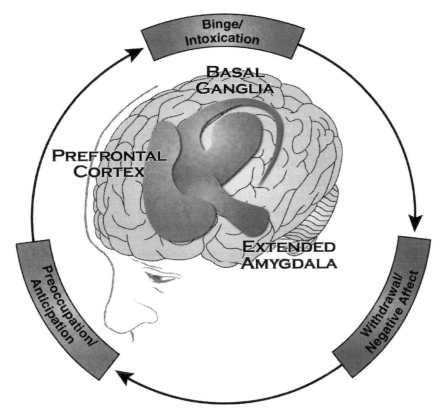

The three stages are linked to and feed on each other, but they also involve different brain regions, circuits (or networks), and neurotransmitters and result in specific kinds of changes in the brain. A person may go through this three-stage cycle over the course of weeks or months or progress through it several times in a day. There may be variation in how people progress through the cycle and the intensity with which they experience each of the stages. Nonetheless, the addiction cycle tends to intensify over time, leading to greater physical and psychological harm.[10]

The following sections describe each of the stages in more detail. But first, it is necessary to explain four behaviors that are central to the addiction cycle: impulsivity, positive reinforcement, negative reinforcement, and compulsivity.

For many people, initial substance use involves an element of impulsivity, or acting without foresight or regard for the consequences. For example, an adolescent may impulsively take a first drink, smoke a cigarette, begin experimenting with marijuana, or succumb to peer pressure to try a party drug. If the experience is pleasurable, this feeling positively reinforces the substance use, making the person more likely to take the substance again.

Another person may take a substance to relieve negative feelings such as stress, anxiety, or depression. In this case, the temporary relief the substance brings from the negative feelings negatively reinforces substance use, increasing the likelihood that the person will use again. Importantly, positive and negative reinforcement need not be driven solely by the effects of the drugs. Many other environmental and social stimuli can reinforce a behavior. For example, the approval of peers positively reinforces substance use for some people. Likewise, if drinking or using drugs with others provides relief from social isolation, substance use behavior could be negatively reinforced.

The positively reinforcing effects of substances tend to diminish with repeated use. This is called tolerance and may lead to use of the substance in greater amounts and/or more frequently in an attempt to experience the initial level of reinforcement. Eventually, in the absence of the substance, a person may experience negative emotions such as stress, anxiety, or depression, or feel physically ill. This is called withdrawal, which often leads the person to use the substance again to relieve the withdrawal symptoms.

As use becomes an ingrained behavior, impulsivity shifts to compulsivity, and the primary drivers of repeated substance use shift from positive reinforcement (feeling pleasure) to negative reinforcement (feeling relief), as the person seeks to stop the negative feelings and physical illness that accompany withdrawal.[15] Eventually, the person begins taking the substance not to get "high," but rather to escape the "low" feelings to which, ironically, chronic drug use has contributed. Compulsive substance seeking is a key characteristic of addiction, as is the loss of control over use. Compulsivity helps to explain why many people with addiction experience relapses after attempting to abstain from or reduce use.

> **KEY TERMS**
>
> **Impulsivity.** An inability to resist urges, deficits in delaying gratification, and unreflective decision-making. It is a tendency to act without foresight or regard for consequences and to prioritize immediate rewards over long-term goals.[1]
>
> **Positive reinforcement.** The process by which presentation of a stimulus such as a drug increases the probability of a response like drug taking.
>
> **Negative reinforcement.** The process by which removal of a stimulus such as negative feelings or emotions increases the probability of a response like drug taking.
>
> **Compulsivity.** Repetitive behaviors in the face of adverse consequences, and repetitive behaviors that are inappropriate to a particular situation. People suffering from compulsions often recognize that the behaviors are harmful, but they nonetheless feel emotionally compelled to perform them. Doing so reduces tension, stress, or anxiety.[1]

The following sections provide more detail about each of the three stages—binge/intoxication, withdrawal/negative affect, and preoccupation/anticipation—and the neurobiological processes underlying them.

Binge/Intoxication Stage: Basal Ganglia

The binge/intoxication stage of the addiction cycle is the stage at which an individual consumes the substance of choice. This stage heavily involves the basal ganglia (Figure 2.4) and its two key brain sub-regions, the nucleus accumbens and the dorsal striatum. In this stage, substances affect the brain in several ways.

Figure 2.4: The Binge/Intoxication Stage and the Basal Ganglia

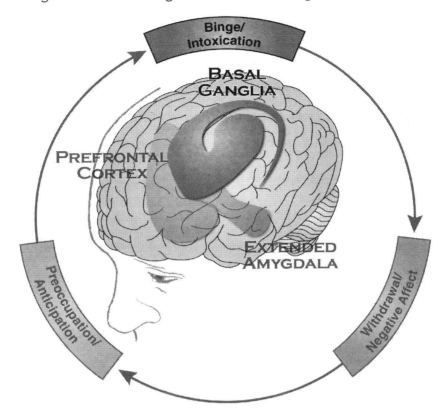

Addictive Substances "Hijack" Brain Reward Systems

All addictive substances produce feelings of pleasure. These "rewarding effects" positively reinforce their use and increase the likelihood of repeated use. The rewarding effects of substances involve activity in the nucleus accumbens, including activation of the brain's dopamine and opioid signaling system. Many studies have shown that neurons that release dopamine are activated, either directly or indirectly, by all addictive substances, but particularly by stimulants such as cocaine, amphetamines, and nicotine (Figure 2.5).[16] In addition, the brain's opioid system, which includes naturally occurring opioid molecules (i.e., endorphins, enkephalins, and dynorphins) and three types of opioid receptors (i.e., mu, delta, and kappa), plays a key role in mediating the rewarding effects of other addictive substances, including opioids and alcohol. Activation of the opioid system by these substances stimulates the nucleus accumbens directly or indirectly through the dopamine system. Brain imaging studies in humans show activation of dopamine and opioid neurotransmitters during alcohol and other substance use (including nicotine).[10,17] Other studies show that antagonists, or inhibitors, of dopamine and opioid receptors can block drug and alcohol seeking in both animals and humans.[14,18,19]

> **KEY TERMS**
>
> **Antagonist.** A chemical substance that binds to and blocks the activation of certain receptors on cells, preventing a biological response. Naloxone is an example of an opioid receptor antagonist.

Cannabinoids such as delta-9-tetrahydrocannabinol (THC), the primary psychoactive component of marijuana, target the brain's internal or endogenous cannabinoid system. This system also contributes to reward by affecting the function of dopamine neurons and the release of dopamine in the nucleus accumbens.

Figure 2.5: Actions of Addictive Substances on the Brain

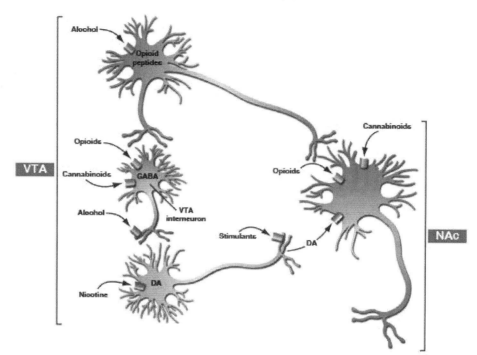

Notes: Figure 2.5 is a simplified schematic of converging acute rewarding actions of addictive substances on the nucleus accumbens (NAc). Dopamine neurons that originate in the ventral tegmental area (VTA) project to the NAc. Opioid peptides act both in the VTA and NAc. Despite diverse initial actions, addictive substances produce some common effects on the VTA and NAc. Stimulants directly increase dopamine (DA) transmission in the NAc. Opioids, alcohol, and inhalants (e.g., the solvent toluene) do the same indirectly. Alcohol also activates the release of opioid peptides. Heroin and prescribed opioid pain relievers directly activate opioid peptide receptors. Nicotine activates dopamine neurons in the VTA. Cannabinoids may act in the VTA to activate dopamine neurons but also act on NAc neurons themselves.

Source: Modified with permission from Nestler, (2005).[16]

Stimuli Associated with Addictive Substances Can Trigger Substance Use

Activation of the brain's reward system by alcohol and drugs not only generates the pleasurable feelings associated with those substances, it also ultimately triggers changes in the way a person responds to stimuli associated with the use of those substances. A person learns to associate the stimuli present while using a substance—including people, places, drug paraphernalia, and even internal states, such as mood—with the substance's rewarding effects. Over time, these stimuli can activate the dopamine system on their own and trigger powerful urges to take the substance. These "wanting" urges are called incentive salience and they can persist even after the rewarding effects of the substance have diminished. As a result, exposure to people, places, or things previously associated with substance use can serve as "triggers" or cues that promote substance seeking and taking, even in people who are in recovery.

Figure 2.6 shows the major neurotransmitter systems involved in the binge/intoxication stage of addiction. In this stage, the neurons in the basal ganglia contribute to the rewarding effects of addictive substances and to incentive salience through the release of dopamine and the brain's natural opioids.

Figure 2.6: Major Neurotransmitter Systems Implicated in the Neuroadaptations Associated with the Binge/Intoxication Stage of Addiction

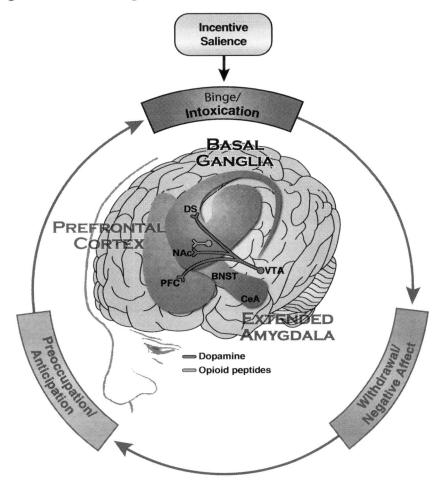

Notes: Blue represents the basal ganglia involved in the Binge/Intoxication stage. Red represents the extended amygdala involved in the Negative Affect/Withdrawal stage. Green represents the prefrontal cortex involved in the Preoccupation/Anticipation stage.

Abbreviations: PFC - prefrontal cortex, DS - dorsal striatum, NAc - nucleus accumbens, BNST - bed nucleus of the stria terminalis, CeA - central nucleus of the amygdala, VTA - ventral tegmental area.

Source: Modified with permission from Koob & Volkow, (2010).[14]

Early studies in animals demonstrated how incentive salience works. For example, after researchers repeatedly gave an animal a stimulant drug (e.g., cocaine) along with a previously neutral stimulus, such as a light or a sound, they found that the neutral stimulus by itself caused the animal to engage in drug-seeking behavior, and it also resulted in dopamine release that had previously occurred only in response to the drug.[20] Even more compelling results were seen when scientists recorded the electrical activity of dopamine-transmitting neurons in animals that had been exposed multiple times to a neutral (non-drug) stimulus followed by a drug. At first, the neurons responded only when they were exposed to the drug. However, over time, the neurons stopped firing in response to the drug and instead fired when they were exposed to the neutral stimulus associated with it. This means that the animals associated the stimulus with the substance and, in anticipation of getting the substance, their brains began releasing dopamine, resulting in a strong motivation to seek the drug.[21,22] Imaging studies in humans have shown similar results. For example, dopamine is released in the brains of people addicted to cocaine when they are exposed to cues they have come to associate with cocaine.[23,24] This effect occurs even though cocaine itself causes less dopamine to be released in these individuals compared to those who are not addicted to cocaine (an effect also seen with other substances).[25]

Together, these studies indicate that stimuli associated with addictive drugs can, by themselves, produce drug-like effects on the brain and trigger drug use. These findings help to explain why individuals with substance use disorders who are trying to maintain abstinence are at increased risk of relapse if they continue to have contact with the people they previously used drugs with or the places where they used drugs.

Substances Stimulate Areas of the Brain Involved in Habit Formation

A second sub-region of the basal ganglia, the dorsal striatum, is involved in another critical component of the binge/intoxication stage: habit formation. The release of dopamine (along with activation of brain opioid systems) and release of glutamate (an excitatory neurotransmitter) can eventually trigger changes in the dorsal striatum.[2,26] These changes strengthen substance-seeking and substance-taking habits as addiction progresses, ultimately contributing to compulsive use.

In Summary: The Binge/Intoxication Stage and the Basal Ganglia

The "reward circuitry" of the basal ganglia (i.e., the nucleus accumbens), along with dopamine and naturally occurring opioids, play a key role in the rewarding effects of alcohol and other substances and the ability of stimuli, or cues, associated with that substance use to trigger craving, substance seeking, and use.

As alcohol or substance use progresses, repeated activation of the "habit circuitry" of the basal ganglia (i.e., the dorsal striatum) contributes to the compulsive substance seeking and taking that are associated with addiction.

The involvement of these reward and habit neurocircuits helps explain the intense desire for the substance (craving) and the compulsive substance seeking that occurs when actively or previously addicted individuals are exposed to alcohol and/or drug cues in their surroundings.

Withdrawal/Negative Affect Stage: Extended Amygdala

The withdrawal/negative affect stage of addiction follows the binge/intoxication stage, and, in turn, sets up future rounds of binge/intoxication. During this stage, a person who has been using alcohol or drugs experiences withdrawal symptoms, which include negative emotions and, sometimes, symptoms of physical illness, when they stop taking the substance. Symptoms of withdrawal may occur with all addictive substances, including marijuana, though they vary in intensity and duration depending on both the type of substance and the severity of use. The negative feelings associated with withdrawal are thought to come from two sources: diminished activation in the reward circuitry of the basal ganglia[14] and activation of the brain's stress systems in the extended amygdala (Figure 2.7).

Figure 2.7: The Withdrawal/Negative Affect Stage and the Extended Amygdala

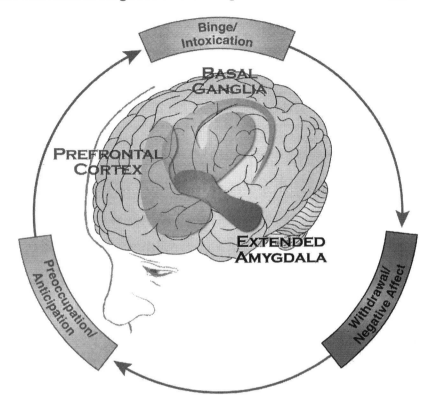

When used over the long-term, all substances of abuse cause dysfunction in the brain's dopamine reward system.[27] For example, brain imaging studies in humans with addiction have consistently shown long-lasting decreases in a particular type of dopamine receptor, the D2 receptor, compared with non-addicted individuals (Figure 2.8).[25,28] Decreases in the activity of the dopamine system have been observed during withdrawal from stimulants, opioids, nicotine, and alcohol. Other studies also show that when an addicted person is given a stimulant, it causes a smaller release of dopamine than when the same dose is given to a person who is not addicted.

These findings suggest that people addicted to substances experience an overall reduction in the sensitivity of the brain's reward system (especially the brain circuits involving dopamine), both to addictive substances and also to natural reinforcers, such as food and sex. This is because natural reinforcers also depend upon the same reward system and circuits. This impairment explains why those who develop a substance use disorder often do not derive the same level of satisfaction or pleasure from once-pleasurable activities. This general loss of reward sensitivity may also account for the compulsive escalation of substance use as addicted individuals attempt to regain the pleasurable feelings the reward system once provided.[15]

Figure 2.8: Time-Related Decrease in Dopamine Released in the Brain of a Cocaine User

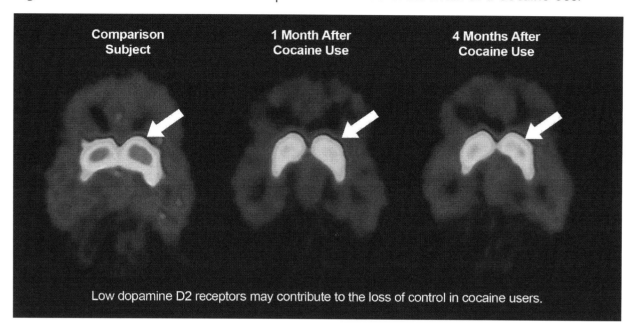

Notes: These fMRI images compare the brain of an individual with a history of cocaine use disorder (middle and right) to the brain of an individual without a history of cocaine use (left). The person who has had a cocaine use disorder has lower levels of the D2 dopamine receptor (depicted in red) in the striatum one month (middle) and four months (right) after stopping cocaine use compared to the non-user. The level of dopamine receptors in the brain of the cocaine user are higher at the 4-month mark (right), but have not returned to the levels observed in the non-user (left).

Source: Modified with permission from Volkow et al., (1993).[29]

At the same time, a second process occurs during the withdrawal stage: activation of stress neurotransmitters in the extended amygdala. These stress neurotransmitters include corticotropin-releasing factor (CRF), norepinephrine, and dynorphin (**Figure 2.9**).[30]

Studies suggest that these neurotransmitters play a key role in the negative feelings associated with withdrawal and in stress-triggered substance use. In animal and human studies, when researchers use special chemicals called antagonists to block activation of the stress neurotransmitter systems, it has the effect of reducing substance intake in response to withdrawal and stress. For example, blocking the activation of stress receptors in the brain reduced alcohol consumption in both alcohol-dependent rats and humans with an alcohol use disorder.[31] Thus, it may be that an additional motivation for drug and alcohol seeking among individuals with substance use disorders is to suppress overactive brain stress systems that produce negative emotions or feelings. Recent research also suggests that neuroadaptations in the endogenous cannabinoid system within the extended amygdala contribute to increased stress reactivity and negative emotional states in addiction.[32]

The desire to remove the negative feelings that accompany withdrawal can be a strong motivator of continued substance use. As noted previously, this motivation is strengthened through negative reinforcement, because taking the substance relieves the negative feelings associated with withdrawal, at least temporarily. Of course, this process is a vicious cycle: Taking drugs or alcohol to lessen the symptoms of withdrawal that occur during a period of abstinence actually causes those symptoms to be even worse the next time a person stops taking the substance, making it even harder to maintain abstinence.

Figure 2.9: Major Neurotransmitter Systems Implicated in the Neuroadaptations Associated with the Withdrawal/Negative Affect Stage of Addiction

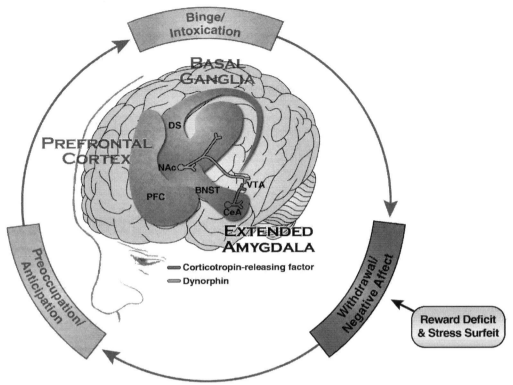

Notes: Not shown is the neurotransmitter norepinephrine which is also activated in the extended amygdala during withdrawal.

Abbreviations: PFC - prefrontal cortex, DS - dorsal striatum, NAc - nucleus accumbens, BNST - bed nucleus of the stria terminalis, CeA - central nucleus of the amygdala, VTA - ventral tegmental area.

Source: Modified with permission from Koob & Volkow, (2010).[14]

In Summary: The Withdrawal/Negative Affect Stage and the Extended Amygdala

This stage of addiction involves a decrease in the function of the brain reward systems and an activation of stress neurotransmitters, such as CRF and dynorphin, in the extended amygdala. Together, these phenomena provide a powerful neurochemical basis for the negative emotional state associated with withdrawal. The drive to alleviate these negative feelings negatively reinforces alcohol or drug use and drives compulsive substance taking.

Preoccupation/Anticipation Stage: Prefrontal Cortex

The preoccupation/anticipation stage of the addiction cycle is the stage in which a person may begin to seek substances again after a period of abstinence. In people with severe substance use disorders, that period of abstinence may be quite short (hours). In this stage, an addicted person becomes preoccupied with using substances again. This is commonly called "craving." Craving has been difficult to measure in human studies and often does not directly link with relapse.

This stage of addiction involves the brain's prefrontal cortex (Figure 2.10) the region that controls executive function: the ability to organize thoughts and activities, prioritize tasks, manage time, make decisions, and regulate one's own actions, emotions, and impulses. Executive function is essential for a person to make appropriate choices about whether or not to use a substance and to override often strong urges to use, especially when the person experiences triggers, such as stimuli associated with that substance (e.g., being at a party where alcohol is served or where people are smoking) or stressful experiences.

Figure 2.10: The Preoccupation/Anticipation Stage and the Prefrontal Cortex

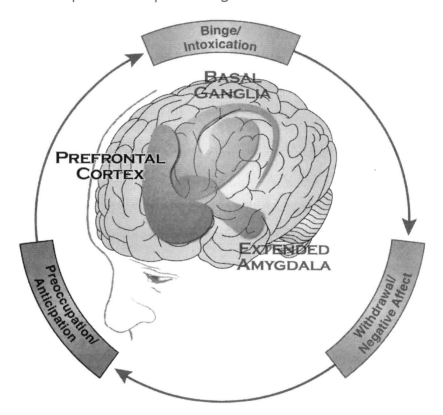

To help explain how the prefrontal cortex is involved in addiction, some scientists divide the functions of this brain region into a "Go system" and an opposing "Stop system."[33] The Go system helps people make decisions, particularly those that require significant attention and those involved with planning. People also engage the Go system when they begin behaviors that help them achieve goals. Indeed, research shows that when substance-seeking behavior is triggered by substance-associated environmental cues (incentive salience), activity in the Go circuits of the prefrontal cortex increases dramatically. This increased activity stimulates the nucleus accumbens to release glutamate, the main excitatory neurotransmitter in the brain. This release, in turn, promotes incentive salience, which creates a powerful urge to use the substance in the presence of drug-associated cues.

The Go system also engages habit-response systems in the dorsal striatum, and it contributes to the impulsivity associated with substance seeking. Habitual responding can occur automatically and subconsciously, meaning a person may not even be aware that they are engaging in such behaviors. The neurons in the Go circuits of the prefrontal cortex stimulate the habit systems of the dorsal striatum through connections that use glutamate (Figure 2.11).

Figure 2.11: Major Neurotransmitter Systems Implicated in the Neuroadaptations Associated with the Preoccupation/Anticipation Stage of Addiction

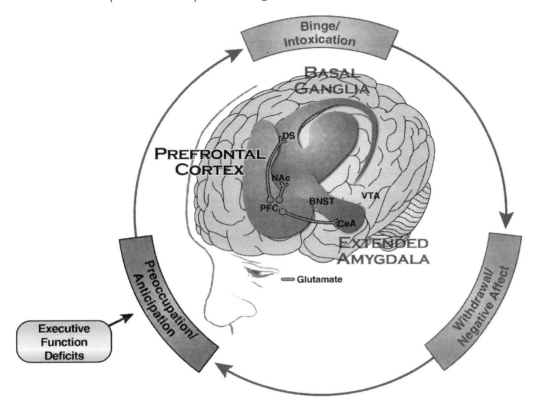

Abbreviations: PFC - prefrontal cortex, DS - dorsal striatum, NAc - nucleus accumbens, BNST - bed nucleus of the stria terminalis, CeA - central nucleus of the amygdala, VTA - ventral tegmental area.

Source: Modified with permission from Koob & Volkow, (2010).[14]

The Stop system inhibits the activity of the Go system. Especially relevant to its role in addiction, this system controls the dorsal striatum and the nucleus accumbens, the areas of the basal ganglia that are involved in the binge/intoxication stage of addiction. Specifically, the Stop system controls habit responses driven by the dorsal striatum, and scientists think that it plays a role in reducing the ability of substance-associated stimuli to trigger relapse—in other words, it inhibits incentive salience.[34]

The Stop system also controls the brain's stress and emotional systems, and plays an important role in relapse triggered by stressful life events or circumstances. Stress-induced relapse is driven by activation of neurotransmitters such as CRF, dynorphin, and norepinephrine in the extended amygdala. As described above, these neurotransmitters are activated during prolonged abstinence during the withdrawal/negative affect stage of addiction. More recent work in animals also implicates disruptions in the brain's cannabinoid system, which also regulates the stress systems in the extended amygdala, in relapse. Studies show that lower activity in the Stop component of the prefrontal cortex is associated with increased activity of stress circuitry involving the extended amygdala, and this increased activity drives substance-taking behavior and relapse.[37]

Brain imaging studies in people with addiction show disruptions in the function of both the Go and Stop circuits.[35-37] For example, people with alcohol, cocaine, or opioid use disorders show impairments in executive function, including disruption of decision-making and behavioral inhibition. These executive function deficits parallel changes in the prefrontal cortex and suggest decreased activity in the Stop system and greater reactivity of the Go system in response to substance-related stimuli.

Indeed, a smaller volume of the prefrontal cortex in abstinent, previously addicted individuals predicts a shorter time to relapse.[38] Studies also show that diminished prefrontal cortex control over the extended amygdala is particularly prominent in humans with post-traumatic stress disorder (PTSD), a condition that is frequently accompanied by drug and alcohol use disorders.[39] These findings bolster support for the role of the prefrontal cortex-extended amygdala circuit in stress-induced relapse, and suggest that strengthening prefrontal cortex circuits could aid substance use disorder treatment.

> ## In Summary: The Preoccupation/Anticipation Stage and the Prefrontal Cortex
>
> This stage of the addiction cycle is characterized by a disruption of executive function caused by a compromised prefrontal cortex. The activity of the neurotransmitter glutamate is increased, which drives substance use habits associated with craving, and disrupts how dopamine influences the frontal cortex.[2] The over-activation of the Go system in the prefrontal cortex promotes habit-like substance seeking, and the under-activation of the Stop system of the prefrontal cortex promotes impulsive and compulsive substance seeking.

To recap, addiction involves a three-stage cycle—binge/intoxication, withdrawal/negative affect, and preoccupation/anticipation—that worsens over time and involves dramatic changes in the brain reward, stress, and executive function systems. Progression through this cycle involves three major regions of the brain: the basal ganglia, the extended amygdala, and the prefrontal cortex, as well as multiple neurotransmitter systems (Figure 2.12). The power of addictive substances to produce positive feelings and relieve negative feelings fuels the development of compulsive use of substances. The combination of increased incentive salience (binge/intoxication stage), decreased reward sensitivity and increased stress sensitivity (withdrawal/negative affect stage), and compromised executive function (preoccupation/anticipation stage) provides an often overwhelming drive for substance seeking that can be unrelenting.

Different Classes of Substances Affect the Brain and Behavior in Different Ways

Although the three stages of addiction generally apply to all addictive substances, different substances affect the brain and behavior in different ways during each stage of the addiction cycle. Differences in the pharmacokinetics of various substances determine the duration of their effects on the body and partly account for the differences in their patterns of use. For example, nicotine has a short half-life, which means smokers need to smoke often to maintain the effect. In contrast, THC, the primary psychoactive compound in marijuana, has a much longer half-life. As a result, marijuana smokers do not typically smoke as frequently as tobacco smokers.[40] Typical patterns of use are described below for the major classes of addictive substances. However, people often use these substances in combination.[41] Additional research is needed to understand how using more than one substance affects the brain and the development and progression of addiction, as well as how use of one substance affects the use of others.

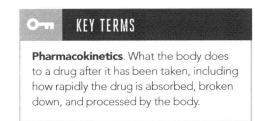

KEY TERMS

Pharmacokinetics. What the body does to a drug after it has been taken, including how rapidly the drug is absorbed, broken down, and processed by the body.

Figure 2.12: The Primary Brain Regions and Neurotransmitter Systems Involved in Each of the Three Stages of the Addiction Cycle

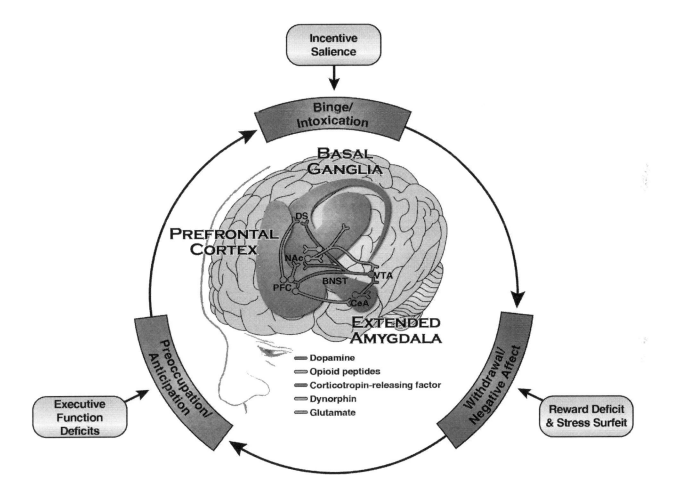

Opioids

Opioids attach to opioid receptors in the brain, which leads to a release of dopamine in the nucleus accumbens, causing euphoria (the high), drowsiness, and slowed breathing, as well as reduced pain signaling (which is why they are frequently prescribed as pain relievers). Opioid addiction typically involves a pattern of: (1) intense intoxication, (2) the development of tolerance, (3) escalation in use, and (4) withdrawal signs that include profound negative emotions and physical symptoms, such as bodily discomfort, pain, sweating, and intestinal distress and, in the most severe cases, seizures. As use progresses, the opioid must be taken to avoid the severe negative effects that occur during withdrawal. With repeated exposure to opioids, stimuli associated with the pleasant effects of the substances (e.g., places, persons, moods, and paraphernalia) and with the negative mental and physical effects of withdrawal can trigger intense craving or preoccupation with use.

Alcohol

When alcohol is consumed it interacts with several neurotransmitter systems in the brain, including the inhibitory neurotransmitter GABA, glutamate, and others that produce euphoria as well as the sedating, motor impairing, and anxiety-reducing effects of alcohol intoxication. Alcohol addiction often involves a similar pattern as opioid addiction, often characterized by periods of binge or heavy drinking followed by withdrawal. As with opioids, addiction to alcohol is characterized by intense craving that is often driven by negative emotional states, positive emotional states, and stimuli that have been associated with drinking, as well as a severe emotional and physical withdrawal syndrome. Many people with severe alcohol use disorder engage in patterns of binge drinking followed by withdrawal for extended periods of time. Extreme patterns of use may evolve into an opioid-like use pattern in which alcohol must be available at all times to avoid the negative consequences of withdrawal.

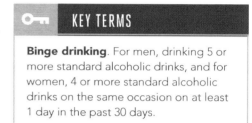

KEY TERMS

Binge drinking. For men, drinking 5 or more standard alcoholic drinks, and for women, 4 or more standard alcoholic drinks on the same occasion on at least 1 day in the past 30 days.

Stimulants

Stimulants increase the amount of dopamine in the reward circuit (causing the euphoric high) either by directly stimulating the release of dopamine or by temporarily inhibiting the removal of dopamine from synapses, the gaps between neurons. These drugs also boost dopamine levels in brain regions responsible for attention and focus on tasks (which is why stimulants like methylphenidate [Ritalin®] or dextroamphetamine [Adderall®] are often prescribed for people with attention deficit hyperactivity disorder). Stimulants also cause the release of norepinephrine, a neurotransmitter that affects autonomic functions like heart rate, causing a user to feel energized.

Addiction to stimulants, such as cocaine and amphetamines (including methamphetamine), typically follows a pattern that emphasizes the binge/intoxication stage. A person will take the stimulant repeatedly during a concentrated period of time lasting for hours or days (these episodes are called binges). The binge is often followed by a crash, characterized by negative emotions, fatigue, and inactivity. Intense craving then follows, which is driven by environmental cues associated with the availability of the substance, as well as by a person's internal state, such as their emotions or mood.

Marijuana (Cannabis)

Like other drugs, marijuana (also called cannabis) leads to increased dopamine in the basal ganglia, producing the pleasurable high. It also interacts with a wide variety of other systems and circuits in the brain that contain receptors for the body's natural cannabinoid neurotransmitters. Effects can be different from user to user, but often include distortions in motor coordination and time perception. Cannabis addiction follows a pattern similar to opioids. This pattern involves a significant binge/

intoxication stage characterized by episodes of using the substance to the point of intoxication. Over time, individuals begin to use the substance throughout the day and show chronic intoxication during waking hours. Withdrawal is characterized by negative emotions, irritability, and sleep disturbances.[40] Although the craving associated with cannabis[42] has been less studied than for other substances, it is most likely linked to both environmental and internal states, similar to those of other addictive substances.[43,44]

Synthetic Drugs

Different classes of chemically synthesized (hence the term synthetic) drugs have been developed, each used in different ways and having different effects in the brain. Synthetic cathinones, more commonly known as "bath salts," target the release of dopamine in a similar manner as the stimulant drugs described above. To a lesser extent, they also activate the serotonin neurotransmitter system, which can affect perception. Synthetic cannabinoids, sometimes referred to as "K2", "Spice", or "herbal incense," somewhat mimic the effects of marijuana but are often much more powerful. Drugs such as MDMA (ecstasy) and lysergic acid diethylamide (LSD) also act on the serotonin neurotransmitter system to produce changes in perception. Fentanyl is a synthetic opioid medication that is used for severe pain management and is considerably more potent than heroin. Prescription fentanyl, as well as illicitly manufactured fentanyl and related synthetic opioids, are often mixed with heroin but are also increasingly used alone or sold on the street as counterfeit pills made to look like prescription opioids or sedatives.

Factors that Increase Risk for Substance Use, Misuse, and Addiction

Not all people use substances, and even among those who use them, not all are equally likely to become addicted. Many factors influence the development of substance use disorders, including developmental, environmental, social, and genetic factors, as well as co-occurring mental disorders. Other factors protect people from developing a substance use disorder or addiction. The relative influence of these risk and protective factors varies across individuals and the lifespan. The following sections discuss some of these factors.

Early Life Experiences

The experiences a person has early in childhood and in adolescence can set the stage for future substance use and, sometimes, escalation to a substance use disorder or addiction. Early life stressors can include physical, emotional, and sexual abuse; neglect; household instability (such as parental substance use and conflict, mental illness, or incarceration of household members);[45] and poverty.[46] Research suggests that the stress caused by these risk factors may act on the same stress circuits in the brain as addictive substances, which may explain why they increase addiction risk.[47]

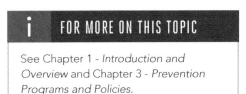

FOR MORE ON THIS TOPIC

See Chapter 1 - *Introduction and Overview* and Chapter 3 - *Prevention Programs and Policies*.

Adolescence is a critical period in the vulnerability to substance use and use disorders, because a hallmark of this developmental period is risk taking and experimentation, which for some young people includes trying alcohol, marijuana, or other drugs. In addition, the brain undergoes significant changes during this life stage, making it particularly vulnerable to substance exposure.[48] Importantly,

NEUROBIOLOGY

the frontal cortex—a region in the front part of the brain that includes the prefrontal cortex—does not fully develop until the early to mid-20s, and research shows that heavy drinking and drug use during adolescence affects development of this critical area of the brain.[49]

About three quarters (74 percent) of 18- to 30-year-olds admitted to treatment programs began using substances at the age of 17 or younger.[50] Individuals who start using substances during adolescence often experience more chronic and intensive use, and they are at greater risk of developing a substance use disorder compared with those who begin use at an older age. In other words, the earlier the exposure, the greater the risk.[51]

Not all adolescents who experiment with alcohol, cigarettes, or other substances go on to develop a substance use disorder, but research suggests that those who do progress to more harmful use may have pre-existing differences in their brains. For example, a brain imaging study of adolescents revealed that the volume of the frontal cortex was smaller in youth who transitioned from no or minimal drinking to heavy drinking over the course of adolescence than it was in youth who did not drink during adolescence.[49] Additional research can shed light on how these differences contribute to the progression from use to a disorder, as well as how changes caused by substance use affect brain function and behavior and whether they can be reversed.

Genetic and Molecular Factors

Genetic factors are thought to account for 40 to 70 percent of individual differences in risk for addiction.[52,53] Although multiple genes are likely involved in the development of addiction, only a few specific gene variants have been identified that either predispose to or protect against addiction. Some of these variants have been associated with the metabolism of alcohol and nicotine, while others involve receptors and other proteins associated with key neurotransmitters and molecules involved in all parts of the addiction cycle.[54] Genes involved in strengthening the connections between neurons and in forming drug memories have also been associated with addiction risk.[55,56] Like other chronic health conditions, substance use disorders are influenced by the complex interplay between a person's genes and environment. Additional research on the mechanisms underlying gene by environment interactions is expected to provide insight into how substance use disorders develop and how they can be prevented and treated.

Use of Multiple Substances and Co-occurring Mental Health Conditions

Many individuals with a substance use disorder also have a mental disorder,[57,58] and some have multiple substance use disorders. For example, according to the 2015 *National Survey on Drug Use and Health* (NSDUH), of the 20.8 million people aged 12 or older who had a substance use disorder during the past year, about 2.7 million (13 percent) had both an alcohol use and an illicit drug use disorder, and 41.2 percent also had a mental illness.[59] Particularly striking is the 3- to 4-fold higher rate of tobacco smoking among patients with schizophrenia and the high prevalence of co-existing alcohol use disorder in those meeting criteria for PTSD. It is estimated that 30-60 percent of patients seeking treatment for alcohol use disorder meet criteria for PTSD,[60,61] and approximately one third of individuals who have experienced PTSD have also experienced alcohol dependence at some point in their lives.[60]

The reasons why substance use disorders and mental disorders often occur together are not clear, and establishing the relationships between these conditions is difficult. Still, three possible explanations deserve attention. One reason for the overlap may be that having a mental disorder increases vulnerability to substance use disorders because certain substances may, at least temporarily, be able to reduce mental disorder symptoms and thus are particularly negatively reinforcing in these individuals. Second, substance use disorders may increase vulnerability for mental disorders,[62-64] meaning that the use of certain substances might trigger a mental disorder that otherwise would have not occurred. For example, research suggests that alcohol use increases risk for PTSD by altering the brain's ability to recover from traumatic experiences.[65,66] Similarly, the use of marijuana, particularly marijuana with a high THC content, might contribute to schizophrenia in those who have specific genetic vulnerabilities.[67] Third, it is also possible that both substance use disorders and mental disorders are caused by shared, overlapping factors, such as particular genes, neurobiological deficits, and exposure to traumatic or stressful life experiences. As these possibilities are not mutually exclusive, the relationship between substance use disorders and mental disorders may result from a combination of these processes.

Regardless of which one might influence the development of the other, mental and substance use disorders have overlapping symptoms, making diagnosis and treatment planning particularly difficult. For example, people who use methamphetamine for a long time may experience paranoia, hallucinations, and delusions that may be mistaken for symptoms of schizophrenia. And, the psychological symptoms that accompany withdrawal, such as depression and anxiety, may be mistaken as simply part of withdrawal instead of an underlying mood disorder that requires independent treatment in its own right. Given the prevalence of co-occurring substance use and mental disorders, it is critical to continue to advance research on the genetic, neurobiological, and environmental factors that contribute to co-occurring disorders and to develop interventions to prevent and treat them.

Biological Factors Contributing to Population-based Differences in Substance Misuse and Substance Use Disorders

Differences Based on Sex

Some groups of people are also more vulnerable to substance misuse and substance use disorders. For example, men tend to drink more than women and they are at higher risk for alcohol use disorder, although the gender differences in alcohol use are declining.[68] Men are also more likely to have other substance use disorders.[69] However, clinical reports suggest that women who use cocaine, opioids, or alcohol progress from initial use to a disorder at a faster rate than do men (called "telescoping").[70-72] Compared with men, women also exhibit greater symptoms of withdrawal from some drugs, such as nicotine. They also report worse negative affects during withdrawal and have higher levels of the stress hormone cortisol.[73]

Sex differences in reaction to addictive substances are not particular to humans. Female rats, in general, learn to self-administer drugs and alcohol more rapidly, escalate their drug taking more quickly, show greater symptoms of withdrawal, and are more likely to resume drug seeking in response to drugs, drug-related cues, or stressors. The one exception is that female rats show less withdrawal symptoms related to alcohol use.[74] Researchers are investigating the neurobiological bases for these differences.

Differences Based on Race and Ethnicity

Research on the neurobiological factors contributing to differential rates of substance use and substance use disorders in particular racial and ethnic groups is much more limited. A study using functional magnetic resonance imaging (fMRI) found that African American smokers showed greater activation of the prefrontal cortex upon exposure to smoking-related cues than did White smokers, an effect that may partly contribute to the lower smoking-cessation success rates observed among African Americans.[75]

Alcohol research with racial and ethnic groups has shown that approximately 36 percent of East Asians carry a gene variant that alters the rate at which members of that racial group metabolize alcohol, causing a buildup of acetaldehyde, a toxic byproduct of alcohol metabolism that produces symptoms such as flushing, nausea, and rapid heartbeat. Although these effects may protect some individuals of East Asian descent from alcohol use disorder, those who drink despite the effects are at increased risk for esophageal[76] and head and neck cancers.[77] Another study found that even low levels of alcohol consumption by Japanese Americans may result in adverse effects on the brain, a finding that may be related to the differences in alcohol metabolism described above.[78] Additional research will help to clarify the interactions between race, ethnicity, and the neuroadaptations that underlie substance misuse and addiction. This work may inform the development of more precise preventive and treatment interventions.

Recommendations for Research

Decades of research demonstrate that chronic substance misuse leads to profound disruptions of brain circuits involved in the experience of pleasure or reward, habit formation, stress, and decision-making. This work has paved the way for the development of a variety of therapies that effectively help people reduce or abstain from alcohol and drug misuse and regain control over their lives. In spite of this progress, our understanding of how substance use affects the brain and behavior is far from complete. Four research areas are specifically emphasized in the text below.

Effects of Substance Use on Brain Circuits and Functions

Continued research is necessary to more thoroughly explain how substance use affects the brain at the molecular, cellular, and circuit levels. Such research has the potential to identify common neurobiological mechanisms underlying substance use disorders, as well as other related mental disorders. This research is expected to reveal new neurobiological targets, leading to new medications and non-pharmacological treatments—such as transcranial magnetic stimulation or vaccines—for the treatment of substance use disorders. A better understanding of the neurobiological mechanisms underlying substance use disorders could also help to inform behavioral interventions. Therefore, basic research that further elucidates the neurobiological framework of substance use disorders and co-occurring mental disorders, as well as research leading to the development of new medications and other therapeutics to treat the underlying neurobiological mechanisms of substance use disorders should be accelerated.

As with other diseases, individuals vary in the development and progression of substance use disorders. Not only are some people more likely to use and misuse substances than are others and to progress from initial use to addiction differently, individuals also differ in their vulnerability to relapse and in how they respond to treatments. For example, some people with substance use disorders are particularly vulnerable to stress-induced relapse, but others may be more likely to resume substance use after being exposed to drug-related cues. Developing a thorough understanding of how neurobiological differences account for variation among individuals and groups will guide the development of more effective, personalized prevention and treatment interventions. Additionally, determining how neurobiological factors contribute to differences in substance misuse and addiction between women and men and among racial and ethnic groups is critical.

Continued advances in neuroscience research will further enhance our understanding of substance use disorders and accelerate the development of new interventions. Data gathered through the National Institutes of Health's Adolescent Brain Cognitive Development study, the largest long-term study of cognitive and brain development in children across the United States, is expected to yield unprecedented information about how substance use affects adolescent brain development. The Human Connectome Project and the Brain Research through Advancing Innovative Neurotechnologies (BRAIN) initiative are poised to spur an explosion of knowledge about the structure and function of brain circuits and how the brain affects behavior. Technologies that can alter the activity of dysfunctional circuits are being explored as possible treatments. Moreover, continued advances in genomics, along with President Obama's Precision Medicine Initiative, a national effort to better understand how individual variability in genes, environment, and lifestyle contribute to disease, are expected to bring us closer to developing individually-tailored preventive and treatment interventions for substance-related conditions.

Neurobiological Effects of Recovery

Little is known about the factors that facilitate or inhibit long-term recovery from substance use disorders or how the brain changes over the course of recovery. Developing a better understanding of the recovery process, and the neurobiological mechanisms that enable people to maintain changes in their substance use behavior and promote resilience to relapse, will inform the development of additional effective treatment and recovery support interventions. Therefore, an investigation of the neurobiological processes that underlie recovery and contribute to improvements in social, educational, and professional functioning is necessary.

Adolescence, Brain Change, and Vulnerability to Substance Use Disorders

Although young people are particularly vulnerable to the adverse effects of substance use, not all adolescents who experiment with alcohol or drugs go on to develop a substance use disorder. Prospective, longitudinal studies are needed to investigate whether pre-existing neurobiological factors contribute to adolescent substance use and the development of substance use disorders, how adolescent substance use affects brain structure and function, and whether the changes in brain structure and function that accompany chronic substance use can recover over time. Studies that follow groups of adolescents over time to learn about the developing human brain should be conducted. These studies should investigate how pre-existing neurobiological factors contribute to substance use, misuse, and addiction, and how adolescent substance use affects brain function and behavior.

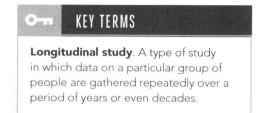

Longitudinal study. A type of study in which data on a particular group of people are gathered repeatedly over a period of years or even decades.

Neurobiological Effects of Polysubstance Use and Emerging Drug Products

Patterns of alcohol and drug use change over time. New drugs or drug combinations, delivery systems, and routes of administration emerge, and with them new questions for public health. For example, concern is growing that increasing use of marijuana extracts with extremely high amounts of THC could lead to higher rates of addiction among marijuana users. Concerns also are emerging about how new products about which little is known, such as synthetic cannabinoids and synthetic cathinones, affect the brain. Additional research is needed to better understand how such products - as well as emerging addictive substances - affect brain function and behavior, and contribute to addiction.

References

1. Berlin, G. S., & Hollander, E. (2014). Compulsivity, impulsivity, and the DSM-5 process. *CNS Spectrums, 19*(1), 62-68.

2. Kalivas, P. W. (2009). The glutamate homeostasis hypothesis of addiction. *Nature Reviews Neuroscience, 10*(8), 561-572.

3. American Psychiatric Association. (2013). *Diagnostic and statistical manual of mental disorders (DSM-5)* (5th ed.). Arlington, VA: American Psychiatric Publishing.

4. McLellan, A. T., Lewis, D. C., O'Brien, C. P., & Kleber, H. D. (2000). Drug dependence, a chronic medical illness: Implications for treatment, insurance, and outcomes evaluation. *JAMA, 284*(13), 1689-1695.

5. Volkow, N. D., Koob, G. F., & McLellan, A. T. (2016). Neurobiologic advances from the brain disease model of addiction. *New England Journal of Medicine, 374*(4), 363-371.

6. Hubbard, R. L., Craddock, S. G., & Anderson, J. (2003). Overview of 5-year followup outcomes in the drug abuse treatment outcome studies (DATOS). *Journal of Substance Abuse Treatment, 25*(3), 125-134.

7. Hser, Y.-I., Hoffman, V., Grella, C. E., & Anglin, M. D. (2001). A 33-year follow-up of narcotics addicts. *Archives of General Psychiatry, 58*(5), 503-508.

8. Vaillant, G. E. (1995). *The natural history of alcoholism revisited.* Cambridge, MA: Harvard University Press.

9. Stone, A. L., Becker, L. G., Huber, A. M., & Catalano, R. F. (2012). Review of risk and protective factors of substance use and problem use in emerging adulthood. *Addictive Behaviors, 37*(7), 747-775.

10. Koob, G. F., & Le Moal, M. (1997). Drug abuse: Hedonic homeostatic dysregulation. *Science, 278*(5335), 52-58.

11. Kalivas, P. W., & Volkow, N. D. (2005). The neural basis of addiction: A pathology of motivation and choice. *The American Journal of Psychiatry, 162*(8), 1403-1413.

12. Davis, M., Walker, D. L., Miles, L., & Grillon, C. (2010). Phasic vs sustained fear in rats and humans: Role of the extended amygdala in fear vs anxiety. *Neuropsychopharmacology, 35*(1), 105-135.

13. Ball, G., Stokes, P. R., Rhodes, R. A., Bose, S. K., Rezek, I., Wink, A.-M., . . . Turkheimer, F. E. (2011). Executive functions and prefrontal cortex: A matter of persistence? *Frontiers in Systems Neuroscience, 5*(3), 1-13.

14. Koob, G. F., & Volkow, N. D. (2010). Neurocircuitry of addiction. *Neuropsychopharmacology, 35*(1), 217–238.

15. Koob, G. F., & Le Moal, M. (2001). Drug addiction, dysregulation of reward, and allostasis. *Neuropsychopharmacology, 24*(2), 97-129.

16. Nestler, E. J. (2005). Is there a common molecular pathway for addiction? *Nature Neuroscience, 8*(11), 1445-1449.

17. Clapp, P., Bhave, S. V., & Hoffman, P. L. (2008). How adaptation of the brain to alcohol leads to dependence: A pharmacological perspective. *Alcohol Research & Health, 31*(4), 310-339.

18. Moreira, F. A., & Dalley, J. W. (2015). Dopamine receptor partial agonists and addiction. *European Journal of Pharmacology, 752*, 112-115.

19. Swift, R. M., & Aston, E. R. (2015). Pharmacotherapy for alcohol use disorder: Current and emerging therapies. *Harvard Review of Psychiatry, 23*(2), 122-133.

20. Uslaner, J. M., Acerbo, M. J., Jones, S. A., & Robinson, T. E. (2006). The attribution of incentive salience to a stimulus that signals an intravenous injection of cocaine. *Behavioural Brain Research, 169*(2), 320-324.

21. Schultz, W., Dayan, P., & Montague, P. R. (1997). A neural substrate of prediction and reward. *Science, 275*(5306), 1593-1599.

22. Phillips, P. E., Stuber, G. D., Heien, M. L., Wightman, R. M., & Carelli, R. M. (2003). Subsecond dopamine release promotes cocaine seeking. *Nature, 422*(6932), 614-618.

23. Volkow, N. D., Wang, G.-J., Telang, F., Fowler, J. S., Logan, J., Childress, A.-R., . . . Wong, C. (2006). Cocaine cues and dopamine in dorsal striatum: Mechanism of craving in cocaine addiction. *The Journal of Neuroscience, 26*(24), 6583-6588.

24. Wong, D. F., Kuwabara, H., Schretlen, D. J., Bonson, K. R., Zhou, Y., Nandi, A., . . . Kumar, A. (2006). Increased occupancy of dopamine receptors in human striatum during cue-elicited cocaine craving. *Neuropsychopharmacology, 31*(12), 2716-2727.

25. Volkow, N. D., Tomasi, D., Wang, G. J., Logan, J., Alexoff, D. L., Jayne, M., . . . Du, C. (2014). Stimulant-induced dopamine increases are markedly blunted in active cocaine abusers. *Molecular Psychiatry, 19*(9), 1037-1043.

26. Belin, D., Jonkman, S., Dickinson, A., Robbins, T. W., & Everitt, B. J. (2009). Parallel and interactive learning processes within the basal ganglia: Relevance for the understanding of addiction. *Behavioural Brain Research, 199*(1), 89-102.

27. Volkow, N. D., & Morales, M. (2015). The brain on drugs: From reward to addiction. *Cell, 162*(4), 712-725.

28. Volkow, N. D., Wang, G.-J., Fowler, J. S., Logan, J., Gatley, S. J., Hitzemann, R., . . . Pappas, N. (1997). Decreased striatal dopaminergic responsiveness in detoxified cocaine-dependent subjects. *Nature, 386*(6627), 830-833.

29. Volkow, N. D., Fowler, J. S., Wang, G. J., Hitzemann, R., Logan, J., Schlyer, D. J., . . . Wolf, A. P. (1993). Decreased dopamine D2 receptor availability is associated with reduced frontal metabolism in cocaine abusers. *Synapse, 14*(2), 169-177.

30. Koob, G. F., & Le Moal, M. (2005). Plasticity of reward neurocircuitry and the 'dark side' of drug addiction. *Nature Neuroscience, 8*(11), 1442-1444.

31. Vendruscolo, L. F., Estey, D., Goodell, V., Macshane, L. G., Logrip, M. L., Schlosburg, J. E., . . . Hunt, H. J. (2015). Glucocorticoid receptor antagonism decreases alcohol seeking in alcohol-dependent individuals. *The Journal of Clinical Investigation, 125*(8), 3193-3197.

32. Parsons, L. H., & Hurd, Y. L. (2015). Endocannabinoid signalling in reward and addiction. *Nature Reviews Neuroscience, 16*(10), 579-594.

33. Koob, G. F., Arends, M. A., & Le Moal, M. (2014). *Drugs, addiction, and the brain.* Waltham, MA: Academic Press.

34. Goldstein, R. Z., & Volkow, N. D. (2011). Dysfunction of the prefrontal cortex in addiction: Neuroimaging findings and clinical implications. *Nature Reviews Neuroscience, 12*(11), 652-669.

35. Crunelle, C. L., Kaag, A. M., van den Munkhof, H. E., Reneman, L., Homberg, J. R., Sabbe, B., . . . van Wingen, G. (2015). Dysfunctional amygdala activation and connectivity with the prefrontal cortex in current cocaine users. *Human Brain Mapping, 36*(10), 4222-4230.

36. Goldstein, R. Z., & Volkow, N. D. (2002). Drug addiction and its underlying neurobiological basis: Neuroimaging evidence for the involvement of the frontal cortex. *American Journal of Psychiatry, 159*(10), 1642-1652.

37. Volkow, N. D., Wang, G.-J., Telang, F., Fowler, J. S., Logan, J., Jayne, M., . . . Wong, C. (2007). Profound decreases in dopamine release in striatum in detoxified alcoholics: Possible orbitofrontal involvement. *The Journal of Neuroscience, 27*(46), 12700-12706.

38. Rando, K., Hong, K.-I., Bhagwagar, Z., Li, C.-S. R., Bergquist, K., Guarnaccia, J., & Sinha, R. (2011). Association of frontal and posterior cortical gray matter volume with time to alcohol relapse: A prospective study. *American Journal of Psychiatry, 168*(2), 183-192.

39. Mahan, A. L., & Ressler, K. J. (2012). Fear conditioning, synaptic plasticity and the amygdala: Implications for posttraumatic stress disorder. *Trends in Neurosciences, 35*(1), 24-35.

40. Koob, G. F., Karde, D. B., Baler, R. D., & Volkow, N. D. (2015). Pathopsychology of addiction. In A. Tasman, J. Kay, J. A. Lieberman, M. B. First, & M. Riba (Eds.), *Psychiatry.* (4th ed., Vol. 1). New York, NY: Wiley-Blackwell.

41. Connor, J. P., Gullo, M. J., White, A., & Kelly, A. B. (2014). Polysubstance use: Diagnostic challenges, patterns of use and health. *Current Opinion in Psychiatry, 27*(4), 269-275.

42. Heishman, S. J., Singleton, E. G., & Liguori, A. (2001). Marijuana craving questionnaire: Development and initial validation of a self-report instrument. *Addiction, 96*(7), 1023-1034.

43. Lundahl, L. H., & Johanson, C. E. (2011). Cue-induced craving for marijuana in cannabis-dependent adults. *Experimental and Clinical Psychopharmacology, 19*(3), 224-230.

44. Buckner, J. D., Zvolensky, M. J., Ecker, A. H., & Jeffries, E. R. (2016). Cannabis craving in response to laboratory-induced social stress among racially diverse cannabis users: The impact of social anxiety disorder. *Journal of Psychopharmacology 30*(4), 363-369.

45. Dube, S. R., Felitti, V. J., Dong, M., Chapman, D. P., Giles, W. H., & Anda, R. F. (2003). Childhood abuse, neglect, and household dysfunction and the risk of illicit drug use: The adverse childhood experiences study. *Pediatrics, 111*(3), 564-572.

46. Najavits, L. M., Hyman, S. M., Ruglass, L. M., Hien, D. A., & Read, J. P. (In press). Substance use disorder and trauma. In S. Gold, J. Cook, & C. Dalenberg (Eds.), *Handbook of trauma psychology.* Washington, DC: American Psychological Association.

47. Teicher, M. H., & Samson, J. A. (2013). Childhood maltreatment and psychopathology: A case for ecophenotypic variants as clinically and neurobiologically distinct subtypes. *American Journal of Psychiatry, 170*(10), 1114-1133.

48. Giedd, J. N., Blumenthal, J., Jeffries, N. O., Castellanos, F. X., Liu, H., Zijdenbos, A., . . . Rapoport, J. L. (1999). Brain development during childhood and adolescence: A longitudinal MRI study. *Nature Neuroscience, 2*(10), 861-863.

49. Squeglia, L. M., Tapert, S. F., Sullivan, E. V., Jacobus, J., Meloy, M. J., Rolfing, T., & Pfefferbaum, A. (2015). Brain development in heavy-drinking adolescents. *American Journal of Psychiatry, 172*(6), 532-542.

50. Substance Abuse and Mental Health Services Administration, & Center for Behavioral Health Statistics and Quality. (2014). *The TEDS Report: Age of substance use initiation among treatment admissions aged 18 to 30*. Rockville, MD: Substance Abuse and Mental Health Services Administration.

51. Hanson, K. L., Medina, K. L., Padula, C. B., Tapert, S. F., & Brown, S. A. (2011). Impact of adolescent alcohol and drug use on neuropsychological functioning in young adulthood: 10-year outcomes. *Journal of Child and Adolescent Substance Abuse, 20*(2), 135-154.

52. Prescott, C. A., & Kendler, K. S. (1999). Genetic and environmental contributions to alcohol abuse and dependence in a population-based sample of male twins. *American Journal of Psychiatry, 156*, 34-40.

53. Schuckit, M. A., Edenberg, H. J., Kalmijn, J., Flury, L., Smith, T. L., Reich, T., . . . Foroud, T. (2001). A genome-wide search for genes that relate to a low level of response to alcohol. *Alcoholism: Clinical and Experimental Research, 25*(3), 323-329.

54. Dick, D. M., & Agrawal, A. (2008). The genetics of alcohol and other drug dependence. *Alcohol Research & Health, 31*(2), 111-119.

55. Drgonova, J., Walther, D., Singhal, S., Johnson, K., Kessler, B., Troncoso, J., & Uhl, G. R. (2015). Altered CSMD1 expression alters cocaine-conditioned place preference: Mutual support for a complex locus from human and mouse models. *PLOS ONE, 10*(7).

56. Zhong, X., Drgonova, J., Li, C. Y., & Uhl, G. R. (2015). Human cell adhesion molecules: Annotated functional subtypes and overrepresentation of addiction-associated genes. *Annals of the New York Academy of Sciences, 1349*(1), 83-95.

57. Grant, B. F., Stinson, F. S., Dawson, D. A., Chou, S. P., Dufour, M. C., Compton, W., . . . Kaplan, K. (2004). Prevalence and co-occurrence of substance use disorders and independent mood and anxiety disorders: Results from the National Epidemiologic Survey on Alcohol and Related Conditions. *Archives of General Psychiatry, 61*(8), 807-816.

58. Grant, B. F., Stinson, F. S., Dawson, D. A., Chou, S. P., Ruan, W. J., & Pickering, R. P. (2004). Co-occurrence of 12-month alcohol and drug use disorders and personality disorders in the United States: Results from the National Epidemiologic Survey on Alcohol and Related Conditions. *Archives of General Psychiatry, 61*(4), 361-368.

59. Center for Behavioral Health Statistics and Quality. (2016). *Results from the 2015 National Survey on Drug Use and Health: Detailed tables*. Rockville, MD: Substance Abuse and Mental Health Services Administration.

60. Chilcoat, H. D., & Menard, C. (2003). Epidemiological investigations: Comorbidity of posttraumatic stress disorder and substance use disorder. In P. Ouimette & P. J. Brown (Eds.), *Trauma and substance abuse: Causes, consequences, and treatment of comorbid disorders.* (pp. 9-28). Washington, DC: American Psychological Association.

61. Kessler, R. C., Berglund, P., Demler, O., Jin, R., Merikangas, K. R., & Walters, E. E. (2005). Lifetime prevalence and age-of-onset distributions of DSM-IV disorders in the National Comorbidity Survey Replication. *Archives of General Psychiatry, 62*(6), 593-602.

62. Jacobsen, L. K., Southwick, S. M., & Kosten, T. R. (2001). Substance use disorders in patients with posttraumatic stress disorder: A review of the literature. *American Journal of Psychiatry, 158*(8), 1184-1190.

63. Leeies, M., Pagura, J., Sareen, J., & Bolton, J. M. (2010). The use of alcohol and drugs to self-medicate symptoms of posttraumatic stress disorder. *Depression and Anxiety, 27*(8), 731-736.

64. Kumari, V., & Postma, P. (2005). Nicotine use in schizophrenia: The self medication hypotheses. *Neuroscience and Biobehavioral Reviews, 29*(6), 1021-1034.

65. Anthenelli, R. M. (2010). Focus on: Comorbid mental health disorders. *Alcohol Research & Health, 33*(1-2), 109-117.

66. Holmes, A., Fitzgerald, P. J., MacPherson, K. P., DeBrouse, L., Colacicco, G., Flynn, S. M., . . . Marcinkiewcz, C. A. (2012). Chronic alcohol remodels prefrontal neurons and disrupts NMDAR-mediated fear extinction encoding. *Nature Neuroscience, 15*(10), 1359-1361.

67. Kelley, M. E., Wan, C. R., Broussard, B., Crisafio, A., Cristofaro, S., Johnson, S., . . . Walker, E. F. (2016). Marijuana use in the immediate 5-year premorbid period is associated with increased risk of onset of schizophrenia and related psychotic disorders. *Schizophrenia Research, 171*(1-3), 62-67.

68. Keyes, K. M., Grant, B. F., & Hasin, D. S. (2008). Evidence for a closing gender gap in alcohol use, abuse, and dependence in the United States population. *Drug and Alcohol Dependence, 93*(1), 21-29.

69. Hasin, D. S., & Grant, B. F. (2015). The National Epidemiologic Survey on Alcohol and Related Conditions (NESARC) Waves 1 and 2: Review and summary of findings. *Social Psychiatry and Psychiatric Epidemiology, 50*(11), 1609-1640.

70. Brady, K. T., & Randall, C. L. (1999). Gender differences in substance use disorders. *Psychiatric Clinics of North America, 22*(2), 241-252.

71. Greenfield, S. F., Back, S. E., Lawson, K., & Brady, K. T. (2010). Substance abuse in women. *Psychiatric Clinics of North America, 33*(2), 339-355.

72. Kosten, T. A., Gawin, F. H., Kosten, T. R., & Rounsaville, B. J. (1993). Gender differences in cocaine use and treatment response. *Journal of Substance Abuse Treatment, 10*(1), 63-66.

73. Chanraud, S., Pitel, A.-L., Müller-Oehring, E. M., Pfefferbaum, A., & Sullivan, E. V. (2013). Remapping the brain to compensate for impairment in recovering alcoholics. *Cerebral Cortex, 23*(1), 97-104.

74. Becker, J. B., & Koob, G. F. (2016). Sex differences in animal models: Focus on addiction. *Pharmacological Reviews, 68*(2), 242-263.

75. Okuyemi, K. S., Powell, J. N., Savage, C. R., Hall, S. B., Nollen, N., Holsen, L. M., . . . Ahluwalia, J. S. (2006). Clinical and imaging study: Enhanced cue-elicited brain activation in African American compared with Caucasian smokers: An fMRI study. *Addiction Biology, 11*(1), 97-106.

76. Brooks, P. J., Enoch, M.-A., Goldman, D., Li, T.-K., & Yokoyama, A. (2009). The alcohol flushing response: An unrecognized risk factor for esophageal cancer from alcohol consumption. *PLOS Medicine, 6*(3).

77. Yokoyama, A., & Omori, T. (2003). Genetic polymorphisms of alcohol and aldehyde dehydrogenases and risk for esophageal and head and neck cancers. *Japanese Journal of Clinical Oncology, 33*(3), 111-121.

78. Fukuda, K., Yuzuriha, T., Kinukawa, N., Murakawa, R., Takashima, Y., Uchino, A., . . . Hirano, M. (2009). Alcohol intake and quantitative MRI findings among community dwelling Japanese subjects. *Journal of the Neurological Sciences, 278*(1), 30-34.

CHAPTER 3.
PREVENTION PROGRAMS AND POLICIES

Chapter 3 Preview

As discussed in earlier chapters, the misuse of alcohol and drugs and substance use disorders has a huge impact on public health in the United States. In 2014, over 43,000 people died from a drug overdose, more than in any previous year on record[2] and alcohol misuse accounts for about 88,000 deaths in the United States each year (including 1 in 10 total deaths among working-age adults).[4] The yearly economic impact of alcohol misuse and alcohol use disorders is estimated at $249 billion ($2.05 per drink) in 2010[6] and the impact of illicit drug use and drug use disorders is estimated at $193 billion–figures that include both direct and indirect costs related to crime, health, and lost productivity.[7] Over half of these alcohol-related deaths and three-quarters of the alcohol-related economic costs were due to binge drinking. In addition, alcohol is involved in about 20 percent of the overdose deaths related to prescription opioid pain relievers.[6]

Substance misuse is also associated with a wide range of health and social problems, including heart disease, stroke, high blood pressure, various cancers (e.g., breast cancer), mental disorders, neonatal abstinence syndrome (NAS), driving under the influence (DUI) and other transportation-related injuries,[8,9] sexual assault and rape,[10,11] unintended pregnancy, sexually transmitted infections,[12] intentional and unintentional injuries,[13] and property crimes.[14]

Given the impact of substance misuse on public health and the increased risk for long-term medical consequences, including substance use disorders, it is critical to prevent substance misuse from starting and to identify those who have already begun to misuse substances and intervene early. Evidence-based prevention interventions, carried out before the need for treatment, are critical because they can delay early use and stop the progression from use to problematic use or to a substance use disorder (including its severest form, addiction), all of which are associated with costly individual, social, and public health consequences.[6,15-17] This chapter will demonstrate that prevention can markedly reduce the burden of disease and related costs. The good news is that there is strong scientific evidence supporting the effectiveness of prevention programs and policies.

> **FOR MORE ON THIS TOPIC**
>
> See Chapter 4 - *Early Intervention, Treatment, and Management of Substance Use Disorders.*

This chapter uses the term evidence-based interventions (EBIs) to refer to programs and policies supported by research. The chapter discusses the predictors of substance use initiation early in life and substance misuse throughout the lifespan, called risk factors, as well as factors that can mitigate those risks, called protective factors. The chapter also includes a system of categorizing prevention strategies defined by the Institute of Medicine (IOM).[18] This discussion is followed by a review of rigorous research on substance use initiation and misuse prevention programs that have demonstrated evidence of effectiveness. The chapter continues with a review of the rigorous research on the effectiveness and population impact of prevention policies, most of which are associated with alcohol misuse, as there is limited scientific literature on policy interventions for other drugs. Detailed reviews of these programs and policies are in <u>Appendix B - Evidence-Based Prevention Programs and Policies</u>. The chapter then describes how communities can build the capacity to implement effective programs and policies community wide to prevent substance use and related harms, and concludes with research recommendations.

KEY FINDINGS*

- Well-supported scientific evidence exists for robust predictors (risk and protective factors) of substance use and misuse from birth through adulthood. These predictors show much consistency across gender, race and ethnicity, and income.

- Well-supported scientific evidence demonstrates that a variety of prevention programs and alcohol policies that address these predictors prevent substance initiation, harmful use, and substance use-related problems, and many have been found to be cost-effective. These programs and policies are effective at different stages of the lifespan, from infancy to adulthood, suggesting that it is never too early and never too late to prevent substance misuse and related problems.

- Communities and populations have different levels of risk, protection, and substance use. Well-supported scientific evidence shows that communities are an important organizing force for bringing effective EBIs to scale. To build effective, sustainable prevention across age groups and populations, communities should build cross-sector community coalitions which assess and prioritize local levels of risk and protective factors and substance misuse problems and select and implement evidence-based interventions matched to local priorities.

- Well-supported scientific evidence shows that federal, state, and community-level policies designed to reduce alcohol availability and increase the costs of alcohol have immediate, positive benefits in reducing drinking and binge drinking, as well as the resulting harms from alcohol misuse, such as motor vehicle crashes and fatalities.

- There is well-supported scientific evidence that laws targeting alcohol-impaired driving, such as administrative license revocation and lower per se legal blood alcohol limits for adults and persons under the legal drinking age, have helped cut alcohol-related traffic deaths per 100,000 in half since the early 1980s.

- As yet, insufficient evidence exists of the effects of state policies to reduce inappropriate prescribing of opioid pain medications.

*The Centers for Disease Control and Prevention (CDC) summarizes strength of evidence as: "Well-supported": when evidence is derived from multiple controlled trials or large-scale population studies; "Supported": when evidence is derived from rigorous but fewer or smaller trials; and "Promising": when evidence is derived from a practical or clinical sense and is widely practiced.[5]

Why We Should Care About Prevention

Beginning in the twentieth century, the major illnesses leading to death shifted from infectious diseases, such as tuberculosis and infections in newborns, to noncommunicable diseases, such as heart disease, diabetes, and cancer. This shift was a result of effective public health interventions, such as improved sanitation and immunizations that reduced the rate of infectious diseases, as well as increased rates of unhealthy behaviors and lifestyles, including smoking, poor nutrition, physical inactivity, and substance misuse. In fact, behavioral health problems such as substance use, violence, risky driving, mental health problems, and risky sexual activity are now the leading causes of death for those aged 15 to 24.[19]

To effectively prevent substance misuse, it is important to understand the nature of the problem, including age of onset. Although people generally start using and misusing substances during adolescence, misuse can begin at any age and can continue to be a problem across the lifespan. As seen in **Figure 3.1**, likelihood of substance use escalates dramatically across adolescence, peaks in a person's twenties, and declines thereafter. For example, the highest prevalence of past month binge drinking and marijuana use occurs at ages 21 and 20, respectively. Other drugs follow similar trajectories, although their use typically begins at a later age.[20] Early substance misuse, including alcohol misuse, is associated with a greater likelihood of developing a substance use disorder later in life.[21,22] Of those who begin using a substance, the percentage of those who develop a substance use disorder, and the rate at which they develop it, varies by substance.

Figure 3.1: Past-Month Alcohol Use, Binge Alcohol Use, and Marijuana Use, by Age: Percentages, 2015 National Survey on Drug and Health (NSDUH)

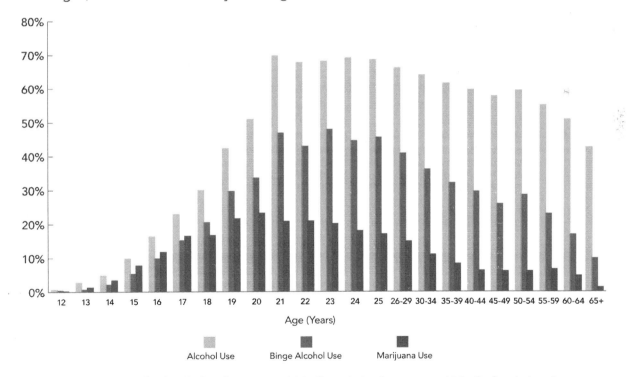

Note: Binge alcohol use is defined as drinking five or more drinks (for males) or four or more drinks (for females) on the same occasion (i.e., at the same time or within a couple of hours of each other) on at least 1 day in the past 30 days.

Source: Center for Behavioral Health Statistics and Quality, (2016).[20]

It is important to note that the vast majority of people in the United States who misuse substances do not have substance use disorders.[20,23] Nonetheless, substance misuse can put individual users and others around them at risk of harm, whether or not they have a disorder. Also, early initiation, substance misuse, and substance use disorders are associated with a variety of negative consequences, including deteriorating relationships, poor school performance, loss of employment, diminished mental health, and increases in sickness and death (e.g., motor vehicle crashes, poisoning, violence, or accidents).[15-17] It is therefore critical to prevent the full spectrum of substance misuse problems in addition to treating those with substance use disorders.

Preventing or reducing early substance use initiation, substance misuse, and the harms related to misuse requires the implementation of effective programs and policies that address substance misuse across the lifespan. The prevention science reviewed in this chapter demonstrates that effective prevention programs and policies exist, and if implemented well, they can markedly reduce substance misuse and related threats to the health of the population. However, evidence-based programs and policies are underutilized. For example, studies have found that many schools and communities are using prevention programs and strategies that have little or no evidence of effectiveness.[24,25] In fact, underuse of effective prevention programs and policies was the impetus for the creation of *Communities That Care* (CTC), a prevention service delivery system that promotes healthy youth development, improves youth outcomes, and reduces substance use and other problem behavior.[26]

At the policy level, research shows that higher alcohol prices reduce alcohol misuse and related harms (e.g., alcohol-related motor vehicle crashes),[27-31] and taxes are one component of price. As of January 1, 2015, 42 states had a beer excise tax of less than $0.50 per gallon, while only four states had an excise tax more than $1.00 per gallon (Table 3.4).[32,33]

Risk and Protective Factors

Longitudinal research has identified predictors of substance use and other behavioral health problems that are targets for preventive interventions.[34-36] Risk and protective factors influence the likelihood that a person will use a substance and whether they will develop a substance use disorder.

Risk and protective factors become influential at different times during development, and they often relate to physiological changes that occur over the course of development or to factors in a person's environment—for example, biological transitions such as puberty or social transitions such as attending a new school, parental divorce or military deployment, or graduation.[37] These factors can be influenced by programs and policies at multiple levels, including the federal, state, community, family, school, and individual levels.[38-41] Targeted programs implemented at the family, school, and individual levels can complement the broader population-level policy interventions, and assist in reducing specific risk factors (Table 3.1) and promoting protective factors (Table 3.2). Although there are exceptions, most

> **KEY TERMS**
>
> **Risk factors.** Factors that increase the likelihood of beginning substance use, of regular and harmful use, and of other behavioral health problems associated with use.
>
> **Protective factors.** Factors that directly decrease the likelihood of substance use and behavioral health problems or reduce the impact of risk factors on behavioral health problems.

risk and protective factors associated with substance use also predict other problems affecting youth, including delinquency, psychiatric conditions, violence, and school dropout. Therefore, programs and policies addressing those common or overlapping predictors of problems have the potential to simultaneously prevent substance misuse as well as other undesired outcomes.[42-44]

Some risk and protective factors appear to have consistent effects across cultural and gender groups, although low-income and disadvantaged populations are generally exposed to more risk factors, including risk factors within the environment, and to fewer protective factors than are other groups in the population. However, research has shown that binge drinking is more common among individuals in higher income households as compared to lower income households.[45] This has implications for the types of prevention programs and policies that might be most successful with disadvantaged populations. Despite the similarities in many identified risk factors across groups, it is important to examine whether there are subpopulation differences in the exposure of groups to risk factors.

Table 3.1: Risk Factors for Adolescent and Young Adult Substance Use

Risk Factors	Definition	Adolescent Substance Use	Young Adult Substance Use
Individual/Peer			
Early initiation of substance use[46,47]	Engaging in alcohol or drug use at a young age.	✔	✔
Early and persistent problem behavior[48,49]	Emotional distress, aggressiveness, and "difficult" temperaments in adolescents.	✔	
Rebelliousness[48,50]	High tolerance for deviance and rebellious activities.	✔	✔
Favorable attitudes toward substance use[51,52]	Positive feelings towards alcohol or drug use, low perception of risk.	✔	✔
Peer substance use[53-55]	Friends and peers who engage in alcohol or drug use.	✔	✔
Genetic predictors[56]	Genetic susceptibility to alcohol or drug use.	✔	✔
Family			
Family management problems (monitoring, rewards, etc.)[57-60]	Poor management practices, including parents' failure to set clear expectations for children's behavior, failure to supervise and monitor children, and excessively severe, harsh, or inconsistent punishment.	✔	✔
Family conflict[61-63]	Conflict between parents or between parents and children, including abuse or neglect.	✔	✔
Favorable parental attitudes[64,65]	Parental attitudes that are favorable to drug use and parental approval of drinking and drug use.	✔	✔
Family history of substance misuse[66,67]	Persistent, progressive, and generalized substance use, misuse, and use disorders by family members.	✔	✔

PREVENTION

Risk Factors	Definition	Adolescent Substance Use	Young Adult Substance Use
School			
Academic failure beginning in late elementary school[68,69]	Poor grades in school.	✔	✔
Lack of commitment to school[70,71]	When a young person no longer considers the role of the student as meaningful and rewarding, or lacks investment or commitment to school.	✔	✔
Community			
Low cost of alcohol[30,72]	Low alcohol sales tax, happy hour specials, and other price discounting.	✔	✔
High availability of substances[73,74]	High number of alcohol outlets in a defined geographical area or per a sector of the population.	✔	✔
Community laws and norms favorable to substance use[75,76]	Community reinforcement of norms suggesting alcohol and drug use is acceptable for youth, including low tax rates on alcohol or tobacco or community beer tasting events.	✔	✔
Media portrayal of alcohol use[77-79]	Exposure to actors using alcohol in movies or television.	✔	
Low neighborhood attachment[80,81]	Low level of bonding to the neighborhood.	✔	
Community disorganization[82,83]	Living in neighborhoods with high population density, lack of natural surveillance of public places, physical deterioration, and high rates of adult crime.	✔	
Low socioeconomic status[84,85]	A parent's low socioeconomic status, as measured through a combination of education, income, and occupation.	✔	
Transitions and mobility[80,86]	Communities with high rates of mobility within or between communities.	✔	

Table 3.2: Protective Factors for Adolescent and Young Adult Substance Use

Protective Factors	Definition	Adolescent Substance Use	Young Adult Substance Use
Individual			
Social, emotional, behavioral, cognitive, and moral competence[87,88]	Interpersonal skills that help youth integrate feelings, thinking, and actions to achieve specific social and interpersonal goals.	✔	✔
Self-efficacy[89,90]	An individual's belief that they can modify, control, or abstain from substance use.	✔	✔
Spirituality[91,92]	Belief in a higher being, or involvement in spiritual practices or religious activities.	✔	✔

Protective Factors	Definition	Adolescent Substance Use	Young Adult Substance Use
Resiliency[88]	An individual's capacity for adapting to change and stressful events in healthy and flexible ways.	✔	✔
Family, School, and Community			
Opportunities for positive social involvement[93,94]	Developmentally appropriate opportunities to be meaningfully involved with the family, school, or community.	✔	✔
Recognition for positive behavior[51]	Parents, teachers, peers and community members providing recognition for effort and accomplishments to motivate individuals to engage in positive behaviors in the future.	✔	✔
Bonding[95-97]	Attachment and commitment to, and positive communication with, family, schools, and communities.	✔	✔
Marriage or committed relationship[98]	Married or living with a partner in a committed relationship who does not misuse alcohol or drugs.		✔
Healthy beliefs and standards for behavior[51,99]	Family, school, and community norms that communicate clear and consistent expectations about not misusing alcohol and drugs.	✔	✔

Note: These tables present some of the key risk and protective factors related to adolescent and young adult substance initiation and misuse.

Types of Prevention Interventions

The IOM has described three categories of prevention interventions: *universal, selective,* and *indicated*.[18] Universal interventions are aimed at all members of a given population (for instance, all children of a certain age); selective interventions are aimed at a subgroup determined to be at high-risk for substance use (for instance, justice-involved youth); indicated interventions are targeted to individuals who are already using substances but have not developed a substance use disorder. Communities must choose from these three types of preventive interventions, but research has not yet been able to suggest an optimal mix. Communities may think it is best to direct services only to those with the highest risk and lowest protection or to those already misusing substances.[100] However, a relatively high percentage of substance misuse-related problems come from people at lower risk, because they are a much larger group within the total population than are people at high-risk. This follows what is known as the Prevention Paradox: "a large number of people at a small risk may give rise to more cases of disease than the small number who are at a high risk."[1] By this logic, providing prevention interventions to everyone (i.e., universal interventions) rather than only to those at highest risk is likely to have greater benefits.[3]

One advantage of a properly implemented universal prevention intervention is that it is likely to reach most or all of the population (for example, school-based interventions are likely to reach all students). Targeted (selective and indicated) approaches are likely to miss a large percentage of their targets, but they provide more intensive services to those who are reached. Because the best mix of interventions has not yet been determined, it is prudent for communities to provide a mix of universal, selective, and indicated preventive interventions.

Universal Prevention Interventions

Universal interventions attempt to reduce specific health problems across all people in a particular population by reducing a variety of risk factors and promoting a broad range of protective factors. Examples of universal interventions include policies—such as the setting of a minimum legal drinking age (MLDA) or reducing the availability of substances in a community—and school-based programs that promote social and emotional competencies to reduce stress, express emotion appropriately, and resist negative social influences. Because they focus on the entire population, universal interventions tend to have the greatest overall impact on substance misuse and related harms relative to interventions focused on individuals alone.[18]

Selective Interventions

Selective interventions are delivered to particular communities, families, or children who, due to their exposure to risk factors, are at increased risk of substance misuse problems. Target audiences for selective interventions may include families living in poverty, the children of depressed or substance-using parents, or children who have difficulties with social skills. Selective interventions typically deliver specialized prevention services to individuals with the goal of reducing identified risk factors, increasing protective factors, or both. Selective programs focus effort and resources on interventions that are intentionally designed for a specific high-risk group.[101] Selective programs have an advantage in that they focus effort and resources on those who are at higher risk for developing behavioral health problems. In so doing, they allow planners to create interventions that are more specifically designed for that audience. However, they are typically not population-based and therefore, compared to population-level interventions, they have more limited reach.

Indicated Interventions

Indicated prevention interventions are directed to those who are already involved in a risky behavior, such as substance misuse, or are beginning to have problems, but who have not yet developed a substance use disorder. Such programs are often intensive and expensive but may still be cost-effective, given the high likelihood of an ensuing expensive disorder or other costly negative consequences in the future.[102]

Evidence-based Prevention Programs

This section identifies universal, selective, and indicated prevention programs that have been shown to successfully reduce the number of people who start using alcohol or drugs or who progress to harmful use. Inclusion of the programs here was based on an extensive review of published research studies. Of the 600 programs considered, 42 met criteria to be included in this *Report*. Studies on programs that included people who already had a substance use or related disorder were excluded. The review used standard literature search procedures which are summarized in detail in Appendix A - Review Process for Prevention Programs.

The vast majority of prevention studies have been conducted on children, adolescents, and young adults, but prevention trials of older populations meeting the criteria were also included. Programs that met the criteria are categorized as follows: Programs for children younger than age 10 (or their families); programs for adolescents aged 10 to 18; programs for individuals ages 18 years and older; and programs coordinated by community coalitions. Due to the number of programs that have proven effective, the following sections highlight just a few of the effective programs from the more comprehensive tables in Appendix B - Evidence-Based Prevention Programs and Policies, which describe the outcomes of all the effective prevention programs. Representative programs highlighted here were chosen for each age group, domain, and level of intervention, and with attention to coverage of specific populations and culturally based population subgroups. It is important to note that screening and brief intervention (SBI) and electronic SBI for reducing alcohol misuse have been recognized as effective strategies for identifying and reducing substance misuse among adults, but these are discussed in detail in Chapter 4 -Early Intervention, Treatment, and Management of Substance Use Disorders as effective early intervention strategies.[103-106]

Interventions for Youth Aged 0 to 10

Few substance use prevention programs for children under the age of 10 have been evaluated for their effect on substance misuse and related problems. Such studies are rare because they require expensive long-term follow-up tracking and assessment to demonstrate an impact on substance initiation or misuse years or decades into the future. Consistent with general strategies to increase protective factors and decrease risk factors, universal prevention interventions for infants, preschoolers, and elementary school students have primarily focused on building healthy parent-child relationships, decreasing aggressive behavior, and building children's social, emotional, and cognitive competence for the transition to school. Both universal and selective programs have shown reductions in child aggression and improvements in social competence and relations with peers and adults (generally predictive of favorable longer-term outcomes), but only a few have studied longer-term effects on substance use.[107,108] Select programs showing positive effects are described below.

Nurse-Family Partnership

Only one program that focused on children younger than age 5—the *Nurse-Family Partnership*—has shown significant reductions in the use of alcohol in the teen years compared with those who did not receive the intervention.[109,110] This selective prevention program uses trained nurses to provide an intensive home visitation intervention for at-risk, first-time mothers during pregnancy. This intervention provides ongoing education and support to improve pregnancy outcomes and infant health and development while strengthening parenting skills.

The Good Behavior Game and Classroom-Centered Intervention

One universal elementary school-based prevention program has shown long-term preventive effects on substance use among a high-risk subgroup, males with high levels of aggression. The *Good Behavior Game* is a classroom behavior management program that rewards children for acting appropriately during instructional times through a team-based award system. Implemented by Grade 1 and 2 teachers, this program significantly lowered rates of alcohol, other substance use, and substance use disorders when the children reached the ages of 19 to 21.[111] The *Classroom-Centered Intervention*, which combined the *Good Behavior Game* with additional models of teacher instruction, also reduced rates of cocaine and heroin use in middle and high school, but it had no preventive effects on alcohol or marijuana initiation.[112,113]

Raising Healthy Children

A number of multicomponent, universal, elementary school programs involving both schools and parents are effective in preventing substance misuse.[114,115] One example is the *Raising Healthy Children* program (also known as *Seattle Social Development Project*) which targets Grades 1 through 6 and combines social and emotional learning, classroom instruction and management training for teachers, and training for parents conducted by school-home coordinators, who work with the children in school and the parents at home, focusing on in-home problem solving and similar workshops. Studies of this program showed reductions in heavy drinking at age 18 (6 years after the intervention)[114,115] and in rates of alcohol and marijuana use.[115]

The Fast Track Program

Two multicomponent selective and universal prevention programs were effective. An example is the *Fast Track Program*, an intensive 10-year intervention that was implemented in four United States locations for children with high rates of aggression in Grade 1. The program includes universal and selective components to improve social competence at school, early reading tutoring, and home visits as well as parenting support groups through Grade 10. Follow-up at age 25 showed that individuals who received the intervention as adolescents decreased alcohol and other substance misuse, with the exception of marijuana use.[116]

Interventions for Adolescents Aged 10 to 18

A variety of universal interventions focused on youth aged 10 to 18 have been shown to affect either the initiation or escalation of substance use.[117-124] In general, school-based programs share a focus on building social, emotional, cognitive, and substance refusal skills and provide children accurate information on rates and amounts of peer substance use.[119,120,124]

School-based Programs

One well-researched and widely used program is *LifeSkills Training*, a school-based program delivered over 3 years.[117] Research has shown that this training delayed early use of alcohol, tobacco, and other substances and reduced rates of use of all substances up to 5 years after the intervention ended. A multicultural model, *keepin'it REAL*, uses student-developed videos and narratives and has shown positive effects on substance use among Mexican American youth in the Southwestern United States.[121] Another example is *Project Toward No Drug Abuse*, which focuses on youth who are at high risk for drug use and violence. It is designed for youth who are attending alternative high schools but can be delivered in traditional high schools as well. The twelve 40-minute interactive sessions have shown positive effects on alcohol and drug misuse.[125]

Family-based Programs

A number of family-focused, universal prevention interventions show substantial preventive effects on substance use.[126-130] For example, *Strengthening Families Program: For Parents and Youth 10–14* (SFP) is a widely used seven-session universal, family-focused program that enhances parenting skills—specifically nurturing, setting limits, and communicating—as well as adolescent substance refusal skills. Across multiple studies conducted in rural United States communities, SFP showed reductions in tobacco, alcohol, and drug use up to 9 years after the intervention (i.e., to age 21) compared with youth who were not assigned to the SFP.[126,130] SFP also shows reductions in prescription drug misuse up to 13 years after the intervention (i.e., to age 25), both on its own and when paired with effective skills-focused school-based prevention.[131,132] *Strong African American Families*, a cultural adaptation of SFP, shows reductions in early initiation and rate of alcohol use for Black or African American rural youth.[127-129]

Three selective programs focus on interventions with families.[133-135] An example is *Familias Unidas*, a family-based intervention for Hispanic or Latino youth. It includes both multi-parent groups (eight weekly 2-hour sessions) and four to ten 1-hour individual family visits and has been shown to lower substance use or delay the start of substance use among adolescents.[133]

A number of selective and indicated interventions successfully prevent substance misuse when delivered to youth aged 10 to 18.[125,136-142] Most of these interventions target students who show early aggressive behavior, delinquency, or early substance use, as these are risk factors for later substance misuse, and some offer both a youth component in the classroom setting and a parent component. An example is *Coping Power*, a 16-month program for children in Grades 5 and 6 who were identified with early aggression. The program, which is designed to build problem-solving and self-regulation skills, has both a parent and a child component and reduces early substance use.[136]

Internet-based Programs

A number of computer- and Internet-based interventions also show positive effects on preventing substance use.[143-146] An example is *I Hear What You're Saying*, which involves nine 45-minute sessions to improve communication, establish family rules, and manage conflict. Specifically focused on mothers and daughters, follow-up results showed lower rates of substance use in an ethnically diverse sample.[143-145] Additionally, *Project Chill*, a brief intervention (30 to 45 minutes) delivered in primary care settings through either a computer or a therapist, reduced the number of youth who started using marijuana.[146]

Programs for Young Adults

Young adulthood is a key developmental period, when individuals are exposed to new social contexts with greater freedom and less social control than they experienced during their high school years. Social roles are changing at the same time that social safety net supports are weakening.[147] In addition, many young adults are undergoing transitions, such as leaving home, leaving the compulsory educational system, beginning college, entering the workforce, and forming families. As a result of all these forces, young adulthood is typically associated with increases in substance use, misuse, and misuse-related consequences.

Numerous studies have examined the effectiveness of brief alcohol interventions for adolescents and young adults. One review examined 185 such experimental studies among adolescents aged 11 to 18 and adults aged 19 to 30. Overall, brief alcohol interventions were associated with significant reductions in alcohol consumption and alcohol-related problems in both adults and adolescents, and in some studies, effects persisted up to one year.[148] The United States Preventive Services Task Force has recommended screening and brief intervention for reducing alcohol misuse among adults, as discussed in Chapter 4 - Early Intervention, Treatment, and Management Of Substance Use Disorders, and the American Academy of Pediatrics recommends that screening and brief interventions for alcohol misuse or use disorders be implemented for adolescent patients as well.[149]

Programs for College Students

Many interventions have been developed to reduce alcohol and marijuana misuse among college students. Several literature reviews of alcohol screening and brief interventions in this population have reported that these interventions reduce college student drinking,[150-154] and several other interventions for college students have shown longer term reductions in substance misuse.[155-165] One analysis reviewed 41 studies with 62 individual or group interventions and found that recipients of interventions experienced reduced alcohol use and fewer alcohol related problems up to four years post intervention.[166] Effective intervention components were personalized feedback, protective strategies to moderate drinking, setting alcohol-related goals, and challenging alcohol expectancies. Interventions with four or more components were most effective. Two example interventions for college students are described below.

Brief Alcohol Screening and Intervention for College Students (BASICS) is an example of a brief motivational intervention for which results have been positive. BASICS is designed to help students reduce alcohol misuse and the negative consequences of their drinking. It consists of two 1-hour interviews, with a brief online assessment after the first session. The first interview gathers information about alcohol consumption patterns and personal beliefs about alcohol, while providing instructions for self-monitoring drinking between sessions. The second interview uses data from the online assessment to develop personalized, normative feedback that reviews negative consequences and risk factors, clarifies perceived risks and benefits of drinking, and provides options for reducing alcohol use and its consequences. Follow-up studies of students who used BASICS have shown reductions in drinking quantity in the general college population, among fraternity members, with heavy drinkers who volunteered to use BASICS, and among those who were mandated to engage in the program from college disciplinary bodies.[106,162,164]

A second intervention, the *Parent Handbook*, focuses on teaching parents how and when to intervene during the critical time between high school graduation and college entry to disrupt the escalation of heavy drinking during the first year of college. The *Parent Handbook* is distributed during the summer before college, and parents receive a booster call to encourage them to read the materials. Research has found that the timing for the *Parent Handbook* is critical. If parents received it during the summer before college, it reduced the odds of students becoming heavy drinkers, but this intervention was not effective if used after the transition to college.[167] One study showed the combination of BASICS, and the *Parent Handbook* significantly reduced alcohol consumption among incoming college students who showed heavy rates of high school drinking.[168]

Many other interventions have been developed for this population that have not shown effects beyond 3 or 6 months after the intervention, and most positive effects are not maintained by 12-month follow-up.[155-159] For example, even though brief motivational interviewing (BMI) interventions have appeared promising, a recent analysis of 17 randomized trials demonstrated little effectiveness among college-aged individuals.[160]

A Resource: The National Institute on Alcohol Abuse and Alcoholism's (NIAAA's) CollegeAIM: Alcohol Intervention Matrix

In an effort to inform colleges and universities of the rapidly growing evidence base of programs and policies that can reduce harmful and underage drinking and related harms by college students, NIAAA has published *CollegeAIM-the College Alcohol Intervention Matrix*.

CollegeAIM reviews nearly 60 interventions, including both individual-level strategies and environmental-level policy strategies. The strategies are ranked by effectiveness (higher, moderate, lower, not effective, and too few studies to evaluate). Implementation costs (lower, mid-range, and higher) and implementation barriers (higher, moderate, and lower) are also ranked, as is public health reach (broad or focused).[169]

Programs in Adult Workplaces

Two programs met this *Report's* criteria for workplace or clinic-based prevention programs;[170-172] others have not shown significant preventive effects longer than 6 months.[173] The successful programs, *Team Awareness* and *Team Resilience*, were delivered in three 2-hour sessions to restaurant workers and led to decreases in heavy drinking and work-related problems. These programs reached approximately 30,000 workers in diverse settings, including military, tribal, and government settings, and with ex-offenders, young restaurant workers, and more.[170,172]

Programs for Older Adults

Only two studies showed preventive effects on alcohol use in older adults.[174,175] One is *Project Share*, which showed reductions in heavy drinking among those aged 60 and older. *Project Share* provided personalized feedback to at-risk older drinkers, which included a personalized patient report, discussion with a physician, and three phone calls from a health educator.[174] A second study, the *Computerized Alcohol-Related Problems Survey* (CARPS) assessed personalized reports of drinking risks and benefits accompanied with education for physicians and patients aged 65 and older. The study found a significant decrease in alcohol misuse, including reductions in the quantity and frequency that older individuals reported drinking.[175]

Economics of Prevention

The Washington State Institute for Public Policy developed a standardized model using scientifically rigorous standards to estimate the costs and benefits associated with various prevention programs. Benefit-per-dollar cost ratios for EBIs ranged from small returns per dollar invested to more than $64 for every dollar invested. These estimates are illustrated below in Table 3.3.

Table 3.3: Cost-Benefit of EBIs Reviewed by the Washington State Institute for Public Policy, 2016

Program	Benefit per Dollar Cost
Nurse-Family Partnership	$1.61
Raising Healthy Children/SSDP	$4.27
Good Behavior Game	$64.18
LifeSkills Training	$17.25
keepin' it REAL	$11.79
Strengthening Families Program 10-14	$5.00
Guiding Good Choices	$2.69
Positive Family Support/ Family Check Up	$0.62
Project Towards No Drug Abuse	$6.54
BASICS	$17.61

*Cost estimates are per participant, based on 2015 United States dollars.

Note: This is a general indication of the potential health and social value of EBIs. It is not possible to estimate specific cost-benefit for every EBI due to challenges in calculating accurate intervention effect sizes, the failure to document costs, the variation of methods used, and few mandates or incentives to complete this research. Reaching a consensus on standards for cost-benefit analyses and making them a routine part of prevention program evaluation could help policymakers choose EBIs that both prevent substance misuse and ensure that investments return benefits over the life course.

Source: Washington State Institute for Public Policy, (2016).[176]

Evidence-based Community Coalition-based Prevention Models

Community-based prevention programs can be effective in helping to address major challenges raised by substance misuse and its consequences. Such programs are often coordinated by local community coalitions composed of representatives from multiple community sectors or organizations (e.g., government, law enforcement, health, education) within a community, as well as private citizens.

These coalitions work to change community-level risk and protective factors and achieve community-wide reductions in substance use by planning and implementing one or more prevention strategies in multiple sectors simultaneously, with the goal of reaching as many members of the community as possible with accurate, consistent messages. For example, interventions may be implemented in family, educational, workplace, health care, law enforcement, and other settings, and they may involve policy interventions and publicly funded social and traditional media campaigns.[28,74,177-179]

A common feature of successful community programs is their reliance on local coalitions to select effective interventions and implement them with fidelity. An important requirement is that coalitions receive proactive training and technical assistance on prevention science and the use of EBIs and that they have clear goals and guidelines. Technical assistance can be provided by independent organizations such as Community Anti-Drug Coalitions of America (CADCA), academic institutions, the program developers, or others with expertise in the substance misuse prevention field. Three examples of effective community-based coalition models are provided below.

Communities That Care

Communities That Care (CTC) creates a broad-based community coalition to assess and prioritize risk and protective factors and substance use rates, using a school survey of all students in Grades 6, 8, 10, and 12. The coalition then chooses and implements EBIs that address their chosen priorities. CTC was tested in a 24-community trial, where 12 communities were randomly assigned to receive the CTC intervention.

Among a panel of students in Grade 5 who were enrolled in the study before the intervention, those in the CTC communities who were compared to the prevention as usual communities had lower rates of alcohol and tobacco initiation at Grades 10 and 12.[26,180-182]

PROmoting School-community-university Partnerships to Enhance Resilience

The PROmoting School-community-university Partnerships to Enhance Resilience (PROSPER) delivery system focuses on community-based collaboration and capacity building that links the land-grant university Cooperative Extension System with the public school system. Local teams select and implement family-focused EBIs in Grade 6 and a school-based EBI in Grade 7. PROSPER has shown reductions through Grade 12 in marijuana, methamphetamine, and inhalant use, and lifetime prescription opioid misuse and prescription drug misuse. Analysis showed greater intervention benefits for youth at higher versus lower risk for most substances.[183,184]

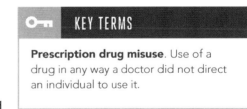

KEY TERMS

Prescription drug misuse. Use of a drug in any way a doctor did not direct an individual to use it.

PREVENTION

Communities That Care - 24 Community Randomized Trials in Colorado, Illinois, Kansas, Maine, Oregon, Utah, and Washington

Agency or Organization:

University of Washington Center for Communities That Care

Purpose:

This evidence-based system provides communities with strategic consultation, training and research-based tools for prevention planning. The CTC system engages entire communities (e.g. youth, parents, elected officials, law enforcement, schools, businesses, etc.) and is tailored to the risks and needs of each defined community population.

> *I think one of the biggest advantages of Communities That Care is that it has really brought together the entire community. When I preach and prepare, and if I'm speaking specifically to something that bears upon the teen culture and teen population, the fact is [with CTC assessment data from the community], I'm able to speak with greater clarity with greater directness and with greater understanding of what they are facing.*
>
> — Adam Kohlstrom, Pastor, Camden, ME

Goals:

1. Promote positive development and healthy behaviors for all children and youth.
2. Prevent problem behaviors, including substance use, delinquency, teen pregnancy, school drop-out, and violence.

Outcomes:

- Following a panel of over 4,000 young people in 24 CTC communities from Grades 5 to 8, researchers found that compared to control communities not using the CTC model, youth in the CTC communities were:
    - 33 percent less likely to begin smoking;
    - 32 percent less likely to begin using alcohol;
    - 33 percent less likely to begin using smokeless tobacco; and
    - 25 percent less likely to initiate delinquent behavior (itself a risk factor for future substance use).

Communities Mobilizing for Change on Alcohol

Community coalition-driven environmental models attempt to reduce substance use by changing the macro-level physical, social, and economic risk and protective factors that influence these behaviors. Most research on environmental interventions has focused on alcohol misuse and related problems, including DUI, injuries, and alcohol use by minors.[185-187] For example, *Communities Mobilizing for Change on Alcohol* (CMCA) implemented coalition-led policy changes aimed at reducing youth access to alcohol, including training for alcohol retailers to reduce sales to minors, increased enforcement of underage drinking laws, measures to reduce availability of alcohol at community events, and media campaigns emphasizing that underage drinking is not acceptable.[188,189] In a randomized trial comparing seven communities in Minnesota and Wisconsin using CMCA with eight communities in states not implementing CMCA, significant reductions in alcohol-related problem behaviors were shown among young adults aged 18 to 20 from the beginning of the initiative to 2.5

years after coalition activities began. The proportion of young adults aged 19 to 20 who reported providing alcohol to other minors declined by 17 percent,[188] and arrests for DUI decreased more for this age group in the intervention compared to the control sites.[189]

Evidence-based Prevention Policies

This section primarily discusses the evidence of effectiveness for policies to reduce alcohol misuse, as well as the more limited body of scientific literature on the effectiveness of policies to prevent the misuse of prescription medications, including pain relievers, tranquilizers, stimulants, and sedatives.

Policies to Reduce Alcohol Misuse and Related Problems

Research has shown that policies focused on reducing alcohol misuse for the general population can effectively reduce alcohol consumption among adults as well as youth, and they can reduce alcohol-related problems including alcohol-impaired driving.[190,191] In addition to discussing a number of effective population-level alcohol policies, this section will also describe policies designed specifically to reduce drinking and driving and underage drinking.

Price and Tax Policies

Evidence indicates that higher prices on alcoholic beverages are associated with reductions in alcohol consumption and alcohol-related problems, including alcohol-impaired driving. Several systematic reviews have linked higher alcohol taxes and prices with reduction in alcohol misuse, including both underage and binge drinking.[28,31,72,192-197] One 2009 review examined 1,003 separate estimates from 112 studies.[72] The authors concluded, "We know of no other prevention intervention to reduce drinking that has the numbers of studies and consistency of effects seen in the literature on alcohol taxes and prices." Similarly, a 2010 review of 73 taxation studies found "consistent evidence that higher alcohol prices and alcohol taxes are associated with reductions in both alcohol misuse and related, subsequent harms."[31] For example, a study found that the price elasticity of binge drinking among individuals aged 18 to 21 was -0.95 for men and -3.54 for women, meaning that a 10.0 percent increase in the price of alcohol is expected to decrease binge drinking by 9.5 percent among men and 35.4 percent among women in that age group.[198]

The effectiveness of increasing alcohol taxes as a strategy for reducing alcohol misuse and related problems has also been acknowledged outside the United States.[28] For example, a 2009 World Health Organization (WHO) review stated that "when other factors are held constant, such as income and the price of other goods, a rise in alcohol prices leads to less alcohol consumption" and "[p]olicies that increase alcohol prices delay the time when young people start to drink, slow their progression towards drinking larger amounts, and reduce their heavy drinking and the volume of alcohol drunk on each occasion."[192] Additionally, studies have found that increasing alcohol taxes is not only cost effective but can result in a net cost savings (i.e., the savings outweigh the costs of the intervention).

PREVENTION

Policies that Affect Access to and Availability of Alcohol

Policies Affecting Alcohol Outlet Density

Research suggests that an increase in the number of retail alcohol outlets in an area—called higher alcohol outlet density—is associated with an increase in alcohol-related problems in that area, such as violence, crime, and injuries.[177,199,200] Four longitudinal studies of communities that reduced the number of alcohol outlets showed consistent and significant reductions in alcohol-related crimes, relative to comparison communities that had not reduced alcohol outlet density.[199,201-203] Although no studies have explicitly analyzed the cost-benefit ratio of this intervention, research suggests that the costs of limiting the number of alcohol outlets is expected to be much smaller than the societal costs of alcohol misuse.[177]

Commercial Host (Dram Shop) Liability Policies

Commercial host (dram shop) liability allows alcohol retailers—such as the owner or server(s) at a bar, restaurant, or other retail alcohol outlet—to be held legally liable for harms resulting from illegal beverage service to intoxicated or underage customers.[204] In a systematic review, 11 studies assessed the association between dram shop laws and alcohol-related health outcomes.[205] The review found a median reduction of 6.4 percent (range was 3.7 percent to 11.3 percent) in alcohol-related motor vehicle fatalities associated with these policies. Two studies on the effects of these laws did not find reductions in binge drinking.

Policies to Reduce Days and Hours of Alcohol Sales

A review of 11 studies of changing days of sale (both at on-premise alcohol outlets such as restaurants and bars, and off-premise outlets such as grocery, liquor, and convenience stores) indicated that increasing the number of days alcohol could be sold was associated with increases in alcohol misuse and alcohol-related harms, while reducing days alcohol is sold was associated with decreases in alcohol-related harms.[206] Similarly, a review of 10 studies (none conducted in the United States) found that increasing hours of sale by two or more hours increased alcohol-related harms, while policies decreasing hours of sale by at least two hours reduced alcohol-related harms.[207] One study found that lifting a ban on Sunday sales of alcohol led to an estimated 41.6 percent increase in alcohol-related fatalities on Sundays during the period from 1995 to 2000, equating to an additional cost of more than $6 million in medical care and lost productivity per year in one state.[208] Banning sales of alcohol on Sundays has been recognized as a cost-effective strategy.

State Policies to Privatize Alcohol Sales

The privatization of alcohol sales involves changing from direct governmental control over the retail sales of one or more types of alcohol, and allowing private, commercial entities to obtain alcohol licenses, typically to sell liquor in convenience, grocery, or other off-premise locations. A systematic review of studies evaluating the impact of privatizing retail alcohol sales found that such policies increased per capita alcohol sales in privatized states by a median of 44.4 percent. Studies show that per capita alcohol sales is known to be a proxy for alcohol misuse.[209,210]

Policies to Reduce Drinking and Driving

Since the early 1980s, alcohol-related traffic deaths in the United States have been cut by more than half (**Figure 3.2**). It has been estimated that reductions in driving after drinking prevented more than 300,000 deaths during this time period.[211] In fact, declines in traffic deaths due to reductions in drinking and driving have exceeded declines from the combined effects of increased use of seat belts, airbags, and motorcycle and bicycle helmets.[212] From 1982 to 2013, alcohol-related traffic deaths decreased by 67 percent, whereas non-alcohol-related traffic deaths decreased by only 14 percent.[213]

Several policies and law enforcement approaches have been found to reduce rates of drinking and driving and related traffic crashes, injuries, and deaths within the general population, among both youth and adults. These DUI policies and enforcement approaches create deterrence by increasing the public's awareness of the consequences of drinking and driving, including the possibility of arrest. Some of these strategies include:

- 0.08 percent criminal per se legal blood alcohol content (BAC) limits, meaning that no further evidence of intoxication beyond a BAC of 0.08 percent is needed for a DUI case;[214-221] and
- Sobriety checkpoints.[222-224]

Figure 3.2: Alcohol- Versus Non-alcohol-related Traffic Deaths, Rate per 100,000, All Ages, United States, 1982-2013

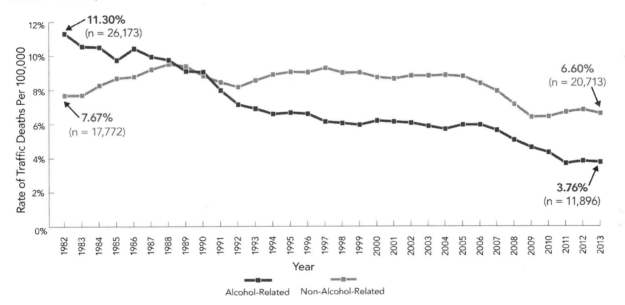

Source: Adapted from Hingson and White, (2014).[213]

PREVENTION

Other proven DUI prevention strategies fall under the rubric of indicated interventions as they target drivers who have been convicted of DUI to reduce recidivism:[223]

- Lower legal blood alcohol limits for people convicted of DUI;[217,223]
- Mandatory ignition interlock laws for all convicted offenders, including first offenders;[223,225,226]
- Mandatory assessment and treatment of persons convicted of DUI;[223]
- DUI courts;[223]
- Continuous 24/7 alcohol monitoring of persons with one or multiple DUI charges;[223] and
- Vehicle impoundment or immobilization.[223]

The Implications of Drinking-Oriented and Driving-Oriented Policies to Reduce Harms

An examination of state-level data on 29 alcohol control policies in all 50 states from 2001-2009[227] divided those policies into two mutually exclusive groups: (1) drinking-oriented policies, intended to regulate alcohol production, sales, and consumption, raise alcohol taxes, and prevent sales to minors; and (2) driving-oriented policies, which are intended to prevent an already intoxicated person from driving. State data on impaired driving from more than 12 million adults during the even years of 2002 through 2010 were evaluated, and four results were reported, two of which are presented here:

- First, the review found that drinking-oriented policies were slightly more effective in reducing impaired driving than driving-oriented policies, though both types of policy changes were independently associated with lower levels of impaired driving.
- Second, drinking-oriented policies appeared to exert their effects by reducing binge drinking, which in turn was associated with a lower likelihood of impaired driving. The authors concluded that most states may have a greater opportunity for adopting and aggressively implementing drinking-oriented policies to reduce overall harms, although there is a need to strengthen driving-oriented policies as well.

Overall, these findings support the importance of implementing a comprehensive range of alcohol policies to effectively reduce alcohol misuse and related harms, including strengthening both drinking-oriented policies and driving-oriented policies.

Policies to Reduce Underage Drinking

Raising the Minimum Legal Drinking Age

Before 1984, only 22 states had a MLDA of 21. To reduce DUIs, Congress passed the National Minimum Drinking Age Act, which threatened to withhold a portion of states' federal highway construction funds if states made the purchase or public possession of alcoholic beverages legal for those under the age of 21. By 1988, all states had adopted age 21 as the MLDA. In the 1982 *Monitoring the Future* annual national survey of middle and high school students, 71.2 percent of high school seniors reported that they drank in the past 30 days and 42 percent reported binge drinking in the past 2 weeks.[228] In 2014, these same statistics were 37.4 percent and 19 percent respectively (**Figure 3.3**).[213] These declines may be partially attributable to the MLDA[214] along with other policy and behavior-change interventions occurring at the same time.

Many studies have shown the benefits of raising the MLDA. A Community Guide review found that raising the MLDA reduced crashes among drivers aged 18 to 20 by a median of 16 percent:[215] A finding replicated in a prospective analysis of the National Highway Traffic Safety Administration's (NHTSA's) Fatality Analysis Reporting System (FARS) examining the ratio of drinking to non-drinking drivers aged 20 and younger. The analysis statistically adjusted for zero tolerance laws, graduated licensing restrictions (e.g., provisional licenses for new drivers that include restrictions on driving at night or with any measurable alcohol in their systems), use/lose laws, administrative license revocation, 0.08% BAC per se laws, per capita beer consumption, unemployment rate, vehicle miles traveled, frequency of sobriety check points, number of licensed drivers, and the ratio of drinking to non-drinking drivers in fatal crashes ages 26 and older.[214] An additional analysis examined national alcohol-related fatal traffic crash data before and after states raised the MLDA to 21. Before those laws were instituted, 61 percent of drivers aged 16 to 20 had a positive BAC compared with 33 percent following institution of those laws.[229] These analyses showed general declines in alcohol-related fatal crashes across age groups, but the declines were highest for drivers aged 16 to 20. Comparing the declines across ages is useful because these older drivers were not the main focus of the MLDA changes.

Figure 3.3: Trends in 2-Week Prevalence of 5 or More Drinks in a Row among 12th Graders, 1980-2015

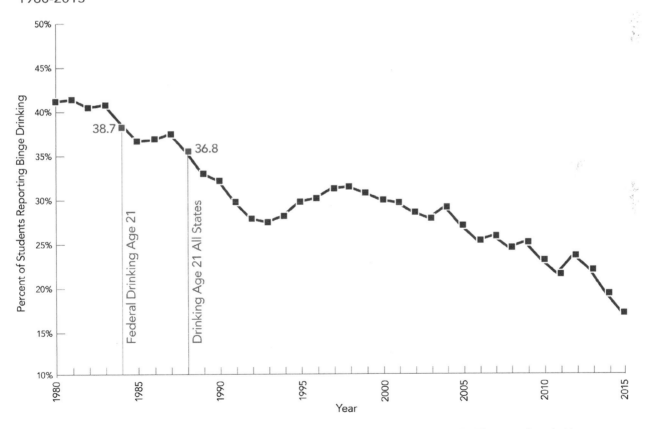

Note: The first vertical bar indicates institution of the MLDA 21 policy change in 7 states in 1984. The second vertical bar indicates federal passage of the MLDA 21 policy in all states in 1988.

Source: Adapted from Hingson and White, (2014).[213]

An extensive review concluded that raising the MLDA to 21 has been directly associated with less frequent drinking, less heavy drinking, and fewer alcohol-related traffic fatalities in the age groups targeted by the law.[178] More specifically, NHTSA estimates that raising the MLDA to 21 may have prevented 30,323 traffic deaths since 1975.[230]

MLDA Compliance Checks

As a complement to the MLDA laws, research has shown the importance of repeated compliance check surveys on alcohol sales to people younger than age 21. These compliance check surveys monitor the percentage of attempts to buy alcohol that result in a sale to a person appearing to be younger than age 21. Alcohol outlet owners are informed in writing whether or not they were observed selling alcohol to underage-appearing individuals, told about the penalties for selling to minors, which can include fines or license suspension, and informed that the surveys will be repeated. A review identified several studies that found these compliance check surveys reduce the percentage of underage alcohol buying attempts and sales of alcohol to youthful-looking decoys by more than 40 percent.[187] This strategy is an effective way to reduce alcohol consumption by minors and can be implemented in conjunction with population level alcohol policies.

Zero Tolerance Laws

All 50 states have passed laws making it illegal for persons younger than age 21 to drive with any measurable BAC. These laws, called zero tolerance laws, were instituted because of the higher fatal crash risk among drivers younger than age 21[215,231] and because of studies showing that lowering the drinking age below age 21 was related to increases in fatal crashes.[232] Another study examined the first eight states to implement zero tolerance laws, comparing each with a nearby state that did not enact such a law.[233] Examining an equal number of years before and after these laws changed, researchers found 20 percent fewer alcohol-related traffic crash deaths in the targeted age groups within the zero tolerance states compared to nearby states without these laws. Similarly, a more recent examination of *Monitoring the Future* survey data for high school seniors in 30 states before and after adoption of zero tolerance laws found that after the laws were enacted, a 19 percent decline in driving after drinking occurred as well as a 23 percent decline in driving after five or more drinks.[234]

Use/Lose Laws

Use/lose laws allow states to suspend a person's driver's license for underage alcohol violations. An examination of the *Youth Risk Behavior Surveillance System* survey data by state (statistically adjusted to account for state differences in age, gender, race, ethnicity, and other factors) from 1999 to 2009 found past-month drinking declined after use/lose laws were instituted.[235] The study also found that after these laws were instituted, survey respondents were half as likely to report driving after drinking compared with before the laws were instituted.

Criminal Social Host Liability Laws

Criminal state social host liability laws require law enforcement to prove intent to provide alcohol to underage guests. Specifically, "social host" refers to adults who knowingly or unknowingly host underage drinking parties on property that they own, lease, or otherwise control. With social host ordinances, law enforcement can hold adults accountable for underage drinking through fines and potentially criminal charges. More than 30 states have some form of social host liability laws. To see the effect of these laws, researchers examined rates of alcohol consumption, binge drinking, and DUI between 1984 and 2004 from the annual *Behavioral Risk Factor Surveillance System*. They also looked at data from the FARS from 1975 to 2005 on alcohol-related versus non-alcohol-related fatal traffic deaths among those aged 18 to 20. After controlling for the state's legal drinking age, several drinking laws, and socioeconomic factors, social host liability laws were independently associated with declines in binge drinking (3 percent), driving after drinking (1.7 percent), and alcohol-related traffic deaths (9 percent).[236]

Civil Social Host Liability Laws

In contrast to state-level criminal social host ordinances, city- or county-level civil liability ordinances allow for a lower burden of proof but still deter underage drinking parties. Through civil social host liability laws, adults can be held responsible for underage drinking parties held on their property, regardless of whether they directly provided alcohol to minors. To date, more than 150 cities or counties have social host liability ordinances in place. The research on this strategy is still emerging, but findings currently show that social host liability reduces alcohol-related motor vehicle crashes as well as other alcohol-related problems.[28,237]

Proposals for Reductions in Alcohol Advertising

Although evidence of a causal relationship is lacking, research has found an association between increased exposure to marketing and increased alcohol consumption among youth.[77] For example, one study found that for every additional advertisement seen by youth per month, they drank one percent more, while for every additional dollar per capita spent on alcohol advertising in a youth's media market, they drank three percent more.[238] Typically, these studies have not controlled for other factors known to influence underage drinking, such as parental attitudes and drinking by peers. Further, studies have yet to determine whether reducing alcohol marketing leads to reductions in youth drinking. One study estimated that a 28 percent decrease in alcohol marketing in the United States could lead to a decrease in the monthly prevalence of adolescent drinking from 25 percent to between 21 and 24 percent.[239] A separate study of alcohol advertising bans concluded that "there is a lack of robust evidence for or against recommending the implementation of alcohol advertising restrictions."[240]

Many Policy Interventions Are Not Consistently Implemented

Despite the evidence discussed in this section, many policies are not consistently implemented in states or communities. For example, commercial host (dram shop) liability laws, which permit alcohol retail establishments to be held responsible for injuries or harms caused by service to intoxicated or underage patrons have not been implemented consistently, have been changed over time, or both. Consequently, as of January 1, 2015, only 20 states had dram shop liability laws with no major limitations; 25 states had these laws but with major limitations (e.g., restrictions on who this liability applied to and the evidence required to determine liability); and six states have no dram shop liability laws at all.[241] These numbers have not changed since 2013 ([Table 3.4](#)).[242]

Policies related to the regulation of alcohol outlet density have changed over time. For example, as of 2013, only 18 states had exclusive local or joint state/local alcohol retail licensing authority, and eight states allowed no local control over alcohol retail licensing.

Additionally, one study analyzed FARS from 1982-2012. The authors compared the ratio of drinking drivers in fatal crashes to non-drinking drivers in fatal crashes among drivers aged 20 and younger and those 26 and older. Using advanced statistical analyses that adjusted for state DUI laws, safety belt laws, economic strength, driving exposure, and beer consumption, the authors identified nine laws designed to reduce underage drinking and driving whose implementation was prospectively, independently, and significantly associated with decreases in the ratio of drinking to non-drinking drivers under age 21 in fatal crashes, including laws prohibiting underage possession and purchase of alcohol; use alcohol lose your license (use/lose) laws; zero tolerance laws; laws requiring bartenders to be aged 21 or older; state responsible beverage/server programs; fake identification state support services for retailers; dram shop liability; and social host civil liability. Those nine laws were estimated to save approximately 1,135 lives annually, yet only five states have enacted all nine laws. The authors estimated that if all states adopted these laws an additional 210 lives could be saved every year.[243]

Table 3.4: Status of Selected Evidence-Based Strategies in States for Preventing Alcohol Misuse and Related Harms

Alcohol Policy (Ratings categories)	Number of states by rating and year of CDC Prevention Status Report					
	Green		Yellow		Red	
	2013	2015	2013	2015	2013	2015
State excise taxes on beer* (Green: ≥$1.00 per gallon; Yellow: $0.50-$0.99 per gallon; Red: <$0.50 per gallon)	3	4	4	4	43	42
State excise taxes on distilled spirits* (Green: ≥$8.00 per gallon; Yellow: $4.00-$7.99 per gallon; Red: <$4.00 per gallon)	3	3	10	11	21	20
State excise taxes on wine* (Green: ≥$2.00 per gallon; Yellow: $1.00-1.99 per gallon; Red: <$1.00 per gallon)	2	2	7	8	30	29
Commercial host (dram shop) liability laws (Green: Commercial host liability with no major limitations; Yellow: Commercial host liability with major limitations; Red: No commercial host liability)	21	20	24	25	6	6
Local authority to regulate alcohol outlet density (Green: Exclusive local or joint state/local alcohol retail licensing; Yellow: Exclusive state alcohol retail licensing but with local zoning authority or other mixed policies; Red: Exclusive state alcohol retail licensing)	18	N/A	24	N/A	8	N/A

Note: *The ratings reflect where each state's tax fell within this range. N/A: Not Applicable.
Sources: Centers for Disease Control and Prevention, (2014)[242] and (2016).[241]

These data suggest that effective alcohol control policies are not being widely implemented in the United States despite the well-documented, scientific evidence on the effectiveness of such policies for reducing alcohol misuse and related harms. To have maximum public health impact, it is critical to implement effective policy interventions that address alcohol misuse and related harms, and that recognize the widespread nature of the problem and the strong relationship between alcohol misuse, particularly binge drinking, and related harms among adults and youth in states.[190,191,244]

Policies to Reduce Other Substance Misuse and Related Problems

Preventing Prescription Drug Misuse

Policies to prevent prescription drug misuse and related harms have only begun to receive research attention. However, some studies have begun to examine the impact of prescription drug monitoring programs (PDMPs) on misuse of prescription medications.[245] These state-initiated policies are designed to curb the rate of inappropriate prescribing of opioid pain relievers through various methods. Data from the U.S. Drug Enforcement Administration's (DEA's) *Automation of Reports and Consolidated Orders System* (ARCOS)[246] showed little impact of these monitoring systems, perhaps because of the variability of the policies controlling different state systems. The ARCOS is an automated, comprehensive drug reporting system which monitors the movement of controlled substances from where they are manufactured through distribution at the retail level, such as hospitals, pharmacies, and practitioners.

Some studies associate state PDMPs with lower rates of prescription drug misuse and altered prescribing practices, although evidence is mixed and inconclusive.[247] One reason for inconsistent findings may be low and variable prescriber utilization of PDMPs. Because mandates are relatively new, their efficacy in increasing PDMP utilization has not been formally studied. However, preliminary data suggest that in some states mandates have contributed to a rapid increase in provider enrollment and utilization of PDMPs and subsequent decreases in prescribing of controlled substances and the number of patients who visit multiple providers seeking the same or similar drugs.[248] Data from Kentucky, Tennessee, New York and Ohio—early adopters of comprehensive PDMP use mandates—indicate substantial increases in queries, reductions in opioid prescribing, and declines in multiple provider episodes (doctor shopping) following implementation.[249] In one of the most rigorous studies to date, Florida's simultaneous institution of a prescription drug monitoring system and "pill mill" control policies was compared to Georgia, a state without either policy. This study demonstrated "modest reductions in total opioid volume, mean morphine milligram equivalent per transaction, and total number of opioid prescriptions dispensed, but no effect on duration of treatment. These reductions were generally limited to patients and prescribers with the highest baseline opioid use and prescribing."[250]

A 2016 study found that the implementation of a PDMP was associated with 1.12 fewer opioid-related overdose deaths per 100,000 people in the year immediately after the program was implemented, and if every state in the United States had a robust PDMP, there would be an estimated 600 fewer overdose deaths per year.[251] However, another study analyzed eight types of laws that restricted the prescribing and dispensing of opioids (including PDMP laws but not including prescriber mandate laws) and found no relationship between the laws and opioid-related outcomes among disabled Medicare beneficiaries, who accounted for nearly 25 percent of opioid overdose deaths in 2008.[252]

Collectively, these early results suggest the potential influence of PDMPs to reduce unsafe controlled substance prescribing and rates of misuse and diversion, but there is a need to conduct additional research on the effectiveness of specific strategies for implementation and use of PDMPs. Multiple efforts to address prescription drug misuse within states occurring in concert with mandatory PDMP legislation may limit the ability to draw causal conclusions about the effectiveness of mandatory use of PDMPs.

The CDC has developed the *CDC Guideline for Prescribing Opioids for Chronic Pain*, which provides research-based recommendations for the prescribing of opioids for pain in patients aged 18 and older in primary care settings. The guideline includes a discussion of when to start opioids for chronic pain, how to select the right opioid and dosage, and how to assess risks and address harms from opioid use.[253] This guideline can help providers reduce opioid misuse and related harms among those with chronic pain.

Adolescent Use of Marijuana

Marijuana use, in adolescents in particular, can cause negative neurological effects. Long-term, regular use starting in the young adult years may impair brain development and functioning. The main chemical in marijuana is delta-9-tetrahydrocannabinol (THC), which, when smoked, quickly passes from the lungs into the bloodstream, which then carries it to organs throughout the body, including the brain.[254] THC disrupts the brain's normal functioning and can lead to problems studying, learning new things, and recalling recent events.[255] One study followed people from age 13 to 38 and found that those who began marijuana use in their teens and developed a persistent cannabis use disorder had up to an eight point drop in IQ, even if they stopped using in adulthood.[256] Frequent marijuana use has also been linked to increased risk of psychosis in individuals with specific pre-existing genetic vulnerabilities.[257,258] And marijuana use—particularly long-term, chronic use or use starting at a young age—can also lead to dependence and addiction.

These effects highlight the importance of prevention. To prevent marijuana use before it starts, or to intervene when use has already begun, parents and other caregivers as well as those with relationships with young people—such as teachers, coaches, and others—should be informed about marijuana's effects in order to provide relevant and accurate information on the dangers and misconceptions of marijuana use. Comprehensive prevention programs focusing on risk and protective factors have shown success preventing marijuana use.[259,260] Evidence-based strategies or best practices in community level prevention efforts can be used to assess, build capacity, plan, implement, and evaluate initiatives.[261]

Prevention Interventions for Specific Populations

An important consideration in any assessment of the overall effectiveness of EBIs is whether and to what extent they work with specific populations, such as Blacks or African Americans, Hispanics or Latino/as, Asians, American Indians or Alaska Natives, Native Hawaiians or Other Pacific Islanders, veterans, or lesbian, gay, bisexual, and transgender (LGBT) populations. The EBIs described in this chapter have been purposely selected because many have been implemented, tested, and found to be effective in diverse populations. It should be noted that while prevention policies have shown impacts for the entire population, and a number of prevention programs at each developmental period have shown positive outcomes with a mix of populations, most studies have not specifically examined their differential effects on racial and ethnic subpopulations. Studies finding significant prevention effects across multiple population subgroups include *LifeSkills Training, keepin' it Real, Nurse Family Partnership, Raising Healthy Children, Good Behavior Game, Classroom-Centered Intervention, Fast Track, SODAs City, I Hear What You're Saying, Project Chill, Positive Family Support, Coping Power, Project Towards No Drug Abuse, Communities That Care, Project Northland,* and *Project STAR.*

> **FOR MORE ON THIS TOPIC**
>
> See Appendix A - *Review Process for Prevention Programs* and Appendix B - *Evidence-Based Prevention Programs and Policies.*

The following programs were found to be equally effective in White and specific racial and ethnic minority populations: *Fast Track*, which is equally effective for White and Black or African American adolescents, *LifeSkills Training*, which is equally effective with White and Black or African American and Hispanic or Latino adolescents, and *keepin' it REAL*, which is equally effective with White and Hispanic or Latino adolescents. In addition, some interventions developed for specific populations have been shown to be effective in those populations, i.e., *Strong African American Families, Familas Unidas* for Hispanics or Latinos, *Bicultural Competence* for American Indian or Alaska Natives, and *PROSPER* for rural communities.

Adaptation of EBIs in Diverse Communities

A goal of prevention and public health professionals is to broadly disseminate all tested-and-effective EBIs, thus making them readily available to communities and consumers.[262] Achieving population-level exposure of an EBI to all population groups—or "going to scale"—raises critical issues of "fit" of the EBI's contents and the needs and preferences of local community residents.[263] Often, some form of local adaptation is necessary when a certain feature of the selected EBI fails to engage a specific group within a local community. However, not all EBIs may work with all community subgroups.[264,265] The sometimes delicate balance that needs to be struck between fidelity to the program as originally designed and tested and the need for adapting it to the needs of specific subgroups is an important issue and requires sophisticated methodology to address. Currently, several cultural adaptations of an original EBI have been developed and tested.[266]

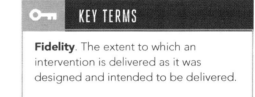

> **KEY TERMS**
>
> **Fidelity**. The extent to which an intervention is delivered as it was designed and intended to be delivered.

Issues regarding the cultural adaptation of EBIs have been reviewed extensively within the past two decades.[266-268] Early studies examined the utility of developing a culturally-focused version of the EBI *LifeSkills Training* to fit the needs of racially and ethnically diverse adolescents living in the New York City area.[269] In general, the challenge involves the viability of implementing an EBI with total fidelity to its protocol, versus adapting it by making adjustments so the EBI is more relevant and responsive to the needs of local community residents.[270] Producing an adapted version of an established EBI may not generalize well enough to create the same effects when implemented with a culturally different group from that used to validate the original intervention. Such limited generalizability might occur if the intervention is insufficiently sensitive, culturally or otherwise, to the unique stressors, resources, cultural traditions, family practices, and other prevailing sociocultural factors that govern the lives of residents from that community.[265]

It is worth noting that the major racial and ethnic populations in the United States—Hispanics or Latinos, Blacks or African Americans, Asians, and American Indians or Alaska Natives—also exhibit significant within-population variations in important sociocultural characteristics.[271] Beyond differential EBI efficacy that may appear by racial or ethnic status—Black or African American versus White, for example—differential efficacy may also be observed by one of several demographic or clinical variables that define any one racial or ethnic group. These variables include gender (male vs. female), age group (younger vs. older), grade level (Grade 8 vs. Grade 10), sexual and gender identity, neighborhood status (problem vs. non-problem), problem severity (moderate vs. high), level of education (middle school vs. high school or greater), level of acculturation (low acculturation, bicultural, high acculturation). It can also include sociocultural needs and preferences that can be incorporated into the culturally adapted prevention intervention.

Given the multiple sources of within-group variation, one dissenting view is that it is impractical to develop many different versions of an original EBI in efforts to respond to the needs of various groups. A contrasting view is that a few selective and directed adaptations may be sufficient to respond to the sociocultural needs of many of these groups "to ensure fit with diverse consumer populations."[265] Clusters of these groups may share common life experiences, such as their identity and identification as a person of color, experiences with discrimination and disempowerment, or the need for cultural validation.[264]

All of these issues create a "Fidelity-Adaptation Dilemma:" How to make necessary local or cultural adaptations that are responsive to the needs of a growing diversity of cultural groups in the United States, while also not compromising the fundamental science-based components or "active ingredients" that drive the effectiveness of the original EBI. As originally formulated, the Fidelity-Adaptation Dilemma framed fidelity and adaptation as diametrically opposed approaches in the implementation of an EBI.[267,268] After more than a decade of analysis and research, this conceptualization appears no longer productive, given that both fidelity and adaptation are now recognized as important for the effective implementation of an EBI, especially when delivered within diverse racial and ethnic communities. The dual aim for resolving the Fidelity-Adaptation Dilemma is to adhere with fidelity to the intervention's theory, principles, goals, and mechanisms of effect for attaining the EBI's intended outcomes, while also making well-reasoned "cultural adaptations" that remedy emerging problems with the EBI's contents and/or activities.[272,273] A partnership between intervention developers, persons delivering the intervention, and potential program participants who can represent the group's concerns, is recommended for developing well-reasoned solutions to remedy specific features of the original EBI that are not working as intended.[121,274] The ultimate aim is to craft needed adaptive adjustments that aptly remedy these emerging problems and that also enhance the efficacy of the intervention in attaining the intended outcomes with local community residents.

Several adaptations use a social participatory approach[274-276] with a community advisory committee that is composed of local leaders who know the local community well.[274] These individuals offer "insider" observations and recommendations that inform substantive deep-structure modifications that can make the original EBI more culturally responsive.[267,277]

Although sufficient evidence has not yet accrued to inform a single best approach for addressing this Fidelity-Adaptation Dilemma, a review of the EBI adaptation literature shows a convergence of specifically prescribed steps for adapting an original EBI.[266] Several models describe these steps in the cultural adaptation and testing of an original EBI.[266] Other approaches have introduced the concept of "adaptive interventions" that aim to tailor the intervention individually based on empirically-developed decision rules.[278,279]

A future goal for effective cultural adaptation would be to identify robust principles and guidelines that can inform and guide the development of cultural adaptations. One emerging principle involves avoiding adaptations that produce detrimental changes, termed "misadaptations," that erode the original EBI's established efficacy for changing intended outcomes.[263] A second emerging principle is to conduct adaptations that enhance consumer engagement based on curriculum activities that are culturally responsive to the needs and preferences of the local community of consumers. Additional research is needed to establish the robustness of these or other emerging principles and to generate clear and functional guidelines that can inform intervention design and implementation to promote both fidelity and adaptive fit. The aim of this adaptation is to maximize intervention effect when delivered to diverse groups of consumers.

EBI adaptation that is based on evidence-based outcomes data constitutes an empirically-based methodology to correct, refine, and enhance an original EBI. From this perspective, these adaptations or modifications transcend fidelity-adaptation issues, advance toward EBI refinement that is conducted systematically, increase efficacy as well as generalizability, and reach and benefit a greater number of those who are most in need of EBIs.

Maximizing Prevention Program and Policy Effectiveness

Although a variety of prevention policies and programs have been shown to reduce substance misuse and consequences of use, many are underutilized. Additionally, many programs are not currently being implemented with sufficient quality to effectively improve public health. For example, although it is difficult to collect data on this issue, research suggests that few family-serving agencies are using EBIs to address child behavioral and emotional problems,[280,281] and surveys of school administrators indicate that only 8 to 10 percent report using EBIs to prevent substance misuse.[282,283] Additionally, research has shown that untested or ineffective prevention programs are used more often than EBIs,[282,283] and, when they are used, EBIs are often poorly implemented, do not serve large numbers of participants, and are not sustained.[284,285] For example, family-based EBIs are often delivered with less intensity and/or to different types of participants than specified by program developers.[286] School officials have reported low rates of implementation fidelity, including failure to deliver all required lessons, content, and activities; to use the required materials; to employ the recommended instructional strategies; to target the appropriate students with lessons; and/or to ensure that all teachers receive training.[24,283,284,287,288] EBIs that are poorly implemented tend to have weak or no effects on participants.[272,289-296] For example, in one study, the *LifeSkills Training* program delivered in middle and junior high schools has shown significant, long-term effects on Grade 12 students' alcohol and marijuana use only among students whose teachers delivered at least 60 percent of the required material.[292]

Research demonstrates that building prevention infrastructure; activating federal, state, local, and tribal stakeholders; ensuring collaboration; and helping communities select, implement, and sustain EBIs[297] is possible and can be done effectively. For example, one large-scale study provided schools and various human service agencies with training and technical assistance to replicate nine EBIs rated as "Model" by the *Blueprints for Healthy Youth Development*.[268] That study indicated that when provided with ongoing support, 74 percent of sites successfully implemented these systems.[298] Evaluations of PROSPER and CTC, which provide community coalitions with prevention infrastructure to choose EBIs that addressed their needs and to implement the chosen EBIs with fidelity, have shown that communities using these delivery systems implement EBIs with high fidelity and sustain them over time.[299-304] In addition, evaluations showed that CTC communities reached more participants with more EBIs compared with communities that did not use this prevention infrastructure support system.[302,303] These and other studies indicate that prevention infrastructure can be generated by taking the actions discussed in the section on **Improving the Dissemination and Implementation of Evidence-based Programs** later in this chapter.

Additionally, strengthening state and local public health capacity will help to increase the surveillance and monitoring of risk and protective factors and substance misuse by adolescents and adults in the general population, including persons who drink to excess but are not dependent on alcohol. It is important to educate and raise awareness about the public health burden of substance misuse and effective program and policy interventions for preventing and reducing substance use across the population.

The History of Substance Use and Misuse Policy Formation and Implementation

The dissemination and implementation of evidence-based prevention programs have been studied extensively; less research has been conducted on evidence-based policy formation and implementation. This section describes three organizations or activities focusing on federal, state, and local policy to reduce substance misuse: Mothers Against Drunk Driving (MADD), CADCA, and the Congressional Sober Truth on Preventing Underage Drinking (STOP) Act.

In the early 1980s, President Ronald Reagan established a bipartisan presidential commission to reduce drunk driving. The commission's first recommended action was to raise the MLDA to 21. In 1984 and with strong support from the newly founded MADD, Congress passed legislation to withhold federal highway construction funds from states that did not raise the MLDA to 21. MADD was also instrumental in supporting the passage of legislation in 1996 to withhold federal highway construction funds from states that did not have zero tolerance laws. They were a key player in 2000 legislation to withhold construction funds from states that did not lower the legal blood alcohol limit to 0.08 percent for adult drivers. Since the early 1980s, more than 2,000 other state laws have been passed to reduce driving after drinking, and MADD has been a major citizen activist force encouraging the passage of many of those laws.

MADD also has prepared and published periodic state and national "report cards" rating each state and the nation's efforts to reduce alcohol-impaired driving.[319] States have been rated on how many of the more than 30 laws scientifically demonstrated to reduce impaired driving had been passed and how many were passed since the previous report card. In one study, these state report cards were found to clearly predict the percent of respondents in each state who reported driving after drinking in the past month.[320] Although the impact of the report cards in accelerating passage of the laws has never been empirically tested, media monitoring of news stories derived from the report cards indicated that at least one third of the United States population has been exposed to media coverage about the report cards.

One study compared characteristics of MADD chapters that had early success in raising the MLDA to 21 to chapters in states that did not raise the age. The analysis found that having chapters headed by people who lost immediate family members through drinking and driving crashes and those with higher percentages of such victim members were the most successful in early passage of MLDA laws. Of note, the size of chapters' financial budget did not predict the passage of these laws.[321]

Although MADD has helped to foster passage of more than 2,000 state-level laws, implementation of those laws is accomplished at the community level. This often requires the existence of trained coalitions focusing on substance use. One such collaboration, CADCA, has played a critical role in training local coalitions in implementing laws, particularly the MLDA law in all 50 states. CADCA's membership includes more than 5,000 community coalitions nationwide that seek to reduce underage drinking and drug use. CADCA has partnered with MADD and federal organizations to develop a manual on how to reduce drinking and driving and underage drinking in communities.[322] CADCA holds its annual leadership meeting in Washington, D.C. so that its members can also meet with congressional representatives to explore better ways to reduce alcohol and drug misuse and underage drinking.

In 2004, the IOM released *Reducing Underage Drinking: A Collective Responsibility*, a report on underage drinking in the United States.[323] Partly in response to this report, Congress passed the STOP Act, which:

- Provided supplemental funding to community programs that were already addressing substance use so that they could also address underage drinking;

- Called on all states to test the BAC in anyone younger than age 21 who died from an injury or overdose;

- Encouraged every state to develop an interagency task force of officials from multiple state governmental departments and private citizens and organizations to develop strategic plans to reduce underage drinking (38 states have established task forces and strategic plans);

- Required the federal government to establish the Interagency Coordinating Committee for the Prevention of Underage Drinking (ICCPUD), comprising the following departments and agencies: Departments of Education, Health and Human Services, Transportation, and Defense; and the Federal Trade Commission. The Committee meets monthly to coordinate federal efforts to reduce underage drinking; and

- Required the federal government through ICCPUD and SAMHSA to provide annual reports to Congress on the magnitude of underage drinking and related problems and what the federal and state governments are doing to prevent and reduce underage drinking.

Improving the Dissemination and Implementation of Evidence-based Programs

The emerging field of dissemination and implementation research seeks to identify ways to increase the use and high-quality implementation of evidence-based programs and address challenges to implementation. This research indicates that the key to achieving significant gains in public health, including reductions in substance use initiation and substance misuse, is to build prevention infrastructure at the local level.[305-307] This means increasing awareness of EBIs among community leaders, service providers, and local citizens. It also means providing tools to help communities select and use EBIs that will be feasible to implement and relevant for their populations.[308-310] When agencies and staff are unaware of, do not support, or lack the ability to select and implement appropriate EBIs with quality, then dissemination, implementation, and sustainability will be hindered.[285,311-313] In contrast, when local systems and agencies learn more about the effectiveness of prevention interventions, have a culture and climate that supports innovation and the use of EBIs, and have the budget and skills needed to plan for and monitor the implementation of EBIs, then effective dissemination and implementation will be fostered.[294,311,312,314-318]

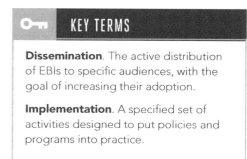

KEY TERMS

Dissemination. The active distribution of EBIs to specific audiences, with the goal of increasing their adoption.

Implementation. A specified set of activities designed to put policies and programs into practice.

Coalition-based systems have been developed to assist communities in building these capacities, and when tested in randomized trials, these systems have been shown to improve community capacity for effective prevention; increase dissemination, implementation, and sustainability of EBIs; and produce community-wide reductions in youth substance use.[324] An important feature of these systems is the provision of community coalitions with multiple training workshops and ongoing technical assistance. Just as organizations require technical assistance to ensure high-quality implementation of specific EBIs, coalitions need technical assistance to support and develop their prevention capacities.[325-328] Each community model has different steps that outline their process; the following four steps are one example of how to build broader implementation of evidence-based prevention.

Step 1. Form Diverse, Representative, Cross-Sector Community Coalitions

Coalitions, or groups of stakeholders working together to achieve a common goal, are a useful mechanism for building and maintaining local prevention infrastructure and capacity.[25,34,324,325,329-331] The first step in building a coalition is to decide on the "community" to be involved in prevention activities, including the geographic area in which services will be delivered, and to identify the organizations, agencies, groups, and individuals whose participation is necessary for success. The more the coalitions represent the community in terms of demographic diversity, organizations expected to deliver services, and groups or individuals expected to receive services, the more likely they are to ensure that EBIs will be supported.[329,332,333] Similarly, such coalitions will be better equipped to implement multiple EBIs across diverse contexts and to a larger percentage of the population, all of which should make population-level improvements more likely.[329] In addition, by sharing information and resources, community coalitions can help minimize duplication of efforts and potentially offer more cost-effective services that are better implemented and more likely to be sustained.[25,334-337]

Step 2. Conduct a Needs Assessment and a Fit Assessment

Needs and fit assessments help coalitions select the right EBIs for their community. The right EBIs are those that address the highest-priority local risk and protective factors the coalition identifies (e.g., the risk factors that are most elevated and the protective factors that are most depressed in the community) and the groups or individuals most in need of services.[330,338] Coalitions conduct needs assessments by gathering data on risk and protective factors, substance misuse, and related problems. For example, in the CTC system, needs assessments rely primarily on data reported by adolescents on school-based, anonymous surveys. These data are reviewed by coalition members and risk factors that are consistently elevated and protective factors that are consistently depressed are identified as targets that need to be addressed by EBIs.[334] The priorities may vary by neighborhood in larger cities or by specific subpopulations (e.g., gender or racial and ethnic groups).[334]

To select the best-fitting EBIs, coalitions need to be familiar with the list of possible interventions that can address their needs, and must consider whether or not they can meet all the implementation requirements of the EBIs.[294,312,339] Consulting a registry of EBIs, such as the *National Registry of Evidence-based Programs and Practices* (NREPP)[340] and the *Blueprints for Healthy Youth Development*[341] or NIAAA's *Alcohol Policy Information System*[342] for alcohol policies, can assist in creating the list of EBIs that meet community needs. These databases compile information about programs that have met rigorous evaluation criteria in a user-friendly format, which makes it easy for communities to learn about and compare intervention costs and requirements.[343,344] The databases also describe the intervention methods and population(s) with which the interventions were tested to help coalitions determine whether the EBI is culturally relevant and compatible with the norms, values, and needs of the local community.

Step 3. Enhance Implementation Fidelity and Implementers' Capacity

Some research suggests that EBIs can never be perfectly replicated in communities and that changes or adaptations to the EBI's content, activities, materials, or methods of delivery will be necessary given the differences between well-controlled research trials and real-world settings.[263,270,345-347] However, research has shown that when EBIs are implemented with fidelity, programs achieve expected results. While culturally relevant adaptations can be expected to increase the relevance of the material, better engage participants, and improve effectiveness, it is clear that poor or inappropriate adaptation can reduce effectiveness.[268,295] For example, an evaluation showed that the effectiveness of the *Nurse-Family Partnership* program was significantly reduced when paraprofessionals rather than registered nurses delivered services in communities that lack registered nurses.[348] These types of inappropriate adaptations emphasize the need for communities to learn as much as they can about EBIs during the fit assessment and select only those interventions that are considered feasible given resources.

Steps to Build Prevention Infrastructure for Effective Community-based Prevention

Conduct a local needs assessment:

- Collect data on levels of substance use;
- Collect data on risk and protective factors related to substance use; and
- Identify and prioritize elevated risk factors and depressed protective factors.

Conduct a resource assessment:

- Assess current prevention programming, including the risk and protective factors addressed by current services, numbers and types of populations served, effectiveness, and implementation quality; and
- Identify potential new services using EBI and policy registries.

Assess the fit of new EBIs with the local community:

- Determine whether or not each potential EBI addresses the identified substance misuse problems and priority risk and protective factors; and
- Assess the degree to which the new EBI is culturally relevant for the local population.

Assess local readiness and capacity to implement EBIs:

- Identify the organization(s) that will deliver each new EBI;
- Assess levels of support for each new EBI among all key personnel; and
- Identify the financial and human resources and all other requirements necessary to implement each EBI.

Select the intervention(s) that is the best fit for the community: The ones that are most likely to be fully supported meet prioritized needs, are culturally relevant, can be well implemented, and can be sustained over the long-term.

Ensure high quality implementation of each new EBI:

- Create a detailed implementation plan;
- Specify participant eligibility criteria, participation goals, and recruitment procedures;
- Create teams to oversee implementation;
- Hire all necessary staff and administrators;
- Ensure that all staff are trained and regularly supervised; and
- Seek regular technical assistance from intervention developers.

Evaluate the impact of the selected interventions: It is critical to systematically collect and analyze information about program activities, participant characteristics, and outcomes.

- Collect data on all aspects of implementation; and
- Regularly review implementation and outcomes data and improve procedures as needed.

In addition to appropriate cultural adaptations, staff competency is critical to successful delivery of EBIs, and coalition members can support local agencies to ensure that they hire staff who have the credentials and experience recommended by developers, and that they receive training in each EBI's theory, content, and methods of delivery.[142,294,312,339,349] Training is an important ingredient in ensuring greater levels of implementation fidelity, especially because the content, activities, and methods of delivery may be new to practitioners.[24,294,295] In general, relatively few professionals responsible for implementing EBIs (including mental health counselors, teachers, psychologists, and social workers) receive training in substance misuse prevention, including knowledge of risk and protective factors that impact alcohol and drug use, the knowledge of EBIs that target these factors, or the importance of implementation fidelity when delivering interventions.[18,350] These topics should be incorporated into undergraduate, graduate, and in-service professional training programs.[351] In the meantime, staff should be supervised and receive coaching and corrective feedback to ensure they are implementing EBIs with quality.[294,295,349,352]

Technical assistance from EBI developers can assist local agencies in staff supervision, and most EBIs offer support in how to monitor implementation activities, overcome challenges when they arise, and integrate EBIs into agency operations.[294,295,353] Although experimental studies are lacking, observational studies have reported that technical assistance, implementation monitoring, and staff feedback help ensure the high-quality delivery and sustainability of EBIs.[268,285,294,312,314,354,355]

Step 4. Plan for Long-Term Sustainability

A lack of funding is a significant barrier to the long-term sustainability of EBIs,[294,308,311,356-359] and it is critical that, even before implementation, agencies and communities consider how each EBI will be integrated into existing systems and funded over time.[304,360] Considering how a new EBI will address local needs can be useful in gaining support.[361]

Recommendations for Research

Although much has been learned in prevention research over the past four decades, much remains to be understood. Future research should develop and evaluate new prevention interventions, both programs and policies, and continue to assess the effectiveness of existing interventions about which little is known. This research will help guide the field toward strategies with the greatest potential for reducing substance misuse and related problems.

Research also is needed to examine the effectiveness of screening and brief interventions for alcohol use in adolescents and for drug use in adolescents and adults; the combinations of evidence-based alcohol policies that most effectively reduce alcohol misuse and related harms; the public health impact of policies to reduce drug misuse; and the effectiveness of strategies to reduce marijuana misuse, driving after drug use, and simultaneous use of alcohol and drugs. In addition, the public health impact of marijuana decriminalization, legalization of medical marijuana, and legalization of recreational marijuana on marijuana, alcohol, and other drug use, as well as policies to reduce prescription drug misuse, should be monitored closely.

Research is needed to develop and test new prevention interventions, both policies and programs, to fill gaps in existing EBIs and to meet emerging public health needs across the lifecourse.

Given that racial and ethnic minority communities are often disproportionately affected by the adverse consequences of substance misuse, culturally-informed research should be conducted to examine ways to increase the cultural relevance, engagement, and effectiveness of prevention interventions for diverse communities. Additionally, studies of these interventions should be replicated and examined to determine the impact of prevention interventions for different cultural groups and contexts.

Consistent standards for evaluating interventions, conducting replication trials, and reporting the results should be developed. Examples of such standards have been developed by the Society for Prevention Research and the United Nations Office on Drugs and Crime.[26,357,362-368] Studies evaluating the effectiveness of interventions for reducing substance misuse should collect data over extended periods of time to track the long-term effects of these interventions on persons of all ages. The impact of environmental interventions on substance misuse should also be followed for at least a year beyond the end of the period of intervention support. The field needs to develop a consensus on standardization of methods of cost-benefit analysis, and increase research on cost-effectiveness evaluations of prevention EBIs.

Evidence is also needed to develop improved strategies for intervention in primary health care settings to prevent the initiation and escalation of adolescent substance use. More research is also needed on linking screening with personalized interventions, improved strategies for effective referral to specialty treatment, and interventions for adolescents that use social media and capitalize on current technologies. Research should also consider the optimal conditions for bringing effective prevention interventions to scale, develop consensus on standardization of methods for cost-benefit analysis, and increase research on cost-effectiveness evaluations of prevention EBIs.

Surveillance of risky drinking, drug use, and related problems needs to be improved. All drivers in fatal crashes should have their blood alcohol content tested and be tested for drug use. All unintentional and intentional injury deaths, including overdoses, should be tested for both alcohol and drugs. Surveillance surveys need to add questions about simultaneous alcohol and drug use and questions about the maximum quantities consumed in a day and frequency of consumption at those levels. Efforts are needed to increase surveillance of the second-hand effects of alcohol and drug use, such as assaults, sexual assaults, motor vehicle crashes, homicides and suicides, and effects of substance use on academic and work performance. Efforts are needed to expand surveillance beyond national and state levels to the level of local communities.

References

1. Rose, G. (1985). Sick individuals and sick populations. *International Journal of Epidemiology, 14*(1), 32-38.

2. Rudd, R. A., Aleshire, N., Zibbel, J. E., & Gladden, R. M. (2016). Increases in drug and opioid overdose deaths — United States, 2000–2014. *MMWR, 64*(50), 1378-1382.

3. Shamblen, S. R., & Derzon, J. H. (2009). A preliminary study of the population-adjusted effectiveness of substance abuse prevention programming: Towards making IOM program types comparable. *The Journal of Primary Prevention, 30*(2), 89-107.

4. Stahre, M., Roeber, J., Kanny, D., Brewer, R. D., & Zhang, X. (2014). Contribution of excessive alcohol consumption to deaths and years of potential life lost in the United States. *Preventing Chronic Disease, 11*(E109).

5. Puddy, R. W., & Wilkins, N. (2011). *Understanding evidence Part 1: Best available research evidence. A guide to the continuum of evidence of effectiveness.* Atlanta, GA: Centers for Disease Control and Prevention.

6. Sacks, J. J., Gonzales, K. R., Bouchery, E. E., Tomedi, L. E., & Brewer, R. D. (2015). 2010 national and state costs of excessive alcohol consumption. *American Journal of Preventive Medicine, 49*(5), e73-e79.

7. National Drug Intelligence Center. (2011). *National drug threat assessment.* Washington, DC: U.S. Department of Justice.

8. Federal Bureau of Investigation (FBI). (2012). Estimated number of arrests: United States, 2012 *Crime in the United States 2012: Uniform crime reports.* Retrieved from https://www.fbi.gov/about-us/cjis/ucr/crime-in-the-u.s/2012/crime-in-the-u.s.-2012/tables/29tabledatadecpdf. Accessed on April 11, 2016.

9. Jewett, A., Shults, R. A., Banerjee, T., & Bergen, G. (2015). Alcohol-impaired driving among adults—United States, 2012. *MMWR, 64*(30), 814-817.

10. Cantor, D., Fisher, B., Chibnall, S., Townsend, R., Lee, H., Bruce, C., & Thomas, C. (2015). *Report on the AAU campus climate survey on sexual assault and sexual misconduct assault and sexual misconduct.* Rockville, MD: The Association of American Universities.

11. Khan, M. R., Berger, A. T., Wells, B. E., & Cleland, C. M. (2012). Longitudinal associations between adolescent alcohol use and adulthood sexual risk behavior and sexually transmitted infection in the United States: Assessment of differences by race. *American Journal of Public Health, 102*(5), 867-876.

12. Baliunas, D., Rehm, J., Irving, H., & Shuper, P. (2010). Alcohol consumption and risk of incident human immunodeficiency virus infection: A meta-analysis. *International Journal of Public Health, 55*(3), 159-166.

13. Maldonado-Molina, M. M., Reingle, J. M., & Jennings, W. G. (2010). Does alcohol use predict violent behaviors? The relationship between alcohol use and violence in a nationally representative longitudinal sample. *Youth Violence and Juvenile Justice.*

14. Popovici, I., Homer, J. F., Fang, H., & French, M. T. (2012). Alcohol use and crime: Findings from a longitudinal sample of US adolescents and young adults. *Alcoholism: Clinical and Experimental Research, 36*(3), 532-543.

15. Dahl, R. E., & Spear, L. P. (2004). Adolescent brain development: A period of vulnerabilities and opportunities. Keynote address. *Annals of the New York Academy of Sciences, 1021*(1), 1-22.

16. Kessler, R. C., Berglund, P., Demler, O., Jin, R., Merikangas, K. R., & Walters, E. E. (2005). Lifetime prevalence and age-of-onset distributions of DSM-IV disorders in the National Comorbidity Survey Replication. *Archives of General Psychiatry, 62*(6), 593-602.

17. Thornberry, T. P., & Krohn, M. D. (2006). *Taking stock of delinquency: An overview of findings from contemporary longitudinal studies.* New York, NY: Springer Science & Business Media.

18. National Research Council and Institute of Medicine. (2009). *Preventing mental, emotional, and behavioral disorders among young people: Progress and possibilities.* Washington, DC: National Academies Press.

19. Centers for Disease Control and Prevention. (2005). *Web-based injury statistics query and reporting system (WISQARS).* Atlanta, GA: National Center for Injury Prevention and Control. Retrieved from http://www.cdc.gov/injury/wisqars/. Accessed on May 14, 2016.

20. Center for Behavioral Health Statistics and Quality. (2016). *Results from the 2015 National Survey on Drug Use and Health: Detailed tables.* Rockville, MD: Substance Abuse and Mental Health Services Administration.

21. DeWit, D. J., Adlaf, E. M., Offord, D. R., & Ogborne, A. C. (2000). Age at first alcohol use: A risk factor for the development of alcohol disorders. *American Journal of Psychiatry, 157*(5), 745-750.

22. Moss, H. B., Chen, C. M., & Yi, H.-y. (2014). Early adolescent patterns of alcohol, cigarettes, and marijuana polysubstance use and young adult substance use outcomes in a nationally representative sample. *Drug and Alcohol Dependence, 136,* 51-62.

23. Esser, M. B., Hedden, S. L., Kanny, D., Brewer, R. D., Gfroerer, J. C., & Naimi, T. S. (2014). Prevalence of alcohol dependence among US adult drinkers, 2009-2011. *Preventing Chronic Disease, 11*(E206).

24. Ennett, S. T., Ringwalt, C. L., Thorne, J., Rohrbach, L. A., Vincus, A., Simons-Rudolph, A., & Jones, S. (2003). A comparison of current practice in school-based substance use prevention programs with meta-analysis findings. *Prevention Science, 4*(1), 1-14.

25. Wandersman, A., & Florin, P. (2003). Community interventions and effective prevention. *American Psychologist, 58*(6-7), 441-448.

26. Hawkins, J. D., Catalano, R. F., Arthur, M. W., Egan, E., Brown, E. C., Abbott, R. D., & Murray, D. M. (2008). Testing Communities That Care: The rationale, design and behavioral baseline equivalence of the community youth development study. *Prevention Science, 9*(3), 178-190.

27. World Health Organization. (2014). *Global status report on noncommunicable diseases 2014.* Geneva, Switzerland: World Health Organization.

28. Babor, T., Caetano, R., Casswell, S., Edwards, G., Giesbrecht, N., Graham, K., . . . Rossow, I. (2010). *Alcohol: No ordinary commodity: Research and public policy* (2nd ed.). New York: Oxford University Press.

29. World Health Organization. (2004). *Global status report on alcohol 2004.* Geneva: World Health Organization, Department of Mental Health and Substance Abuse

30. Chaloupka, F. J., Grossman, M., & Saffer, H. (2002). The effects of price on alcohol consumption and alcohol-related problems. *Alcohol Research and Health, 26*(1), 22-34.

31. Elder, R. W., Lawrence, B., Ferguson, A., Naimi, T. S., Brewer, R. D., Chattopadhyay, S. K., ... Task Force on Community Preventive Services. (2010). The effectiveness of tax policy interventions for reducing excessive alcohol consumption and related harms. *American Journal of Preventive Medicine, 38*(2), 217-229.

32. Alcohol Policy Information System. (n.d.). Alcohol beverages taxes: Beer. Retrieved from https://alcoholpolicy.niaaa.nih.gov/Taxes_Beer.html. Accessed on June 8, 2016.

33. Drenkard, S. (2015). How high are beer taxes in your state? Retrieved from http://taxfoundation.org/blog/how-high-are-beer-taxes-your-state. Accessed on June 29, 2016.

34. Catalano, R. F., Fagan, A. A., Gavin, L. E., Greenberg, M. T., Irwin, C. E., Ross, D. A., & Shek, D. T. (2012). Worldwide application of prevention science in adolescent health. *The Lancet, 379*(9826), 1653-1664.

35. Stone, A. L., Becker, L. G., Huber, A. M., & Catalano, R. F. (2012). Review of risk and protective factors of substance use and problem use in emerging adulthood. *Addictive Behaviors, 37*(7), 747-775.

36. Viner, R. M., Ozer, E. M., Denny, S., Marmot, M., Resnick, M., Fatusi, A., & Currie, C. (2012). Adolescence and the social determinants of health. *The Lancet, 379*(9826), 1641-1652.

37. Masten, A. S. (2004). Regulatory processes, risk, and resilience in adolescent development. *Annals of the New York Academy of Sciences, 1021*(1), 310-319.

38. Shek, D. T. L., Sun, R. C. F., & Merrick, J. (2012). Positive youth development constructs: Conceptual review and application. *The Scientific World Journal, 2012*.

39. Seligman, M. E. P., Berkowitz, M. W., Catalano, R. F., Damon, W., Eccles, J. S., Gillham, J. E., ... Penn, D. L. (2005). The positive perspective on youth development. In Evans D L, Foa E B, Gur R E, Hendin H, O'Brien C P, Seligman M E P, & W. B. T (Eds.), *Treating and preventing adolescent mental health disorders: What we know and what we don't know.* (pp. 498-527). New York, NY: Oxford University Press.

40. Catalano, R. F., Hawkins, J. D., & Toumbourou, J. W. (2014). Positive youth development in the United States: History, efficacy, and links to moral and character education. In Nucci L, Narvaez D, & K. T (Eds.), *Handbook of moral and character education.* (2 ed., pp. 459-483). New York, NY and London, UK: Routledge.

41. Catalano, R. F., Berglund, M. L., Ryan, J. A., Lonczak, H. S., & Hawkins, J. D. (2002). Positive youth development in the United States: Research findings on evaluations of positive youth development programs. *Prevention & Treatment, 5*(1).

42. Botvin, G. J., & Griffin, K. W. (2002). Life skills training as a primary prevention approach for adolescent drug abuse and other problem behaviors. *International Journal of Emergency Mental Health, 4*(1), 41-47.

43. Flay, B. R., Graumlich, S., Segawa, E., Burns, J. L., & Holliday, M. Y. (2004). Effects of 2 prevention programs on high-risk behaviors among African American youth: A randomized trial. *Archives of Pediatrics & Adolescent Medicine, 158*(4), 377-384.

44. Schweinhart, L. J., Montie, J., Xiang, Z., Barnett, W. S., Belfield, C. R., & Nores, M. (2005). *Lifetime effects: The High/Scope Perry Preschool study through age 40. (Monographs of the High/Scope Educational Research Foundation, 14).* Ypsilanti, MI: High/Scope Press.

45. Kanny, D., Liu, Y., Brewer, R., Garvin, W., & Balluz, L. (2010). Vital signs: Binge drinking among high school students and adults-United States, 2009. *MMWR, 59*(39), 1274-1279.

46. Grant, B. F., Stinson, F. S., & Harford, T. C. (2001). Age at onset of alcohol use and DSM-IV alcohol abuse and dependence: A 12-year follow-up. *Journal of Substance Abuse, 13*(4), 493-504.

47. Zucker, R. A., Donovan, J. E., Masten, A. S., Mattson, M. E., & Moss, H. B. (2008). Early developmental processes and the continuity of risk for underage drinking and problem drinking. *Pediatrics, 121*(Supplement 4), S252-S272.

48. Shedler, J., & Block, J. (1990). Adolescent drug use and psychological health: A longitudinal inquiry. *American Psychologist, 45*(5), 612-630.

49. Brook, J. S., Brook, D. W., Gordon, A. S., Whiteman, M., & Cohen, P. (1990). The psychosocial etiology of adolescent drug use: A family interactional approach. *Genetic, Social, and General Psychology Monographs, 116*(2), 111-267.

50. Zucker, R. A. (2008). Anticipating problem alcohol use developmentally from childhood into middle adulthood: What have we learned? *Addiction, 103*(s1), 100-108.

51. Guo, J., Hawkins, J. D., Hill, K. G., & Abbott, R. D. (2001). Childhood and adolescent predictors of alcohol abuse and dependence in young adulthood. *Journal of Studies on Alcohol, 62*(6), 754-762.

52. Jackson, K. M., Sher, K. J., & Schulenberg, J. E. (2005). Conjoint developmental trajectories of young adult alcohol and tobacco use. *Journal of Abnormal Psychology, 114*(4), 612-626.

53. Chassin, L., Pitts, S. C., & Prost, J. (2002). Binge drinking trajectories from adolescence to emerging adulthood in a high-risk sample: Predictors and substance abuse outcomes. *Journal of Consulting and Clinical Psychology, 70*(1), 67-78.

54. Sher, K. J., & Rutledge, P. C. (2007). Heavy drinking across the transition to college: Predicting first-semester heavy drinking from precollege variables. *Addictive Behaviors, 32*(4), 819-835.

55. Brook, J. S., Kessler, R. C., & Cohen, P. (1999). The onset of marijuana use from preadolescence and early adolescence to young adulthood. *Development and Psychopathology, 11*(4), 901-914.

56. Goldman, D., Oroszi, G., & Ducci, F. (2005). The genetics of addictions: Uncovering the genes. *Nature Reviews Genetics, 6*(7), 521-532.

57. King, K. M., & Chassin, L. (2004). Mediating and moderated effects of adolescent behavioral undercontrol and parenting in the prediction of drug use disorders in emerging adulthood. *Psychology of Addictive Behaviors, 18*(3), 239-249.

58. Kosterman, R., Hawkins, J. D., Guo, J., Catalano, R. F., & Abbott, R. D. (2000). The dynamics of alcohol and marijuana initiation: Patterns and predictors of first use in adolescence. *American Journal of Public Health, 90*(3), 360-366.

59. Arria, A. M., Kuhn, V., Caldeira, K. M., O'Grady, K. E., Vincent, K. B., & Wish, E. D. (2008). High school drinking mediates the relationship between parental monitoring and college drinking: A longitudinal analysis. *Substance Abuse Treatment, Prevention, and Policy, 3*(1).

60. Ghandour, L. A. (2009). *Young adult alcohol involvement: The role of parental monitoring, child disclosure, and parental knowledge during childhood.* Ann Arbor, MI: ProQuest.

61. Kilpatrick, D. G., Acierno, R., Saunders, B., Resnick, H. S., Best, C. L., & Schnurr, P. P. (2000). Risk factors for adolescent substance abuse and dependence: Data from a national sample. *Journal of Consulting and Clinical Psychology, 68*(1), 19-30.

62. Maggs, J. L., Patrick, M. E., & Feinstein, L. (2008). Childhood and adolescent predictors of alcohol use and problems in adolescence and adulthood in the National Child Development Study. *Addiction, 103*(s1), 7-22.

63. Penning, M., & Barnes, G. E. (1982). Adolescent marijuana use: A review. *International Journal of the Addictions, 17*(5), 749-791.

64. Brook, J. S., Whiteman, M., Gordon, A. S., & Cohen, P. (1986). Some models and mechanisms for explaining the impact of maternal and adolescent characteristics on adolescent stage of drug use. *Developmental Psychology, 22*(4), 460-467.

65. McDermott, D. (1984). The relationship of parental drug use and parents' attitude concerning adolescent drug use to adolescent drug use. *Adolescence, 19*(73), 89-97.

66. Chassin, L., Flora, D. B., & King, K. M. (2004). Trajectories of alcohol and drug use and dependence from adolescence to adulthood: The effects of familial alcoholism and personality. *Journal of Abnormal Psychology, 113*(4), 483-498.

67. Hill, S. Y., Steinhauer, S. R., Locke-Wellman, J., & Ulrich, R. (2009). Childhood risk factors for young adult substance dependence outcome in offspring from multiplex alcohol dependence families: A prospective study. *Biological Psychiatry, 66*(8), 750-757.

68. Hundleby, J. D., & Mercer, G. W. (1987). Family and friends as social environments and their relationship to young adolescents' use of alcohol, tobacco, and marijuana. *Journal of Marriage and the Family, 49*(1), 151-164.

69. O'Donnell, J., Hawkins, J. D., Catalano, R. F., Abbott, R. D., & Day, L. E. (1995). Preventing school failure, drug use, and delinquency among low-income children: Long-term intervention in elementary schools. *American Journal of Orthopsychiatry, 65*(1), 87-100.

70. Najaka, S. S., Gottfredson, D. C., & Wilson, D. B. (2001). A meta-analytic inquiry into the relationship between selected risk factors and problem behavior. *Prevention Science, 2*(4), 257-271.

71. Bond, L., Butler, H., Thomas, L., Carlin, J., Glover, S., Bowes, G., & Patton, G. (2007). Social and school connectedness in early secondary school as predictors of late teenage substance use, mental health, and academic outcomes. *Journal of Adolescent Health, 40*(4), 357-357.

72. Wagenaar, A. C., Salois, M. J., & Komro, K. A. (2009). Effects of beverage alcohol price and tax levels on drinking: A meta-analysis of 1003 estimates from 112 studies. *Addiction, 104*(2), 179-190.

73. Scribner, R., Mason, K., Theall, K., Simonsen, N., Schneider, S. K., Towvim, L. G., & DeJong, W. (2008). The contextual role of alcohol outlet density in college drinking. *Journal of Studies on Alcohol and Drugs, 69*(1), 112-120.

74. Weitzman, E. R., Folkman, A., Folkman, M. P., & Wechsler, H. (2003). The relationship of alcohol outlet density to heavy and frequent drinking and drinking-related problems among college students at eight universities. *Health & Place, 9*(1), 1-6.

75. Read, J. P., Wood, M. D., Davidoff, O. J., McLacken, J., & Campbell, J. F. (2002). Making the transition from high school to college: The role of alcohol-related social influence factors in students' drinking. *Substance Abuse, 23*(1), 53-65.

76. Perkins, H. (2003). *The social norms approach to preventing school and college age substance abuse: A handbook for educators, counselors, and clinicians.* San Francisco, CA: Jossey-Bass.

77. Anderson, P., De Bruijn, A., Angus, K., Gordon, R., & Hastings, G. (2009). Impact of alcohol advertising and media exposure on adolescent alcohol use: A systematic review of longitudinal studies. *Alcohol and Alcoholism, 44*(3), 229-243.

78. Hanewinkel, R., & Sargent, J. D. (2009). Longitudinal study of exposure to entertainment media and alcohol use among German adolescents. *Pediatrics, 123*(3), 989-995.

79. Jernigan, D., Noel, J., Landon, J., Thornton, N., & Lobstein, T. (2016). Alcohol marketing and youth alcohol consumption: A systematic review of longitudinal studies published since 2008. *Addiction.*

80. Hemphill, S. A., Heerde, J. A., Herrenkohl, T. I., Patton, G. C., Toumbourou, J. W., & Catalano, R. F. (2011). Risk and protective factors for adolescent substance use in Washington State, the United States and Victoria, Australia: A longitudinal study. *Journal of Adolescent Health, 49*(3), 312-320.

81. Beyers, J. M., Toumbourou, J. W., Catalano, R. F., Arthur, M. W., & Hawkins, J. D. (2004). A cross-national comparison of risk and protective factors for adolescent substance use: The United States and Australia. *Journal of Adolescent Health, 35*(1), 3-16.

82. Elliott, D. S., Wilson, W. J., Huizinga, D., Sampson, R. J., Elliott, A., & Rankin, B. (1996). The effects of neighborhood disadvantage on adolescent development. *Journal of Research in Crime and Delinquency, 33*(4), 389-426.

83. Sampson, R. J. (1997). Collective regulation of adolescent misbehavior validation results from eighty Chicago neighborhoods. *Journal of Adolescent Research, 12*(2), 227-244.

84. Herting, J. R., & Guest, A. M. (1985). Components of satisfaction with local areas in the metropolis. *The Sociological Quarterly, 26*(1), 99-116.

85. Hawkins, J. D., Arthur, M. W., & Catalano, R. F. (1995). Preventing substance abuse. *Crime and Justice: A Review of Research, 19,* 343-428.

86. Sampson, R. J., & Lauritsen, J. L. (1994). Violent victimization and offending: Individual-, situational-, and community-level risk factors. In A. J. Reiss Jr., J. A. Roth, & N. R. Council (Eds.), *Understanding and Preventing Violence.* (Vol. 3, pp. 1-114).

87. Botvin, G. J., Schinke, S. P., Epstein, J. A., Diaz, T., & Botvin, E. M. (1995). Effectiveness of culturally focused and generic skills training approaches to alcohol and drug abuse prevention among minority adolescents: Two-year follow-up results. *Psychology of Addictive Behaviors, 9*(3), 183-194.

88. Masten, A. S., Best, K. M., & Garmezy, N. (1990). Resilience and development: Contributions from the study of children who overcome adversity. *Development and Psychopathology, 2*(04), 425-444.

89. DiClemente, C. C., Fairhurst, S. K., & Piotrowski, N. A. (1995). Self-efficacy and addictive behaviors. *Self-efficacy, adaptation, and adjustment.* (pp. 109-141). New York, NY: Springer.

90. Locke, E. A., Frederick, E., Lee, C., & Bobko, P. (1984). Effect of self-efficacy, goals, and task strategies on task performance. *Journal of Applied Psychology, 69*(2), 241-251.

91. Jackson, K. M., Sher, K. J., & Schulenberg, J. E. (2008). Conjoint developmental trajectories of young adult substance use. *Alcoholism: Clinical and Experimental Research, 32*(5), 723-737.

92. White, H. R., Fleming, C. B., Kim, M. J., Catalano, R. F., & McMorris, B. J. (2008). Identifying two potential mechanisms for changes in alcohol use among college-attending and non-college-attending emerging adults. *Developmental Psychology, 44*(6), 1625-1639.

93. Chalk, R., & Phillips, D. A. (1997). *Youth development and neighborhood influences: Challenges and opportunities.* Washington, DC: National Academies Press.

94. Darling, N., & Steinberg, L. (1993). Parenting style as context: An integrative model. *Psychological Bulletin, 113*(3), 487-496.

95. Hill, K. G., Hawkins, J. D., Catalano, R. F., Abbott, R. D., & Guo, J. (2005). Family influences on the risk of daily smoking initiation. *Journal of Adolescent Health, 37*(3), 202-210.

96. Locke, T. F., & Newcomb, M. (2004). Child maltreatment, parent alcohol-and drug-related problems, polydrug problems, and parenting practices: A test of gender differences and four theoretical perspectives. *Journal of Family Psychology, 18*(1), 120-134.

97. Kaufmann, D. R., Wyman, P. A., Forbes-Jones, E. L., & Barry, J. (2007). Prosocial involvement and antisocial peer affiliations as predictors of behavior problems in urban adolescents: Main effects and moderating effects. *Journal of Community Psychology, 35*(4), 417-434.

98. Duncan, G. J., Wilkerson, B., & England, P. (2006). Cleaning up their act: The effects of marriage and cohabitation on licit and illicit drug use. *Demography, 43*(4), 691-710.

99. Hawkins, J. D., Catalano, R. F., Morrison, D. M., O'Donnell, J., Abbott, R. D., & Day, L. E. (1992). The Seattle Social Development Project: Effects of the first four years on protective factors and problem behaviors. In J. McCord & R. E. Tremblay (Eds.), *Preventing antisocial behavior: Interventions from birth through adolescence.* (pp. 139-161). New York: Guilford Press.

100. Durlak, J. A. (1995). *School-based prevention programs for children and adolescents* (Vol. 34). Thousand Oaks, CA: Sage Publications.

101. Rutter, M., Bishop, D., Pine, D., Scott, S., Stevenson, J. S., Taylor, E. A., & Thapar, A. (2015). *Rutter's child and adolescent psychiatry* (6th ed.). Oxford, UK: John Wiley & Sons, Ltd.

102. Lee, S., Aos, S., Drake, E., Pennucci, A., Miller, M., & Anderson, L. (2012). *Return on investment: Evidence-based options to improve statewide outcomes.* (Document No. 12-04-1201). Olympia, WA: Washington State Institute for Public Policy.

103. Whitlock, E. P., Polen, M. R., Green, C. A., Orleans, T., & Klein, J. (2004). Behavioral counseling interventions in primary care to reduce risky/harmful alcohol use by adults: A summary of the evidence for the US Preventive Services Task Force. *Annals of Internal Medicine, 140*(7), 557-568.

104. Kaner, E. F., Beyer, F., Dickinson, H. O., Pienaar, E., Campbell, F., Schlesinger, C., . . . Burnand, B. (2007). Effectiveness of brief alcohol interventions in primary care populations. *Cochrane Database Systematic Reviews*(2).

105. Tansil, K. A., Esser, M. B., Sandhu, P., Reynolds, J. A., Elder, R. W., Williamson, R. S., & et al. (In press). Electronic screening and brief intervention (e-SBI) to reduce excessive alcohol consumption and related harms: A Community Guide systematic review. *American Journal of Preventive Medicine.*

106. Jonas, D. E., Garbutt, J. C., Brown, J. M., Amick, H. R., Brownley, K. A., Council, C. L., . . . Richmond, E. M. (2012). *Screening, behavioral counseling, and referral in primary care to reduce alcohol misuse.* (AHRQ Publication No. 12-EHC055-EF). Rockville, MD: Agency for Healthcare Research and Quality.

107. Spoth, R., Greenberg, M., & Turrisi, R. (2008). Preventive interventions addressing underage drinking: State of the evidence and steps toward public health impact. *Pediatrics, 121*(Suppl 4), S311-S336.

108. Greenberg, M. T., & Riggs, N. R. (2015). Prevention of mental disorders and promotion of competence In A. Thapar, D. S. Pine, J. F. Leckman, S. Scott, M. J. Snowling, & E. A. Taylor (Eds.), *Rutter's Child and Adolescent Psychiatry* (6th ed., pp. 215-226). Oxford, UK: John Wiley & Sons Ltd.

109. Olds, D., Henderson Jr, C. R., Cole, R., Eckenrode, J., Kitzman, H., Luckey, D., . . . Powers, J. (1998). Long-term effects of nurse home visitation on children's criminal and antisocial behavior: 15-year follow-up of a randomized controlled trial. *JAMA 280*(14), 1238-1244.

110. Kitzman, H. J., Olds, D. L., Cole, R. E., Hanks, C. A., Anson, E. A., Arcoleo, K. J., . . . Holmberg, J. R. (2010). Enduring effects of prenatal and infancy home visiting by nurses on children: follow-up of a randomized trial among children at age 12 years. *Archives of Pediatrics & Adolescent Medicine, 164*(5), 412-418.

111. Kellam, S. G., Wang, W., Mackenzie, A. C. L., Brown, C. H., Ompad, D. C., Or, F., . . . Windham, A. (2014). The impact of the Good Behavior Game, a universal classroom-based preventive intervention in first and second grades, on high-risk sexual behaviors and drug abuse and dependence disorders into young adulthood. *Prevention Science, 15*(1), S6-S18.

112. Furr-Holden, C. D. M., Ialongo, N. S., Anthony, J. C., Petras, H., & Kellam, S. G. (2004). Developmentally inspired drug prevention: Middle school outcomes in a school-based randomized prevention trial. *Drug and Alcohol Dependence, 73*(2), 149-158.

113. Liu, W., Lynne-Landsman, S. D., Petras, H., Masyn, K., & Ialongo, N. (2013). The evaluation of two first-grade preventive interventions on childhood aggression and adolescent marijuana use: A latent transition longitudinal mixture model. *Prevention Science, 14*(3), 206-217.

114. Hawkins, J. D., Kosterman, R., Catalano, R. F., Hill, K. G., & Abbott, R. D. (2005). Promoting positive adult functioning through social development intervention in childhood: Long-term effects from the Seattle Social Development Project. *Archives of Pediatrics & Adolescent Medicine, 159*(1), 25-31.

115. Brown, E. C., Catalano, R. F., Fleming, C. B., Haggerty, K. P., & Abbott, R. D. (2005). Adolescent substance use outcomes in the Raising Healthy Children project: A two-part latent growth curve analysis. *Journal of Consulting and Clinical Psychology, 73*(4), 699-710.

116. Dodge, K. A., Bierman, K. L., Coie, J. D., Greenberg, M. T., Lochman, J. E., McMahon, R. J., & Pinderhughes, E. E. (2014). Impact of early intervention on psychopathology, crime, and well-being at age 25. *American Journal of Psychiatry, 172*(1), 59-70.

117. Botvin, G. J., Griffin, K. W., & Nichols, T. D. (2006). Preventing youth violence and delinquency through a universal school-based prevention approach. *Prevention Science, 7*(4), 403-408.

118. Faggiano, F., Vigna-Taglianti, F., Burkhart, G., Bohrn, K., Cuomo, L., Gregori, D., . . . Varona, L. (2010). The effectiveness of a school-based substance abuse prevention program: 18-month follow-up of the EU-Dap cluster randomized controlled trial. *Drug and Alcohol Dependence, 108*(1-2), 56-64.

119. McBride, N., Midford, R., Farringdon, F., & Phillips, M. (2000). Early results from a school alcohol harm minimization study: The School Health and Alcohol Harm Reduction Project. *Addiction, 95*(7), 1021-1042.

120. McBride, N., Farringdon, F., Midford, R., Meuleners, L., & Phillips, M. (2004). Harm minimization in school drug education: Final results of the School Health and Alcohol Harm Reduction Project (SHAHRP). *Addiction, 99*(3), 278-291.

121. Hecht, M. L., Marsiglia, F. F., Elek, E., Wagstaff, D. A., Kulis, S., Dustman, P., & Miller-Day, M. (2003). Culturally grounded substance use prevention: An evaluation of the keepin'it REAL curriculum. *Prevention Science, 4*(4), 233-248.

122. Hecht, M. L., Graham, J. W., & Elek, E. (2006). The drug resistance strategies intervention: Program effects on substance use. *Health Communication, 20*(3), 267-276.

123. Kulis, S., Marsiglia, F. F., Sicotte, D., & Nieri, T. (2007). Neighborhood effects on youth substance use in a southwestern city. *Sociological Perspectives, 50*(2), 273-301.

124. Schinke, S. P., Tepavac, L., & Cole, K. C. (2000). Preventing substance use among Native American youth: Three-year results. *Addictive Behaviors, 25*(3), 387-397.

125. Sussman, S., Dent, C. W., & Stacy, A. W. (2002). Project Towards No Drug Abuse: A review of the findings and future directions. *American Journal of Health Behavior, 26*(5), 354-365.

126. Spoth, R. L., Trudeau, L. S., Guyll, M., & Shin, C. (2012). Benefits of universal intervention effects on a youth protective shield 10 years after baseline. *Journal of Adolescent Health, 50*(4), 414-417.

127. Brody, G. H., Murry, V. M., Chen, Y.-f., Kogan, S. M., & Brown, A. C. (2006). Effects of family risk factors on dosage and efficacy of a family-centered preventive intervention for rural African Americans. *Prevention Science, 7*(3), 281-291.

128. Brody, G. H., Murry, V. M., Kogan, S. M., Gerrard, M., Gibbons, F. X., Molgaard, V., . . . Wills, T. A. (2006). The Strong African American Families Program: A cluster-randomized prevention trial of long-term effects and a mediational model. *Journal of Consulting and Clinical Psychology, 74*(2), 356-366.

129. Brody, G. H., Chen, Y.-F., Kogan, S. M., Murry, V. M., & Brown, A. C. (2010). Long-term effects of the Strong African American Families program on youths' alcohol use. *Journal of Consulting and Clinical Psychology, 78*(2), 281-285.

130. Spoth, R., Trudeau, L., Guyll, M., Shin, C., & Redmond, C. (2009). Universal intervention effects on substance use among young adults mediated by delayed adolescent substance initiation. *Journal of Consulting and Clinical Psychology, 77*(4), 620-632.

131. Spoth, R. L., Clair, S., Shin, C., & Redmond, C. (2006). Long-term effects of universal preventive interventions on methamphetamine use among adolescents. *Archives of Pediatrics and Adolescent Medicine, 160*(9), 876-882.

132. Spoth, R., Trudeau, L., Shin, C., Ralston, E., Redmond, C., Greenberg, M., & Feinberg, M. (2013). Longitudinal effects of universal preventive intervention on prescription drug misuse: Three randomized controlled trials with late adolescents and young adults. *American Journal of Public Health, 103*(4), 665-672.

133. Pantin, H., Prado, G., Lopez, B., Huang, S., Tapia, M. I., Schwartz, S. J., . . . Branchini, J. (2009). A randomized controlled trial of Familias Unidas for Hispanic adolescents with behavior problems. *Psychosomatic Medicine, 71*(9), 987-995.

134. Dishion, T. J., & Andrews, D. W. (1995). Preventing escalation in problem behaviors with high-risk young adolescents: Immediate and 1-year outcomes. *Journal of Consulting and Clinical Psychology, 63*(4), 538-548.

135. Kim, H. K., & Leve, L. D. (2011). Substance use and delinquency among middle school girls in foster care: A three-year follow-up of a randomized controlled trial. *Journal of Consulting and Clinical Psychology, 79*(6), 740-750.

136. Lochman, J. E., & Wells, K. C. (2003). Effectiveness of the Coping Power Program and of classroom intervention with aggressive children: Outcomes at a 1-year follow-up. *Behavior Therapy, 34*(4), 493-515.

137. Conrod, P. J., Castellanos-Ryan, N., & Strang, J. (2010). Brief, personality-targeted coping skills interventions and survival as a non–drug user over a 2-year period during adolescence. *Archives of General Psychiatry, 67*(1), 85-93.

138. Conrod, P. J., Castellanos-Ryan, N., & Mackie, C. (2011). Long-term effects of a personality-targeted intervention to reduce alcohol use in adolescents. *Journal of Consulting and Clinical Psychology, 79*(3), 296-306.

139. Conrod, P. J., O'Leary-Barrett, M., Newton, N., Topper, L., Castellanos-Ryan, N., Mackie, C., & Girard, A. (2013). Effectiveness of a selective, personality-targeted prevention program for adolescent alcohol use and misuse: A cluster randomized controlled trial. *JAMA Psychiatry, 70*(3), 334-342.

140. Mahu, I. T., Doucet, C., O'Leary-Barrett, M., & Conrod, P. J. (2015). Can cannabis use be prevented by targeting personality risk in schools? 24-month outcome of the adventure trial on cannabis use: A cluster randomized controlled trial. *Addiction, 110*(10), 1625-1633.

141. Lammers, J., Goossens, F., Conrod, P., Engels, R., Wiers, R. W., & Kleinjan, M. (2015). Effectiveness of a selective intervention program targeting personality risk factors for alcohol misuse among young adolescents: Results of a cluster randomized controlled trial. *Addiction, 110*(7), 1101-1109.

142. Roberts-Gray, C., Gingiss, P. M., & Boerm, M. (2007). Evaluating school capacity to implement new programs. *Evaluation and Program Planning, 30*(3), 247-257.

143. Schinke, S. P., Fang, L., & Cole, K. C. (2009). Preventing substance use among adolescent girls: 1-year outcomes of a computerized, mother–daughter program. *Addictive Behaviors, 34*(12), 1060-1064.

144. Schinke, S. P., Fang, L., & Cole, K. C. (2009). Computer-delivered, parent-involvement intervention to prevent substance use among adolescent girls. *Preventive Medicine, 49*(5), 429-435.

145. Schinke, S. P., Schwinn, T. M., Di Noia, J., & Cole, K. C. (2004). Reducing the risks of alcohol use among urban youth: Three-year effects of a computer-based intervention with and without parent involvement. *Journal of Studies on Alcohol, 65*(4), 443-449.

146. Walton, M. A., Resko, S., Barry, K. L., Chermack, S. T., Zucker, R. A., Zimmerman, M. A., . . . Blow, F. C. (2014). A randomized controlled trial testing the efficacy of a brief cannabis universal prevention program among adolescents in primary care. *Addiction, 109*(5), 786-797.

147. Park, M. J., Mulye, T. P., Adams, S. H., Brindis, C. D., & Irwin, C. E. (2006). The health status of young adults in the United States. *Journal of Adolescent Health, 39*(3), 305-317.

148. Tanner-Smith, E. E., & Lipsey, M. W. (2015). Brief alcohol interventions for adolescents and young adults: A systematic review and meta-analysis. *Journal of Substance Abuse Treatment, 51,* 1-18.

149. Levy, S. J., Williams, J. F., & Committee on Substance Use and Prevention. (2016). Substance use screening, brief intervention, and referral to treatment. *Pediatrics, 138*(1).

150. Larimer, M. E., & Cronce, J. M. (2007). Identification, prevention, and treatment revisited: Individual-focused college drinking prevention strategies 1999-2006. *Addictive Behaviors, 32*(11), 2439-2468.

151. Carey, K. B., et al. (2007). Individual-level interventions to reduce college student drinking: A 1557 meta-analytic review. *Addictive Behaviors, 32*(11), 2469-2494.

152. Cronce, J. M., & Larimer, M. E. (2011). Individual-focused approaches to the prevention of college student drinking. *34*(2), 210-221.

153. Seigers, D. K., & Carey, K. B. (2010). Screening and brief interventions for alcohol use in college health centers: A review. *Journal of American College Health, 59*(3), 151-158.

154. Fachini, A., Aliane, P. P., Martinez, E. Z., & Furtado, E. F. (2012). Efficacy of brief alcohol screening intervention for college students (BASICS): A meta-analysis of randomized controlled trials. *Substance Abuse Treatment, Prevention, and Policy, 7*(40).

155. Carey, K. B., Scott-Sheldon, L. A., Elliott, J. C., Garey, L., & Carey, M. P. (2012). Face-to-face versus computer-delivered alcohol interventions for college drinkers: A meta-analytic review, 1998 to 2010. *Clinical Psychology Review, 32*(8), 690-703.

156. Henson, J. M., Pearson, M. R., & Carey, K. B. (2015). Defining and characterizing differences in college alcohol intervention efficacy: A growth mixture modeling application. *Journal of Consulting and Clinical Psychology, 83*(2), 370-381.

157. Lee, C. M., Kilmer, J. R., Neighbors, C., Atkins, D. C., Zheng, C., Walker, D. D., & Larimer, M. E. (2013). Indicated prevention for college student marijuana use: A randomized controlled trial. *Journal of Consulting and Clinical Psychology, 81*(4), 702-709.

158. Samson, J. E., & Tanner-Smith, E. E. (2015). Single-session alcohol interventions for heavy drinking college students: A systematic review and meta-analysis. *Journal of Studies on Alcohol and Drugs, 76*(4), 530-543.

159. Scott-Sheldon, L. A., Terry, D. L., Carey, K. B., Garey, L., & Carey, M. P. (2012). Efficacy of expectancy challenge interventions to reduce college student drinking: A meta-analytic review. *Psychology of Addictive Behaviors, 26*(3), 393-405.

160. Huh, D., Mun, E. Y., Larimer, M. E., White, H. R., Ray, A. E., Rhew, I. C., . . . Atkins, D. C. (2015). Brief motivational interventions for college student drinking may not be as powerful as we think: An individual participant-level data meta-analysis. *Alcoholism: Clinical and Experimental Research, 39*(5), 919-931.

161. Baer, J. S., Kivlahan, D. R., Blume, A. W., McKnight, P., & Marlatt, G. A. (2001). Brief intervention for heavy-drinking college students: 4-year follow-up and natural history. *American Journal of Public Health, 91*(8), 1310-1316.

162. Marlatt, G. A., Baer, J. S., Kivlahan, D. R., Dimeff, L. A., Larimer, M. E., Quigley, L. A., . . . Williams, E. (1998). Screening and brief intervention for high-risk college student drinkers: Results from a 2-year follow-up assessment. *Journal of Consulting and Clinical Psychology, 66*(4), 604-615.

163. Larimer, M. E., Turner, A. P., Anderson, B. K., Fader, J. S., Kilmer, J. R., Palmer, R. S., & Cronce, J. M. (2001). Evaluating a brief alcohol intervention with fraternities. *Journal of Studies on Alcohol, 62*(3), 370-380.

164. Terlecki, M. A., Buckner, J. D., Larimer, M. E., & Copeland, A. L. (2015). Randomized controlled trial of brief alcohol screening and intervention for college students for heavy-drinking mandated and volunteer undergraduates: 12-month outcomes. *Psychology of Addictive Behaviors, 29*(1), 2-16.

165. Wood, M. D., Fairlie, A. M., Fernandez, A. C., Borsari, B., Capone, C., Laforge, R., & Carmona-Barros, R. (2010). Brief motivational and parent interventions for college students: A randomized factorial study. *Journal of Consulting and Clinical Psychology, 78*(3), 349-361.

166. Scott-Sheldon, L. A. J., Carey, K. B., Elliott, J. C., Garey, L., & Carey, M. P. (2014). Efficacy of alcohol interventions for first-year college students: A meta-analytic review of randomized controlled trials. *Journal of Consulting and Clinical Psychology, 82*(2), 177-188.

167. Turrisi, R., Mallett, K. A., Cleveland, M. J., Varvil-Weld, L., Abar, C., Scaglione, N., & Hultgren, B. (2013). Evaluation of timing and dosage of a parent-based intervention to minimize college students' alcohol consumption. *Journal of Studies on Alcohol and Drugs, 74*(1), 30-40.

168. Turrisi, R., Larimer, M. E., Mallett, K. A., Kilmer, J. R., Ray, A. E., Mastroleo, N. R., . . . Montoya, H. (2009). A randomized clinical trial evaluating a combined alcohol intervention for high-risk college students. *Journal of Studies on Alcohol and Drugs, 70*(4), 555-567.

169. National Institute on Alcohol Abuse and Alcoholism. (2015). *Planning alcohol interventions using NIAAA's College AIM: Alcohol Intervention Matrix.* (NIH Publication No. 15-AA-8017). Rockville, MD: National Institute on Alcohol Abuse and Alcoholism.

170. Snow, D. L., Swan, S. C., & Wilton, L. (2003). A workplace coping-skills intervention to prevent alcohol abuse. In J. B. Bennett & W. E. K. Lehman (Eds.), *Preventing workplace substance abuse: Beyond drug testing to wellness.* (pp. 57-96). Washington, DC: American Psychological Association.

171. Longabaugh, R., Woolard, R. E., Nirenberg, T. D., Minugh, A. P., Becker, B., Clifford, P. R., . . . Gogineni, A. (2001). Evaluating the effects of a brief motivational intervention for injured drinkers in the emergency department. *Journal of Studies on Alcohol, 62*(6), 806-816.

172. Broome, K. M., & Bennett, J. B. (2011). Reducing heavy alcohol consumption in young restaurant workers. *Journal of Studies on Alcohol and Drugs, 72*(1), 117-124.

173. Ames, G. M., & Bennett, J. B. (2011). Prevention interventions of alcohol problems in the workplace: A review and guiding framework. *Alcohol Research: Current Reviews, 34*(2), 175-187.

174. Ettner, S. L., Xu, H., Duru, O. K., Ang, A., Tseng, C.-H., Tallen, L., . . . Moore, A. A. (2014). The effect of an educational intervention on alcohol consumption, at-risk drinking, and health care utilization in older adults: The Project SHARE study. *Journal of Studies on Alcohol and Drugs, 75*(3), 447-457.

175. Fink, A., Elliott, M. N., Tsai, M., & Beck, J. C. (2008). An evaluation of an intervention to assist primary care physicians in screening and educating older patients who use alcohol: Erratum. *Journal of the American Geriatrics Society, 56*(6), 1165-1165.

176. Washington State Institute for Public Policy. (2016). Benefit-cost results. Retrieved from http://www.wsipp.wa.gov/BenefitCost?topicId=. Accessed on September 26, 2016.

177. Campbell, C. A., Hahn, R. A., Elder, R., Brewer, R., Chattopadhyay, S., Fielding, J., . . . Middleton, J. C. (2009). The effectiveness of limiting alcohol outlet density as a means of reducing excessive alcohol consumption and alcohol-related harms. *American Journal of Preventive Medicine, 37*(6), 556-569.

178. DeJong, W., & Blanchette, J. (2014). Case closed: Research evidence on the positive public health impact of the age 21 minimum legal drinking age in the United States. *Journal of Studies on Alcohol and Drugs, Suppl 17*, 108-115.

179. Mosher, J. F., & Jernigan, D. H. (1989). New directions in alcohol policy. *Annual Review of Public Health, 10*(1), 245-279.

180. Hawkins, J. D., Kosterman, R., Catalano, R. F., Hill, K. G., & Abbott, R. D. (2008). Effects of social development intervention in childhood 15 years later. *Archives of Pediatrics and Adolescent Medicine, 162*(12), 1133-1141.

181. Hawkins, J. D., Oesterle, S., Brown, E. C., Abbott, R. D., & Catalano, R. F. (2014). Youth problem behaviors 8 years after implementing the Communities That Care prevention system: A community-randomized trial. *JAMA Pediatrics, 168*(2), 122-129.

182. Hawkins, J. D., Oesterle, S., Brown, E. C., Monahan, K. C., Abbott, R. D., Arthur, M. W., & Catalano, R. F. (2012). Sustained decreases in risk exposure and youth problem behaviors after installation of the Communities That Care prevention system in a randomized trial. *Archives of Pediatrics & Adolescent Medicine, 166*(2), 141-148.

183. Spoth, R., Greenberg, M., Bierman, K., & Redmond, C. (2004). PROSPER community–university partnership model for public education systems: Capacity-building for evidence-based, competence-building prevention. *Prevention Science, 5*(1), 31-39.

184. Spoth, R., Redmond, C., Shin, C., Greenberg, M., Feinberg, M., & Schainker, L. (2013). PROSPER community–university partnership delivery system effects on substance misuse through 6 1/2 years past baseline from a cluster randomized controlled intervention trial. *Preventive Medicine, 56*(3), 190-196.

185. Wagenaar, A. C., & Perry, C. L. (1994). Community strategies for the reduction of youth drinking: Theory and application. *Journal of Research on Adolescence, 4*(2), 319-345.

186. Pentz, M. A. (2000). Institutionalizing community-based prevention through policy change. *Journal of Community Psychology, 28*(3), 257-270.

187. Elder, R. W., Lawrence, B. A., Janes, G., Brewer, R. D., Toomey, T. L., Hingson, R. W., . . . Fielding, J. (2007). Enhanced enforcement of laws prohibiting sale of alcohol to minors: Systematic review of effectiveness for reducing sales and underage drinking. *Transportation Research Circular, 2007*(E-C123), 181-188.

188. Wagenaar, A. C., Murray, D. M., Gehan, J. P., Wolfson, M., Forster, J. L., Toomey, T. L., . . . Jones-Webb, R. (2000). Communities Mobilizing For Change on Alcohol: Outcomes from a randomized community trial. *Journal of Studies on Alcohol, 61*(1), 85-94.

189. Wagenaar, A. C., Murray, D. M., & Toomey, T. L. (2000). Communities Mobilizing for Change on Alcohol (CMCA): Effects of a randomized trial on arrests and traffic crashes. *Addiction, 95*(2), 209-217.

190. Nelson, T. F., Naimi, T. S., Brewer, R. D., & Wechsler, H. (2005). The state sets the rate: The relationship among state-specific college binge drinking, state binge drinking rates, and selected state alcohol control policies. *American Journal of Public Health, 95*(3), 441-446.

191. Xuan, Z., Blanchette, J. G., Nelson, T. F., Nguyen, T. H., Hadland, S. E., Oussayef, N. L., . . . Naimi, T. S. (2015). Youth drinking in the United States: Relationships with alcohol policies and adult drinking. *Pediatrics, 136*(1), 18-27.

192. World Health Organization. (2009). *Evidence for the effectiveness and cost-effectiveness of interventions to reduce alcohol-related harm.* Copenhagen, Denmark: WHO Regional Office for Europe.

193. Xu, X., & Chaloupka, F. J. (2011). The effects of prices on alcohol use and its consequences. *Alcohol Research and Health, 34*(2), 236-245.

194. Rabinovich, L., Brutscher, P.-B., de Vries, H., Tiessen, J., Clift, J., & Reding, A. (2009). *The affordability of alcoholic beverages in the European Union: Understanding the link between alcohol affordability, consumption and harms.* Santa Monica, CA: RAND Corporation.

195. Fogarty, J. (2006). The nature of the demand for alcohol: Understanding elasticity. *British Food Journal, 108*(4), 316-332.

196. Wagenaar, A. C., Tobler, A. L., & Komro, K. A. (2010). Effects of alcohol tax and price policies on morbidity and mortality: A systematic review. *American Journal of Public Health, 100*(11), 2270-2278.

197. Gallet, C. A. (2007). The demand for alcohol: A meta-analysis of elasticities. *Australian Journal of Agricultural and Resource Economics, 51*(2), 121-135.

198. Kenkel, D. S. (1993). Drinking, driving, and deterrence: The effectiveness and social costs of alternative policies. *The Journal of Law & Economics, 36*(2), 877-913.

199. Xu, Y., Yu, Q., Scribner, R., Theall, K., Scribner, S., & Simonsen, N. (2012). Multilevel spatiotemporal change-point models for evaluating the effect of an alcohol outlet control policy on changes in neighborhood assaultive violence rates. *Spatial and Spatio-temporal Epidemiology, 3*(2), 121-128.

200. Anderson, P., Chisholm, D., & Fuhr, D. C. (2009). Effectiveness and cost-effectiveness of policies and programmes to reduce the harm caused by alcohol. *The Lancet, 373*(9682), 2234-2246.

201. Zhang, X., Hatcher, B., Clarkson, L., Holt, J., Bagchi, S., Kanny, D., & Brewer, R. (2015). Changes in density of on-premises alcohol outlets and impact on violent crime, Atlanta, Georgia, 1997–2007. *Preventing Chronic Disease, 12*(E84).

202. Gruenewald, P. J., & Remer, L. (2006). Changes in outlet densities affect violence rates. *Alcoholism: Clinical and Experimental Research, 30*(7), 1184-1193.

203. Yu, Q., Scribner, R., Carlin, B., Theall, K., Simonsen, N., Ghosh-Dastidar, B., . . . Mason, K. (2008). Multilevel spatio-temporal dual changepoint models for relating alcohol outlet destruction and changes in neighbourhood rates of assaultive violence. *Geospatial Health, 2*(2), 161-172.

204. Mosher, J. F. (1979). Dram shop liability and the prevention of alcohol-related problems. *Journal of Studies on Alcohol, 40*(9), 773-798.

205. Rammohan, V., Hahn, R. A., Elder, R., Brewer, R., Fielding, J., Naimi, T. S., . . . Services, T. F. o. C. P. (2011). Effects of dram shop liability and enhanced overservice law enforcement initiatives on excessive alcohol consumption and related harms: Two Community Guide systematic reviews. *American Journal of Preventive Medicine, 41*(3), 334-343.

206. Middleton, J. C., Hahn, R. A., Kuzara, J. L., Elder, R., Brewer, R., Chattopadhyay, S., . . . Lawrence, B. (2010). Effectiveness of policies maintaining or restricting days of alcohol sales on excessive alcohol consumption and related harms. *American Journal of Preventive Medicine, 39*(6), 575-589.

207. Hahn, R. A., Kuzara, J. L., Elder, R., Brewer, R., Chattopadhyay, S., Fielding, J., . . . Lawrence, B. (2010). Effectiveness of policies restricting hours of alcohol sales in preventing excessive alcohol consumption and related harms. *American Journal of Preventive Medicine, 39*(6), 590-604.

208. McMillan, G. P., & Lapham, S. (2006). Effectiveness of bans and laws in reducing traffic deaths: Legalized Sunday packaged alcohol sales and alcohol-related traffic crashes and crash fatalities in New Mexico. *American Journal of Public Health, 96*(11), 1944-1948.

209. Community Preventive Services Task Force. (2012). Recommendations on privatization of alcohol retail sales and prevention of excessive alcohol consumption and related harms. *American Journal of Preventive Medicine, 42*(4), 428-429.

210. Cook, P. J. (2012). Alcohol retail privatization. *American Journal of Preventive Medicine, 42*(4), 430-432.

211. Fell, J. C., & Voas, R. B. (2006). Mothers Against Drunk Driving (MADD): The first 25 years. *Traffic Injury Prevention, 7*(3), 195-212.

212. Cummings, P., Rivara, F. P., Olson, C. M., & Smith, K. M. (2006). Changes in traffic crash mortality rates attributed to use of alcohol, or lack of a seat belt, air bag, motorcycle helmet, or bicycle helmet, United States, 1982–2001. *Injury Prevention, 12*(3), 148-154.

213. Hingson, R., & White, A. (2014). New research findings since the 2007 Surgeon General's Call to Action to Prevent and Reduce Underage Drinking: A review. *Journal of Studies on Alcohol and Drugs, 75*(1), 158-169.

214. Fell, J. C., Fisher, D. A., Voas, R. B., Blackman, K., & Tippetts, A. S. (2009). The impact of underage drinking laws on alcohol-related fatal crashes of young drivers. *Alcoholism: Clinical and Experimental Research, 33*(7), 1208-1219.

215. Shults, R. A., Elder, R. W., Sleet, D. A., Nichols, J. L., Alao, M. O., Carande-Kulis, V. G., . . . Task Force on Community Preventive Services. (2001). Reviews of evidence regarding interventions to reduce alcohol-impaired driving. *American Journal of Preventive Medicine, 21*(4), 66-88.

216. Johnson, D., & Fell, J. (1995). *The impact of lowering the illegal BAC limit to .08 in five states in the US.* Paper presented at the 39th Proceedings of the Association for the Advancement of Automotive Medicine (AAAM). Retrieved from http://casr.adelaide.edu.au/T95/paper/s15p1.html. Accessed on April 12, 2016.

217. Hingson, R., Heeren, T., & Winter, M. (2000). Effects of recent 0.08% legal blood alcohol limits on fatal crash involvement. *Injury Prevention, 6*(2), 109-114.

218. Dee, T. S. (2001). Does setting limits save lives? The case of 0.08 BAC laws. *Journal of Policy Analysis and Management, 20*(1), 111-128.

219. Voas, R. B., Taylor, E., Baker, T. K., & Tippetts, P. S. (2000). *Effectiveness of the Illinois 0.08% law.* Washington, DC: National Highway Traffic Safety Administration.

220. Hingson, R., Heeren, T., & Winter, M. (1996). Lowering state legal blood alcohol limits to 0.08%: The effect on fatal motor vehicle crashes. *American Journal of Public Health, 86*(9), 1297-1299.

221. Voas, R. B., & Tippetts, A. S. (1999). *The relationship of alcohol safety laws to drinking drivers in fatal crashes.* (0001-4575). Washington, DC: National Highway Traffic Safety Administration.

PREVENTION

222. Bergen, G., Pitan, A., Qu, S., Shults, R. A., Chattopadhyay, S. K., Elder, R. W., . . . Nichols, J. L. (2014). Publicized sobriety checkpoint programs: A Community Guide systematic review. *American Journal of Preventive Medicine, 46*(5), 529-539.

223. Goodwin, A., Kirley, B., Sandt, L., Hall, W., Thomas, L., O'Brien, N., & Summerlin, D. (2013). *Countermeasures that work: A highway safety countermeasure guide for state highway safety offices* (7th ed.). (Report No. DOT HS 811 727). Washington, DC: National Highway Traffic Safety Administration.

224. Lenk, K. M., Nelson, T. F., Toomey, T. L., Jones-Webb, R., & Erickson, D. J. (2016). Sobriety checkpoint and open container laws in US: Associations with reported drinking-driving. *Traffic Injury Prevention.*

225. Elder, R. W., Voas, R., Beirness, D., Shults, R. A., Sleet, D. A., Nichols, J. L., . . . Services, T. F. o. C. P. (2011). Effectiveness of ignition interlocks for preventing alcohol-impaired driving and alcohol-related crashes: A Community Guide systematic review. *American Journal of Preventive Medicine, 40*(3), 362-376.

226. Kaufman, E. J., & Wiebe, D. J. (2016). Impact of state ignition interlock laws on alcohol-involved crash deaths in the United States. *American Journal of Public Health, 106*(5), 865-871.

227. Xuan, Z., Blanchette, J. G., Nelson, T. F., Heeren, T. C., Nguyen, T. H., & Naimi, T. S. (2015). Alcohol policies and impaired driving in the United States: Effects of driving-vs. drinking-oriented policies. *The International Journal of Alcohol and Drug Research, 4*(2), 119-130.

228. Miech, R. A., Johnston, L. D., O'Malley, P. M., Bachman, J. G., & Schulenberg, J. E. (2015). *Monitoring the Future national survey results on drug use, 1975-2014: Volume I, secondary school students* (Vol. 1). Ann Arbor, MI: Institute for Social Research, The University of Michigan.

229. McCartt, A. T., Hellinga, L. A., & Kirley, B. B. (2010). The effects of minimum legal drinking age 21 laws on alcohol-related driving in the United States. *Journal of Safety Research, 41*(2), 173-181.

230. National Highway Traffic Safety Administration. (2015). *Traffic safety facts 2014: A compilation of motor vehicle crash data from the fatality analysis reporting system and the general estimates system.* Washington, DC: National Highway Traffic Safety Administration.

231. Voas, R. B., Torres, P., Romano, E., & Lacey, J. H. (2012). Alcohol-related risk of driver fatalities: An update using 2007 data. *Journal of Studies on Alcohol and Drugs, 73*(3), 341-350.

232. Carpenter, C., & Dobkin, C. (2011). The minimum legal drinking age and public health. *The Journal of Economic Perspectives, 25*(2), 133-156.

233. Hingson, R., Heeren, T., & Winter, M. (1994). Lower legal blood alcohol limits for young drivers. *Public Health Reports, 109*(6), 738-744.

234. Wagenaar, A. C., O'Malley, P. M., & LaFond, C. (2001). Lowered legal blood alcohol limits for young drivers: Effects on drinking, driving, and driving-after-drinking behaviors in 30 states. *American Journal of Public Health, 91*(5), 801-804.

235. Cavazos-Rehg, P. A., Krauss, M. J., Spitznagel, E. L., Chaloupka, F. J., Schootman, M., Grucza, R. A., & Bierut, L. J. (2012). Associations between selected state laws and teenagers' drinking and driving behaviors. *Alcoholism: Clinical and Experimental Research, 36*(9), 1647-1652.

236. Dills, A. K. (2010). Social host liability for minors and underage drunk-driving accidents. *Journal of Health Economics, 29*(2), 241-249.

237. Paschall, M. J., Grube, J. W., Thomas, S., Cannon, C., & Treffers, R. (2012). Relationships between local enforcement, alcohol availability, drinking norms, and adolescent alcohol use in 50 California cities. *Journal of Studies on Alcohol and Drugs, 73*(4), 657-665.

238. Snyder, L. B., Milici, F. F., Slater, M., Sun, H., & Strizhakova, Y. (2006). Effects of alcohol advertising exposure on drinking among youth. *Archives of Pediatrics & Adolescent Medicine, 160*(1), 18-24.

239. Saffer, H., & Dave, D. (2006). Alcohol advertising and alcohol consumption by adolescents. *Health Economics, 15*(6), 617-637.

240. Siegfried, N., Pienaar, D. C., Ataguba, J. E., Volmink, J., Kredo, T., Jere, M., & Parry, C. D. (2014). Restricting or banning alcohol advertising to reduce alcohol consumption in adults and adolescents. *Cochrane Database of Systematic Reviews*(11).

241. Centers for Disease Control and Prevention. (2016). Prevention status reports: Alcohol-related harms. Retrieved from http://www.cdc.gov/psr/national-summary/arh.html. Accessed on September 2, 2016.

242. Centers for Disease Control and Prevention. (2014). Prevention status reports 2013: Excessive alcohol use. Retrieved from http://www.cdc.gov/psr/2013/alcohol/index.html. Accessed on September 2, 2016.

243. Fell, J. C., Scherer, M., Thomas, S., & Voas, R. B. (2016). Assessing the impact of twenty underage drinking laws. *Journal of Studies on Alcohol and Drugs, 77*(2), 249-260.

244. Nelson, D. E., Naimi, T. S., Brewer, R. D., & Nelson, H. A. (2009). State alcohol-use estimates among youth and adults, 1993–2005. *American Journal of Preventive Medicine, 36*(3), 218-224.

245. Paulozzi, L. J., Kilbourne, E. M., & Desai, H. A. (2011). Prescription drug monitoring programs and death rates from drug overdose. *Pain Medicine, 12*(5), 747-754.

246. Office of Diversion Control, & Drug Enforcement Administration. (2015). Automation of reports and consolidated orders system (ARCOS). Retrieved from http://www.deadiversion.usdoj.gov/arcos/. Accessed

247. Haffajee, R. L., Jena, A. B., & Weiner, S. G. (2015). Mandatory use of prescription drug monitoring programs. *JAMA, 313*(9), 891-892.

248. Haegerich, T. M., Paulozzi, L. J., Manns, B. J., & Jones, C. M. (2014). What we know, and don't know, about the impact of state policy and systems-level interventions on prescription drug overdose. *Drug and Alcohol Dependence, 145*, 34-47.

249. Prescription Drug Monitoring Program Center of Excellence. (2016). *COE Briefing: PDMP prescriber use mandates: Characteristics, current status, and outcomes in selected states.* Waltham, MA: Brandeis University.

250. Rutkow, L., Chang, H.-Y., Daubresse, M., Webster, D. W., Stuart, E. A., & Alexander, G. C. (2015). Effect of Florida's prescription drug monitoring program and pill mill laws on opioid prescribing and use. *JAMA Internal Medicine, 175*(10), 1642-1649.

251. Patrick, S. W., Fry, C. E., Jones, T. F., & Buntin, M. B. (2016). Implementation of prescription drug monitoring programs associated with reductions in opioid-related death rates. *Health Affairs*.

252. Meara, E., Horwitz, J. R., Powell, W., McClelland, L., Zhou, W., O'Malley, A. J., & Morden, N. E. (2016). State legal restrictions and prescription-opioid use among disabled adults. *New England Journal of Medicine, 375*(1), 44-53.

253. Dowell, D., Haegerich, T. M., & R., C. (2016). CDC guideline for prescribing opioids for chronic pain - United States. *MMWR, 65*(1), 1-49.

254. National Institute on Drug Abuse. (2016). DrugFacts: Marijuana. Retrieved from https://www.drugabuse.gov/publications/drugfacts/marijuana. Accessed on June 20, 2016.

255. Crean, R. D., Crane, N. A., & Mason, B. J. (2011). An evidence based review of acute and long-term effects of cannabis use on executive cognitive functions. *Journal of Addiction Medicine, 5*(1), 1-15.

256. Mehmedic, Z., Chandra, S., Slade, D., Denham, H., Foster, S., Patel, A. S., . . . ElSohly, M. A. (2010). Potency trends of Δ9-THC and other cannabinoids in confiscated cannabis preparations from 1993 to 2008. *Journal of Forensic Sciences, 55*(5), 1209-1217.

257. Di Forti, M., Iyegbe, C., Sallis, H., Kolliakou, A., Falcone, M. A., Paparelli, A., . . . Marques, T. R. (2012). Confirmation that the AKT1 (rs2494732) genotype influences the risk of psychosis in cannabis users. *Biological Psychiatry, 72*(10), 811-816.

258. Caspi, A., Moffitt, T. E., Cannon, M., McClay, J., Murray, R., Harrington, H., . . . Braithwaite, A. (2005). Moderation of the effect of adolescent-onset cannabis use on adult psychosis by a functional polymorphism in the catechol-O-methyltransferase gene: longitudinal evidence of a gene X environment interaction. *Biological Psychiatry, 57*(10), 1117-1127.

259. Center for the Application of Prevention Technologies. (2014). *Prevention programs that address youth marijuana use.* Rockville, MD: Substance Abuse and Mental Health Services Administration.

260. Mason, W. A., Fleming, C. B., & Haggerty, K. P. (In press). Prevention of marijuana misuse: School-, family-, and community-based approaches. In M. T. Compton (Ed.), *Marijuana and mental health.* Arlington, VA: American Psychiatric Publishing.

261. Substance Abuse and Mental Health Administration. (2016). Practicing effective prevention. Retrieved from http://www.samhsa.gov/capt/practicing-effective-prevention. Accessed on June 27, 2016.

262. Spoth, R., Rohrbach, L. A., Greenberg, M., Leaf, P., Brown, C. H., Fagan, A., . . . Society for Prevention Research Type 2 Translational Task Force. (2013). Addressing core challenges for the next generation of type 2 translation research and systems: The translation science to population impact (TSci impact) framework. *Prevention Science, 14*(4), 319-351.

263. Castro, F. G., Barrera Jr, M., & Steiker, L. K. H. (2010). Issues and challenges in the design of culturally adapted evidence-based interventions. *Annual Review of Clinical Psychology, 6,* 213-239.

264. Burlew, A. K., Copeland, V. C., Ahuama-Jonas, C., & Calsyn, D. A. (2013). Does cultural adaptation have a role in substance abuse treatment? *Social Work in Public Health, 28*(3-4), 440-460.

265. Lau, A. S. (2006). Making the case for selective and directed cultural adaptations of evidence-based treatments: Examples from parent training. *Clinical Psychology: Science and Practice, 13*(4), 295-310.

266. Barrera Jr, M., Castro, F. G., Strycker, L. A., & Toobert, D. J. (2013). Cultural adaptations of behavioral health interventions: A progress report. *Journal of Consulting and Clinical Psychology, 81*(2), 196-205.

267. Castro, F. G., Barrera Jr, M., & Martinez Jr, C. R. (2004). The cultural adaptation of prevention interventions: Resolving tensions between fidelity and fit. *Prevention Science, 5*(1), 41-45.

268. Elliott, D. S., & Mihalic, S. (2004). Issues in disseminating and replicating effective prevention programs. *Prevention Science, 5*(1), 47-53.

269. Botvin, G. J., Schinke, S. P., Epstein, J. A., & Diaz, T. (1994). Effectiveness of culturally focused and generic skills training approaches to alcohol and drug abuse prevention among minority youths. *Psychology of Addictive Behaviors, 9*(3), 116-127.

270. Kumpfer, K. L., Alvarado, R., Smith, P., & Bellamy, N. (2002). Cultural sensitivity and adaptation in family-based prevention interventions. *Prevention Science, 3*(3), 241-246.

271. Castro, F. G., Kellison, J. G., & Corbin, W. R. (2014). Prevention of substance abuse in ethnic minority youth. In F. Leong (Ed.), *Handbook of multicultural psychology* (Vol. 2). Washington, DC: American Psychological Association.

272. Pettigrew, J., Graham, J. W., Miller-Day, M., Hecht, M. L., Krieger, J. L., & Shin, Y. J. (2015). Adherence and delivery: Implementation quality and program outcomes for the seventh-grade keepin'it REAL program. *Prevention Science, 16*(1), 90-99.

273. Colby, M., Hecht, M. L., Miller-Day, M., Krieger, J. L., Syvertsen, A. K., Graham, J. W., & Pettigrew, J. (2013). Adapting school-based substance use prevention curriculum through cultural grounding: A review and exemplar of adaptation processes for rural schools. *American Journal of Community Psychology, 51*(1-2), 190-205.

274. Donovan, D. M., Daley, D. C., Brigham, G. S., Hodgkins, C. C., Perl, H. I., & Floyd, A. S. (2011). How practice and science are balanced and blended in the NIDA clinical trials network: The bidirectional process in the development of the STAGE-12 protocol as an example. *The American Journal of Drug and Alcohol Abuse, 37*(5), 408-416.

275. Parsai, M. B., Castro, F. G., Marsiglia, F. F., Harthun, M. L., & Valdez, H. (2011). Using community based participatory research to create a culturally grounded intervention for parents and youth to prevent risky behaviors. *Prevention Science, 12*(1), 34-47.

276. Calsyn, D. A., Burlew, A. K., Hatch-Maillette, M. A., Wilson, J., Beadnell, B., & Wright, L. (2012). Real Men Are Safe–culturally adapted: Utilizing the Delphi process to revise Real Men Are Safe for an ethnically diverse group of men in substance abuse treatment. *AIDS Education and Prevention, 24*(2), 117-131.

277. Kumpfer, K. L., Xie, J., & O'Driscoll, R. (2012). Effectiveness of a culturally adapted strengthening families program 12–16 years for high-risk Irish families. *Child & Youth Care Forum, 41*(2), 173-195.

278. Collins, L. M. (2014). Optimizing family intervention programs: The multiphase optimization strategy (MOST). In S. M. McHale, P. Amato, & A. Booth (Eds.), *Emerging Methods in Family Research.* (Vol. 4, pp. 231-244). New York, NY: Springer.

279. Wingood, G. M., & DiClemente, R. J. (2008). The ADAPT-ITT model: A novel method of adapting evidence-based HIV Interventions. *Journal of Acquired Immune Deficiency Syndromes, 47*(Suppl 1), S40-S46.

280. Kumpfer, K. L., & Alvarado, R. (2003). Family-strengthening approaches for the prevention of youth problem behaviors. *American Psychologist, 58*(6-7), 457-465.

281. Prinz, R. J., & Sanders, M. R. (2007). Adopting a population-level approach to parenting and family support interventions. *Clinical Psychology Review, 27*(6), 739-749.

282. Ringwalt, C., Hanley, S., Vincus, A. A., Ennett, S. T., Rohrbach, L. A., & Bowling, J. M. (2008). The prevalence of effective substance use prevention curricula in the Nation's high schools. *The Journal of Primary Prevention, 29*(6), 479-488.

283. Crosse, S., Williams, B., Hagen, C. A., Harmon, M., Ristow, L., DiGaetano, R., ... Derzon, J. H. (2011). *Prevalence and implementation fidelity of research-based prevention programs in public schools: Final report.* Washington, DC: U.S. Department of Education, Office of Planning, Evaluation and Policy Development, Policy and Program Studies Service.

284. Gottfredson, D. C., & Gottfredson, G. D. (2002). Quality of school-based prevention programs: Results from a national survey. *Journal of Research in Crime and Delinquency, 39*(1), 3-35.

285. Rohrbach, L. A., Grana, R., Sussman, S., & Valente, T. W. (2006). Type II translation: Transporting prevention interventions from research to real-world settings. *Evaluation & the Health Professions, 29*(3), 302-333.

286. Gottfredson, D., Kumpfer, K., Polizzi-Fox, D., Wilson, D., Puryear, V., Beatty, P., & Vilmenay, M. (2006). The strengthening Washington D.C. families project: A randomized effectiveness trial of family-based prevention. *Prevention Science, 7*(1), 57-74.

287. Hallfors, D., & Godette, D. (2002). Will the "Principles of Effectiveness" improve prevention practice? Early findings from a diffusion study. *Health Education Research, 17*(4), 461-470.

288. Ringwalt, C. L., Ennett, S., Johnson, R., Rohrbach, L. A., Simons-Rudolph, A., Vincus, A., & Thorne, J. (2003). Factors associated with fidelity to substance use prevention curriculum guides in the nation's middle schools. *Health Education & Behavior, 30*(3), 375-391.

289. Tobler, N. S. (1986). Meta-analysis of 143 adolescent drug prevention programs: Quantitative outcome results of program participants compared to a control or comparison group. *Journal of Drug Issues, 16*(4), 537-567.

290. Derzon, J. H., Sale, E., Springer, J. F., & Brounstein, P. (2005). Estimating intervention effectiveness: Synthetic projection of field evaluation results. *The Journal of Primary Prevention, 26*(4), 321-343.

291. Pentz, M. A., Trebow, E. A., Hansen, W. B., MacKinnon, D. P., Dwyer, J. H., Johnson, C. A., ... Cormack, C. (1990). Effects of program implementation on adolescent drug use behavior: The Midwestern Prevention Project (MPP). *Evaluation Review, 14*(3), 264-289.

292. Botvin, G. J., Baker, E., Dusenbury, L., Botvin, E. M., & Diaz, T. (1995). Long-term follow-up results of a randomized drug abuse prevention trial in a white middle-class population. *JAMA, 273*(14), 1106-1112.

293. Weitzman, E. R., Nelson, T. F., Lee, H., & Wechsler, H. (2004). Reducing drinking and related harms in college: Evaluation of the "A Matter of Degree" program. *American Journal of Preventive Medicine, 27*(3), 187-196.

294. Fixsen, D. L., Naoom, S. F., Blase, K. A., & Friedman, R. M. (2005). *Implementation research: A synthesis of the literature.* (FMHI Publication #231). Tampa, FL: University of South Florida, Louis de la Parte Florida Mental Health Institute, The National Implementation Research Network.

295. Durlak, J. A., & DuPre, E. P. (2008). Implementation matters: A review of research on the influence of implementation on program outcomes and the factors affecting implementation. *American Journal of Community Psychology, 41*(3-4), 327-350.

296. Neta, G., Glasgow, R. E., Carpenter, C. R., Grimshaw, J. M., Rabin, B. A., Fernandez, M. E., & Brownson, R. C. (2014). A framework for enhancing the value of research for dissemination and implementation. *American Journal of Public Health, 105*(1), 49-57.

297. Fagan, A. A., Hawkins, J. D., & Catalano, R. F. (2011). Engaging communities to prevent underage drinking. *Alcohol Research & Health, 34*(2), 167-174.

298. Mihalic, S. F., & Irwin, K. (2003). Blueprints for violence prevention: From research to real-world settings—factors influencing the successful replication of model programs. *Youth Violence and Juvenile Justice, 1*(4), 307-329.

299. Spoth, R., Guyll, M., Lillehoj, C. J., Redmond, C., & Greenberg, M. (2007). PROSPER study of evidence-based intervention implementation quality by community–university partnerships. *Journal of Community Psychology, 35*(8), 981-999.

300. Spoth, R., Guyll, M., Redmond, C., Greenberg, M., & Feinberg, M. (2011). Six-year sustainability of evidence-based intervention implementation quality by community-university partnerships: The PROSPER study. *American Journal of Community Psychology, 48*(3-4), 412-425.

301. Spoth, R., Clair, S., Greenberg, M., Redmond, C., & Shin, C. (2007). Toward dissemination of evidence-based family interventions: Maintenance of community-based partnership recruitment results and associated factors. *Journal of Family Psychology, 21*(2), 137-146.

302. Fagan, A. A., Arthur, M. W., Hanson, K., Briney, J. S., & Hawkins, J. D. (2011). Effects of Communities That Care on the adoption and implementation fidelity of evidence-based prevention programs in communities: Results from a randomized controlled trial. *Prevention Science, 12*(3), 223-234.

303. Fagan, A. A., Hanson, K., Briney, J. S., & Hawkins, J. D. (2012). Sustaining the utilization and high quality implementation of tested and effective prevention programs using the Communities That Care prevention system. *American Journal of Community Psychology, 49*(3-4), 365-377.

304. Cooper, B. R., Bumbarger, B. K., & Moore, J. E. (2015). Sustaining evidence-based prevention programs: Correlates in a large-scale dissemination initiative. *Prevention Science, 16*(1), 145-157.

305. Glasgow, R. E., Vinson, C., Chambers, D., Khoury, M. J., Kaplan, R. M., & Hunter, C. (2012). National Institutes of Health approaches to dissemination and implementation science: Current and future directions. *American Journal of Public Health, 102*(7), 1274-1281.

306. Institute of Medicine (IOM) and National Research Council (NRC). (2014). *Strategies for scaling effective family-focused preventive interventions to promote children's cognitive, affective, and behavioral health: Workshop summary*. Washington, DC: The National Academies Press.

307. Tabak, R. G., Khoong, E. C., Chambers, D. A., & Brownson, R. C. (2012). Bridging research and practice: Models for dissemination and implementation research. *American Journal of Preventive Medicine, 43*(3), 337-350.

308. Shediac-Rizkallah, M. C., & Bone, L. R. (1998). Planning for the sustainability of community-based health programs: Conceptual frameworks and future directions for research, practice and policy. *Health Education Research, 13*(1), 87-108.

309. Altman, D. G. (1995). Sustaining interventions in community systems: On the relationship between researchers and communities. *Health Psychology, 14*(6), 526-536.

310. Backer, T. E., & Guerra, N. G. (2011). Mobilizing communities to implement evidence-based practices in youth violence prevention: The state of the art. *American Journal of Community Psychology, 48*(1-2), 31-42.

311. Greenhalgh, T., Robert, G., Macfarlane, F., Bate, P., & Kyriakidou, O. (2004). Diffusion of innovations in service organizations: Systematic review and recommendations. *Milbank Quarterly, 82*(4), 581-629.

312. Damschroder, L. J., Aron, D. C., Keith, R. E., Kirsh, S. R., Alexander, J. A., & Lowery, J. C. (2009). Fostering implementation of health services research findings into practice: A consolidated framework for advancing implementation science. *Implementation Science, 4*(50), 1-15.

313. Rogers, E. M. (1995). *Diffusion of innovations* (4th ed.). New York, NY: Free Press.

314. Meyers, D. C., Durlak, J. A., & Wandersman, A. (2012). The quality implementation framework: A synthesis of critical steps in the implementation process. *American Journal of Community Psychology, 50*(3-4), 462-480.

315. Flaspohler, P., Duffy, J., Wandersman, A., Stillman, L., & Maras, M. A. (2008). Unpacking prevention capacity: An intersection of research-to-practice models and community-centered models. *American Journal of Community Psychology, 41*(3-4), 182-196.

316. Backer, T. E. (1995). Assessing and enhancing readiness for change: Implications for technology transfer. In T. E. Backer, S. L. David, & G. Soucy (Eds.), *Reviewing the behavioral science knowledge base on technology transfer.* (Vol. 155, pp. 21-41). Rockville, MD: National Institute on Drug Abuse.

317. Edwards, R. W., Jumper-Thurman, P., Plested, B. A., Oetting, E. R., & Swanson, L. (2000). Community readiness: Research to practice. *Journal of Community Psychology, 28*(3), 291-307.

318. Foster-Fishman, P. G., & Watson, E. R. (2012). The ABLe change framework: A conceptual and methodological tool for promoting systems change. *American Journal of Community Psychology, 49*(3-4), 503-516.

319. Mothers Against Drunk Driving. (2002). *Rating the states: An assessment of the nation's attention to the problem of drunk driving & underage drinking.* Irving, TX: Mothers Against Drunk Driving.

320. Shults, R. A., Sleet, D. A., Elder, R. W., Ryan, G. W., & Sehgal, M. (2002). Association between state level drinking and driving countermeasures and self reported alcohol impaired driving. *Injury Prevention, 8*(2), 106-110.

321. Wolfson, M. (1995). The legislative impact of social movement organizations: The anti-drunken driving movement and the 21-year-old drinking age. *Social Science Quarterly, 76*(2), 311-327.

322. Community Anti-Drug Coalitions of America. (n.d.). *Strategizer 54 - A community's call to action: Underage drinking and impaired driving.* Alexandria, VA: Community Anti-Drug Coalitions of America.

323. Bonnie, R. J., & O'Connell, M. E. (Eds.). (2004). *Reducing underage drinking: A collective responsibility.* Washington, DC: National Academies Press.

324. Fagan, A. A., & Hawkins, J. D. (2012). Community-based substance use prevention. In B. C. Welsh & D. P. Farrington (Eds.), *The Oxford handbook on crime prevention* (pp. 247-268). New York, NY: Oxford University Press.

325. Chinman, M., Hannah, G., Wandersman, A., Ebener, P., Hunter, S. B., Imm, P., & Sheldon, J. (2005). Developing a community science research agenda for building community capacity for effective preventive interventions. *American Journal of Community Psychology, 35*(3-4), 143-157.

326. Feinberg, M. E., Ridenour, T. A., & Greenberg, M. T. (2008). The longitudinal effect of technical assistance dosage on the functioning of Communities That Care prevention boards in Pennsylvania. *The Journal of Primary Prevention, 29*(2), 145-165.

327. Rhoades, B. L., Bumbarger, B. K., & Moore, J. E. (2012). The role of a state-level prevention support system in promoting high-quality implementation and sustainability of evidence-based programs. *American Journal of Community Psychology, 50*(3-4), 386-401.

328. Leeman, J., Calancie, L., Hartman, M. A., Escoffery, C. T., Herrmann, A. K., Tague, L. E., . . . Samuel-Hodge, C. (2015). What strategies are used to build practitioners' capacity to implement community-based interventions and are they effective? A systematic review. *Implementation Science, 10*(80).

329. Foster-Fishman, P. G., Berkowitz, S. L., Lounsbury, D. W., Jacobson, S., & Allen, N. A. (2001). Building collaborative capacity in community coalitions: A review and integrative framework. *American Journal of Community Psychology, 29*(2), 241-261.

330. Arthur, M. W., & Blitz, C. (2000). Bridging the gap between science and practice in drug abuse prevention through needs assessment and strategic community planning. *Journal of Community Psychology, 28*(3), 241-255.

331. Spoth, R. L., & Greenberg, M. T. (2005). Toward a comprehensive strategy for effective practitioner–scientist partnerships and larger-scale community health and well-being. *American Journal of Community Psychology, 35*(3-4), 107-126.

332. Kreuter, M. W., Lezin, N. A., & Young, L. A. (2000). Evaluating community-based collaborative mechanisms: Implications for practitioners. *Health Promotion Practice, 1*(1), 49-63.

333. Florin, P., Mitchell, R., & Stevenson, J. (1993). Identifying training and technical assistance needs in community coalitions: A developmental approach. *Health Education Research, 8*(3), 417-432.

334. Hawkins, J. D., Catalano, R. F., & Arthur, M. W. (2002). Promoting science-based prevention in communities. *Addictive Behaviors, 27*(6), 951-976.

335. Woolf, S. H. (2008). The power of prevention and what it requires. *JAMA, 299*(20), 2437-2439.

336. Stevenson, J. F., & Mitchell, R. E. (2003). Community-level collaboration for substance abuse prevention. *The Journal of Primary Prevention, 23*(3), 371-404.

337. Butterfoss, F. D., Goodman, R. M., & Wandersman, A. (1993). Community coalitions for prevention and health promotion. *Health Education Research, 8*(3), 315-330.

338. Hawkins, J. D., Van Horn, M. L., & Arthur, M. W. (2004). Community variation in risk and protective factors and substance use outcomes. *Prevention Science, 5*(4), 213-220.

339. Gingiss, P. M., Roberts-Gray, C., & Boerm, M. (2006). Bridge-It: A system for predicting implementation fidelity for school-based tobacco prevention programs. *Prevention Science, 7*(2), 197-207.

340. Substance Abuse and Mental Health Services Administration. National registry of evidence-based programs and practices (NREPP). Retrieved from http://www.samhsa.gov/nrepp. Accessed on March 11, 2016.

341. Mihalic, S. F., & Elliott, D. S. (2015). Evidence-based programs registry: Blueprints for Healthy Youth Development. *Evaluation and Program Planning, 48*, 124-131.

342. National Institute on Alcohol Abuse and Alcoholism. (n.d.). Alcohol policy information system. Retrieved from http://www.alcoholpolicy.niaaa.nih.gov/. Accessed on March 4, 2016.

343. Wandersman, A., Duffy, J., Flaspohler, P., Noonan, R., Lubell, K., Stillman, L., . . . Saul, J. (2008). Bridging the gap between prevention research and practice: The interactive systems framework for dissemination and implementation. *American Journal of Community Psychology, 41*(3-4), 171-181.

344. Fagan, A. A., & Mihalic, S. (2003). Strategies for enhancing the adoption of school-based prevention programs: Lessons learned from the Blueprints for Violence Prevention replications of the Life Skills Training program. *Journal of Community Psychology, 31*(3), 235-253.

345. Moore, J. E., Bumbarger, B. K., & Cooper, B. R. (2013). Examining adaptations of evidence-based programs in natural contexts. *The Journal of Primary Prevention, 34*(3), 147-161.

346. Hoagwood, K., Burns, B. J., Kiser, L., Ringeisen, H., & Schoenwald, S. K. (2001). Evidence-based practice in child and adolescent mental health services. *Psychiatric Services, 52*(9), 1179-1189.

347. Backer, T. E. (2001). *Finding the balance: Program fidelity and adaptation in substance abuse prevention: A state-of-the-art review.* Rockville, MD: Substance Abuse and Mental Health Services Administration, Center for Substance Abuse Prevention.

348. Olds, D. L., Robinson, J., O'Brien, R., Luckey, D. W., Pettitt, L. M., Henderson, C. R., . . . Hiatt, S. (2002). Home visiting by paraprofessionals and by nurses: A randomized, controlled trial. *Pediatrics, 110*(3), 486-496.

349. Dusenbury, L., Brannigan, R., Falco, M., & Hansen, W. B. (2003). A review of research on fidelity of implementation: Implications for drug abuse prevention in school settings. *Health Education Research, 18*(2), 237-256.

350. Institute of Medicine, & Committee on Crossing the Quality Chasm. (2006). *Improving the quality of health care for mental and substance-use conditions.* Washington, DC: National Academies Press.

351. Hawkins, J. D., Shapiro, V. B., & Fagan, A. A. (2010). Disseminating effective community prevention practices: Opportunities for social work education. *Research on Social Work Practice, 20*(5), 518-527.

352. Becker, K. D., Bradshaw, C. P., Domitrovich, C., & Ialongo, N. S. (2013). Coaching teachers to improve implementation of the good behavior game. *Administration and Policy in Mental Health and Mental Health Services Research, 40*(6), 482-493.

353. Spoth, R., & Greenberg, M. (2011). Impact challenges in community science-with-practice: Lessons from PROSPER on transformative practitioner-scientist partnerships and prevention infrastructure development. *American Journal of Community Psychology, 48*(1-2), 106-119.

354. Elias, M. J., Zins, J. E., Graczyk, P. A., & Weissberg, R. P. (2003). Implementation, sustainability, and scaling up of social-emotional and academic innovations in public schools. *School Psychology Review, 32*(3), 303-319.

355. Kershner, S., Flynn, S., Prince, M., Potter, S. C., Craft, L., & Alton, F. (2014). Using data to improve fidelity when implementing evidence-based programs. *Journal of Adolescent Health, 54*(3), S29-S36.

356. Brownson, R. C., Allen, P., Jacob, R. R., Harris, J. K., Duggan, K., Hipp, P. R., & Erwin, P. C. (2015). Understanding mis-implementation in public health practice. *American Journal of Preventive Medicine, 48*(5), 543-551.

357. Johnson, K., Hays, C., Center, H., & Daley, C. (2004). Building capacity and sustainable prevention innovations: A sustainability planning model. *Evaluation and Program Planning, 27*(2), 135-149.

358. Proctor, E., Luke, D., Calhoun, A., McMillen, C., Brownson, R., McCrary, S., & Padek, M. (2015). Sustainability of evidence-based healthcare: Research agenda, methodological advances, and infrastructure support. *Implementation Science, 10*(88).

359. Stirman, S. W., Kimberly, J., Cook, N., Calloway, A., Castro, F., & Charns, M. (2012). The sustainability of new programs and innovations: A review of the empirical literature and recommendations for future research. *Implementation Science, 7*(17), 1-19.

360. Feinberg, M. E., Bontempo, D. E., & Greenberg, M. T. (2008). Predictors and level of sustainability of community prevention coalitions. *American Journal of Preventive Medicine, 34*(6), 495-501.

361. Tibbits, M. K., Bumbarger, B. K., Kyler, S. J., & Perkins, D. F. (2010). Sustaining evidence-based interventions under real-world conditions: Results from a large-scale diffusion project. *Prevention Science, 11*(3), 252-262.

362. Testa, M., Hoffman, J. H., Livingston, J. A., & Turrisi, R. (2010). Preventing college women's sexual victimization through parent based intervention: A randomized controlled trial. *Prevention Science, 11*(3), 308-318.

363. United Nations Office of Drugs and Crime. (2013). *International standards on drug use prevention.* Vienna, Austria: United Nations. Retrieved from http://www.unodc.org/unodc/en/prevention/prevention-standards.html. Accessed on April 6, 2016.

364. Flay, B. R., Biglan, A., Boruch, R. F., Castro, F. G., Gottfredson, D., Kellam, S., . . . Ji, P. (2005). Standards of evidence: Criteria for efficacy, effectiveness and dissemination. *Prevention Science, 6*(3), 151-175.

365. Gottfredson, D. C., Cook, T. D., Gardner, F. E., Gorman-Smith, D., Howe, G. W., Sandler, I. N., & Zafft, K. M. (2015). Standards of evidence for efficacy, effectiveness, and scale-up research in prevention science: Next generation. *Prevention Science, 16*(7), 893-926.

366. Hingson, R., McGovern, T., Howland, J., Heeren, T., Winter, M., & Zakocs, R. C. (1996). Reducing alcohol-impaired driving in Massachusetts: The Saving Lives program. *American Journal of Public Health, 86*(6), 791-797.

367. Wolfson, M., Champion, H., McCoy, T. P., Rhodes, S. D., Ip, E. H., Blocker, J. N., . . . Durant, R. H. (2012). Impact of a randomized campus/community trial to prevent high-risk drinking among college students. *Alcoholism: Clinical and Experimental Research, 36*(10), 1767-1778.

368. Treno, A. J., Gruenewald, P. J., Lee, J. P., & Remer, L. G. (2007). The Sacramento Neighborhood Alcohol Prevention Project: Outcomes from a community prevention trial. *Journal of Studies on Alcohol and Drugs, 68*(2), 197-207.

CHAPTER 4.
EARLY INTERVENTION, TREATMENT, AND MANAGEMENT OF SUBSTANCE USE DISORDERS

Chapter 4 Preview

A substance use disorder is a medical illness characterized by clinically significant impairments in health, social function, and voluntary control over substance use.[2] Substance use disorders range in severity, duration, and complexity from mild to severe. In 2015, 20.8 million people aged 12 or older met criteria for a substance use disorder. While historically the great majority of treatment has occurred in specialty substance use disorder treatment programs with little involvement by primary or general health care, a shift is occurring toward the delivery of treatment services in general health care practice. For those with mild to moderate substance use disorders, treatment through the general health care system may be sufficient, while those with severe substance use disorders (addiction) may require specialty treatment.

The good news is that a spectrum of effective strategies and services are available to identify, treat, and manage substance use problems and substance use disorders. Research shows that the most effective way to help someone with a substance use problem who may be at risk for developing a substance

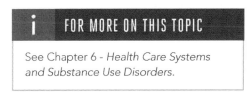

FOR MORE ON THIS TOPIC

See Chapter 6 - *Health Care Systems and Substance Use Disorders.*

use disorder is to intervene early, before the condition can progress. With this recognition, screening for substance misuse is increasingly being provided in general health care settings, so that emerging problems can be detected and early intervention provided if necessary. The addition of services to address substance use problems and disorders in mainstream health care has extended the continuum of care, and includes a range of effective, evidence-based medications, behavioral therapies, and supportive services. However, a number of barriers have limited the widespread adoption of these services, including lack of resources, insufficient training, and workforce shortages.[5] This is particularly true for the treatment of those with co-occurring substance use and physical or mental disorders.[6,7]

TREATMENT

This chapter provides an overview of the scientific evidence supporting the effectiveness of treatment interventions, therapies, services, and medications available to identify, treat, and manage substance use problems and disorders.

KEY FINDINGS*

- Well-supported scientific evidence shows that substance use disorders can be effectively treated, with recurrence rates no higher than those for other chronic illnesses such as diabetes, asthma, and hypertension. With comprehensive continuing care, recovery is now an achievable outcome.

- Only about 1 in 10 people with a substance use disorder receive any type of specialty treatment. The great majority of treatment has occurred in specialty substance use disorder treatment programs with little involvement by primary or general health care. However, a shift is occurring to mainstream the delivery of early intervention and treatment services into general health care practice.

- Well-supported scientific evidence shows that medications can be effective in treating serious substance use disorders, but they are under-used. The U.S. Food and Drug Administration (FDA) has approved three medications to treat alcohol use disorders and three others to treat opioid use disorders. However, an insufficient number of existing treatment programs or practicing physicians offer these medications. To date, no FDA-approved medications are available to treat marijuana, cocaine, methamphetamine, or other substance use disorders, with the exception of the medications previously noted for alcohol and opioid use disorders.

- Supported scientific evidence indicates that substance misuse and substance use disorders can be reliably and easily identified through screening and that less severe forms of these conditions often respond to brief physician advice and other types of brief interventions. Well-supported scientific evidence shows that these brief interventions work with mild severity alcohol use disorders, but only promising evidence suggests that they are effective with drug use disorders.

- Well-supported scientific evidence shows that treatment for substance use disorders—including inpatient, residential, and outpatient—are cost-effective compared with no treatment.

- The primary goals and general management methods of treatment for substance use disorders are the same as those for the treatment of other chronic illnesses. The goals of treatment are to reduce key symptoms to non-problematic levels and improve health and functional status; this is equally true for those with co-occurring substance use disorders and other psychiatric disorders. Key components of care are medications, behavioral therapies, and recovery support services (RSS).

- Well-supported scientific evidence shows that behavioral therapies can be effective in treating substance use disorders, but most evidence-based behavioral therapies are often implemented with limited fidelity and are under-used. Treatments using these evidence-based practices have shown better results than non-evidence-based treatments and services.

- Promising scientific evidence suggests that several electronic technologies, like the adoption of electronic health records (EHRs) and the use of telehealth, could improve access, engagement, monitoring, and continuing supportive care of those with substance use disorders.

*The Centers for Disease Control and Prevention (CDC) summarizes strength of evidence as: "Well-supported": when evidence is derived from multiple controlled trials or large-scale population studies; "Supported": when evidence is derived from rigorous but fewer or smaller trials; and "Promising": when evidence is derived from a practical or clinical sense and is widely practiced.[8]

Continuum of Treatment Services

Substance use disorders typically emerge during adolescence and often (but not always) progress in severity and complexity with continued substance misuse.[9,10] Currently, substance use disorders are classified diagnostically into three severity categories: mild, moderate, and severe.[2]

Substance use disorder treatment is designed to help individuals stop or reduce harmful substance misuse, improve their health and social function, and manage their risk for relapse. In this regard, substance use disorder treatment is effective and has a positive economic impact. Research shows that treatment also improves individuals' productivity,[11] health,[11,12] and overall quality of life.[13-15] In addition, studies show that every dollar spent on substance use disorder treatment saves $4 in health care costs and $7 in criminal justice costs.[11]

Mild substance use disorders can be identified quickly and reliably in many medical and social settings. These common but less severe disorders often respond to brief motivational interventions and/or supportive monitoring, referred to as guided self-change.[16] In contrast, severe, complex, and chronic substance use disorders often require specialty substance use disorder treatment and continued post-treatment support to achieve full remission and recovery. To address the spectrum of substance use problems and disorders, a continuum of care provides individuals an array of service options based on need, including prevention, early intervention, treatment, and recovery support (**Figure 4.1**). Traditionally, the vast majority of treatment for substance use disorders has been provided in specialty substance use disorder treatment programs, and these programs vary substantially in their clinical objectives and in the frequency, intensity, and setting of care delivery.

> **KEY TERMS**
>
> **Substance Use Disorder Treatment.** A service or set of services that may include medication, counseling, and other supportive services designed to enable an individual to reduce or eliminate alcohol and/or other drug use, address associated physical or mental health problems, and restore the patient to maximum functional ability.[3]
>
> **Continuum of Care.** An integrated system of care that guides and tracks a person over time through a comprehensive array of health services appropriate to the individual's need. A continuum of care may include prevention, early intervention, treatment, continuing care, and recovery support.[4]

TREATMENT

Figure 4.1: Substance Use Status and Substance Use Care Continuum

Positive Physical, Social, and Mental Health	Substance Misuse	Substance Use Disorder
A state of physical, mental, and social well-being, free from substance misuse, in which an individual is able to realize his or her abilities, cope with the normal stresses of life, work productively and fruitfully, and make a contribution to his or her community.	The use of any substance in a manner, situation, amount, or frequency that can cause harm to the user and/or to those around them.	Clinically and functionally significant impairment caused by substance use, including health problems, disability, and failure to meet major responsibilities at work, school, or home; substance use disorders are measured on a continuum from mild, moderate, to severe based on a person's number of symptoms.

Substance Use Status Continuum

◄─────────────────────────────────►

Substance Use Care Continuum

Enhancing Health	Primary Prevention	Early Intervention	Treatment	Recovery Support
Promoting optimum physical and mental health and well-being, free from substance misuse, through health mmunications and access to health care services, income and economic security, and workplace certainty.	Addressing individual and environmental risk factors for substance use through evidence-based programs, policies, and strategies.	Screening and detecting substance use problems at an early stage and providing brief intervention, as needed.	Intervening through medication, counseling, and other supportive services to eliminate symptoms and achieve and maintain sobriety, physical, spiritual, and mental health and maximum functional ability. Levels of care include: • Outpatient services; • Intensive Outpatient/ Partial Hospitalization Services; • Residential/ Inpatient Services; and • Medically Managed Intensive Inpatient Services.	Removing barriers and providing supports to aid the long-term recovery process. Includes a range of social, educational, legal, and other services that facilitate recovery, wellness, and improved quality of life.

This chapter describes the early intervention and treatment components of the continuum of care, the major behavioral, pharmacological, and service components of care, services available, and emerging treatment technologies:

- *Early Intervention,* for addressing substance misuse problems or mild disorders and helping to prevent more severe substance use disorders.

- *Treatment engagement and harm reduction interventions,* for individuals who have a substance use disorder but who may not be ready to enter treatment, help engage individuals in treatment and reduce the risks and harms associated with substance misuse.

- *Substance use disorder treatment,* an individualized set of evidence-based clinical services designed to improve health and function, including medications and behavioral therapies.

- *Emerging treatment technologies* are increasingly being used to support the assessment, treatment, and maintenance of continuing contact with individuals with substance use disorders.

Early Intervention: Identifying and Engaging Individuals At Risk for Substance Misuse and Substance Use Disorders

Early intervention services can be provided in a variety of settings (e.g., school clinics, primary care offices, mental health clinics) to people who have problematic use or mild substance use disorders.[17] These services are usually provided when an individual presents for another medical condition or social service need and is not seeking treatment for a substance use disorder. The goals of early intervention are to reduce the harms associated with substance misuse, to reduce risk behaviors before they lead to injury,[18] to improve health and social function, and to prevent progression to a disorder and subsequent need for specialty substances use disorder services.[17,18] Early intervention consists of providing information about substance use risks, normal or safe levels of use, and strategies to quit or cut down on use and use-related risk behaviors, and facilitating patient initiation and engagement in treatment when needed. Early intervention services may be considered the bridge between prevention and treatment services. For individuals with more serious substance misuse, intervention in these settings can serve as a mechanism to engage them into treatment.[17]

Populations Who Should Receive Early Intervention

Early intervention should be provided to both adolescents and adults who are at risk of or show signs of substance misuse or a mild substance use disorder.[17] One group typically in need of early intervention is people who binge drink: people who have consumed at least 5 (for men) or 4 (for women) drinks on a single occasion at least once in the past 30 days.[19] Recent national survey data suggest that over 66 million individuals aged 12 or older can be classified as binge drinkers.[19] Of particular concern are the 1.4 million binge drinkers aged 12 to 17, who may be at higher risk for future substance use disorders because of their young age.[19]

Other groups who are likely to benefit from early intervention are people who use substances while driving and women who use substances while pregnant. In 2015, an estimated 214,000 women consumed alcohol while pregnant, and an estimated 109,000 pregnant women used illicit drugs.[19]

Available research shows that brief, early interventions, given by a respected care provider, such as a nurse, nurse educator, or physician, in the context of usual medical care (for example, a routine medical exam or care for an injury or illness) can educate and motivate many individuals who are misusing substances to understand and acknowledge their risky behavior and to reduce their substance use.[20,21]

Regardless of the substance, the first step to early intervention is screening to identify behaviors that put the individual at risk for harm or for developing a substance use disorder. Positive screening results should then be followed by brief advice or counseling tailored to the specific problems and interests of the individual and delivered in a non-judgmental manner, emphasizing both the importance of reducing substance use and the individual's ability to accomplish this goal.[17] Later follow-up monitoring should assess whether the screening and brief intervention were effective in reducing the substance use below risky levels or whether the person needs formal treatment.

Components of Early Intervention

One structured approach to delivering early intervention to people showing signs of substance misuse and/or early signs of a substance use disorder is through screening and brief intervention (SBI).[22]

Research has shown that several methods of SBI are effective in decreasing "at-risk" substance use and that they work for a variety of populations and in a variety of health care settings.[22,23] As mentioned earlier, this research has demonstrated positive effects for reducing alcohol use;[24,25] the research with SBI among those with other substance use disorders has shown mixed results.[26-29]

In addition, research shows that SBI can be cost-effective. For example, a randomized study compared SBI to screening alone for alcohol and drug use disorders among patients covered by Medicaid in eight emergency medicine clinics in the State of Washington. A year later, investigators compared total Medicaid expenditures between the two groups and found that the costs per member, per month for the SBI group were $185 to $192 lower than the costs for the screening-only group. This added up to a savings of more than $2,200 per patient in one year.[30]

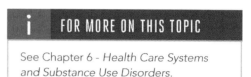

FOR MORE ON THIS TOPIC

See Chapter 6 - *Health Care Systems and Substance Use Disorders.*

SBI: Screening

Ideally, substance misuse screening should occur for all individuals who present in health care settings, including primary, urgent, psychiatric, and emergency care. Professional organizations, including the American College of Obstetricians and Gynecologists, the American Medical Association, the American Academy of Family Physicians, and the American Academy of Pediatrics recommend universal and ongoing screening for substance use and mental health issues for adults and adolescents.[31-36] Such screening practices can help identify the severity of the individual's substance use and whether substance use disorder treatment may be necessary.

Within these contexts, substance misuse can be reliably identified through dialogue, observation, medical tests, and screening instruments.[37] Several validated screening instruments have been developed to help non-specialty providers identify individuals who may have, or be at risk for, a substance use disorder.

Table 4.1 provides examples of available substance use screening tools, how they are used, and for which age groups. In addition to these tools, single-item screens for presence of drug use ("How many times in the past year have you used an illegal drug or used a prescription medication for nonmedical reasons?") and for alcohol use ("How many times in the past year have you had X or more drinks in a day?", where X is 5 for men and 4 for women) have been validated and shown in primary care to accurately identify individuals at risk for or experiencing a substance use disorder.[38-42]

Table 4.1: Evidence-Based Screening Tools for Substance Use

Screening Tool	Substance Type		Age Group	
	Alcohol	Drugs	Adolescents	Adults
Alcohol Screening and Brief Intervention for Adolescents and Youth: A Practitioner's Guide	✔		✔	
Alcohol Use Disorders Identification Test (AUDIT)	✔			✔
Alcohol Use Disorders Identification Test-C (AUDIT-C)	✔			✔
Brief Screener for Tobacco, Alcohol, and Other Drugs (BSTAD)	✔	✔	✔	
CRAFFT	✔	✔	✔	
CRAFFT (Part A)	✔	✔	✔	
Drug Abuse Screen Test (DAST-10)		✔		✔
DAST-20: Adolescent version		✔	✔	
Helping Patients Who Drink Too Much: A Clinicians' Guide	✔		✔	✔
NIDA Drug Use Screening Tool	✔	✔		✔
NIDA Drug Use Screening Tool: Quick Screen	✔	✔	See APA Adapted NM ASSIST tools	✔
Opioid Risk Tool		✔		✔
S2BI	✔	✔	✔	

Source: National Institute on Drug Abuse, (2015).[43]

SBI: Brief Interventions

Brief interventions (or brief advice) range from informal counseling to structured therapies. They often include feedback to the individual about their level of use relative to safe limits, as well as advice to aid the individual in decision-making.[17]

Motivational interviewing (MI) is a client-centered counseling style that addresses a person's ambivalence to change. A counselor uses a conversational approach to help their client discover their interest in changing their substance using behavior. The counselor asks the client to express their desire for change and any ambivalence they might have and then begins to work with the client on a plan to change their behavior and to make a commitment to the change process. The main purpose of MI is to examine and resolve ambivalence, and the counselor is intentionally directive in pursuing this goal.[44] It is effective in reducing the substance misuse of patients who come to medical settings for other health-related conditions.[45] In these settings, individuals who receive MI are more likely to adhere to a treatment plan and, subsequently, to have better outcomes.[24,46]

SAMHSA SBIRT Education

SAMHSA offers free SBIRT Continuing Medical Education and Continuing Education courses for providers.

Adding Referral to Treatment When Necessary

When an individual's substance use problem meets criteria for a substance use disorder, and/or when brief interventions do not produce change, it may be necessary to motivate the patient to engage in specialized treatment. This is called Screening, Brief Intervention, and Referral to Treatment (SBIRT). In such cases, the care provider makes a referral for a clinical assessment followed by a clinical treatment plan developed with the individual that is tailored to meet the person's needs.[47] Effective referral processes should incorporate strategies to motivate patients to accept the referral. Although the screening and brief intervention components of SBIRT are the same as SBI, referral to treatment helps the individual access, select, and navigate barriers to substance use disorder treatment.

The literature on the effectiveness of drug-focused brief intervention in primary care and emergency departments is less clear, with some studies finding no improvements among those receiving brief interventions.[48,49] However, at least one study found significant reductions in subsequent drug use.[50] Even if brief interventions are not found to be sufficient to address patients' drug use disorders, general health care settings still have an important role to play in addressing drug use disorders, by providing medication-assisted treatment (MAT), providing more robust monitoring and care coordination, and actively promoting engagement in specialty substance use disorder treatment.

Trials evaluating different types of screening and brief interventions for drug use in a range of settings and on a range of patient characteristics are lacking. Recently, efforts have been made to adapt SBIRT for adolescents and for all groups with substance use disorders.[51,52] The results of preliminary studies are promising,[20,53] but gaps in knowledge about SBIRT for adolescents still need to be filled.[54]

Treatment Engagement: Reaching and Reducing Harm Among Those Who Need Treatment

Populations Who Need Treatment but Are Not Receiving It

Despite the fact that substance use disorders are widespread, only a small percentage of people receive treatment. Results from the 2015 *National Survey of Drug Use and Health* (NSDUH) reveal that only about 2.2 million people with a substance use disorder, or about 1 in 10 affected individuals, received any type of treatment in the year before the survey was administered.[19] This "treatment gap" is a large and costly concern for individuals, families, and communities. Of those who needed treatment but did not receive treatment, over 7 million were women and more than 1 million were adolescents aged 12 to 17.[19] Some racial and ethnic groups experience disparities in entering and receiving substance use disorder treatment services.[55] For example, approximately 13 million of those who did not receive treatment were non-Hispanic or non-Latino Whites, about 3 million were Hispanics or Latinos, and about 3 million were non-Hispanic Blacks or African Americans.[19] Among all individuals who met criteria for a substance use disorder, alcohol was by far the most prevalent substance reported, followed by marijuana, misuse of prescription pain relievers, cocaine, and methamphetamines, and about 1 in

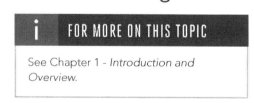

FOR MORE ON THIS TOPIC

See Chapter 1 - *Introduction and Overview*.

10 reported use of multiple substances.[19] Additionally, over 8 million individuals, or about 40 percent of those with a substance use disorder, also had a mental disorder diagnosed in the year before the survey.[19] Nonetheless, only 6.8 percent of these individuals received treatment for both conditions, and 52.0 percent received no treatment at all.[19] Many individuals with substance use disorders also have related physical health problems. Substance use can contribute to medical issues, such as an increased risk of liver, lung, or cardiovascular disease, as well as infectious diseases such as Hepatitis B or C, and HIV/AIDS, and can worsen these health outcomes.[56]

Reasons for Not Seeking Treatment

There are many reasons people do not seek treatment. The most common reason is that they are unaware that they need treatment; they have never been told they have a substance use disorder or they do not consider themselves to have a problem. This is one reason why screening for substance use disorders in general health care settings is so important. In addition, among those who do perceive that they need substance use disorder treatment, many still do not seek it. For these individuals, the most common reasons given are:[19]

- Not ready to stop using (40.7 percent). A common clinical feature associated with substance use disorders is an individual's tendency to underestimate the severity of their problem and to over-estimate their ability to control it. This is likely due to substance-induced changes in the brain circuits that control impulses, motivation, and decision making.

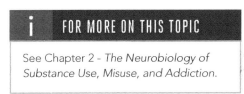

FOR MORE ON THIS TOPIC

See Chapter 2 - *The Neurobiology of Substance Use, Misuse, and Addiction.*

- Do not have health care coverage/could not afford (30.6 percent).
- Might have a negative effect on job (16.4 percent) or cause neighbors/community to have a negative opinion (8.3 percent).
- Do not know where to go for treatment (12.6 percent) or no program has the type of treatment desired (11.0 percent).
- Do not have transportation, programs are too far away, or hours are inconvenient (11.8 percent).

The costs of care and lack of insurance coverage are particularly important issues for people with substance use disorders. The 2015 NSDUH found that among individuals who needed and made an effort to get treatment but did not receive specialty substance use treatment, 30.0 percent reported that they did not have insurance coverage and could not afford to pay for treatment.[19] Thus, a way to reduce health disparities is to increase the number of people who have health insurance. However, even if an individual is insured, the payor may not cover some types or components of substance use disorder treatments, particularly medications.[57,58] These challenges are magnified further for those who live in rural areas, where substance use disorder treatment services can be distant and thus difficult to reach, as well as expensive because of travel time and cost.[58]

Strategies to Reduce Harm

Strategies to reduce the harms associated with substance use have been developed as a way to engage people in treatment and to address the needs of those who are not yet ready to participate in treatment. Harm reduction programs provide public health-oriented, evidence-based, and cost-effective services to prevent and reduce substance use-related risks among those actively using substances,[59] and substantial evidence supports their effectiveness.[60,61] These programs work with populations who may not be ready to stop substance use – offering individuals strategies to reduce risks while still using substances. Strategies include outreach and education programs, needle/syringe exchange programs, overdose prevention education, and access to naloxone to reverse potentially lethal opioid overdose.[59,62] These strategies are designed to reduce substance misuse and its negative consequences for the users and those around them, such as transmission of HIV and other infectious diseases.[63] They also seek to help individuals engage in treatment to reduce, manage, and stop their substance use when appropriate.

Outreach and Education

Outreach activities seek to identify those with active substance use disorders who are not in treatment and help them realize that treatment is available, accessible, and necessary. Outreach and engagement methods may include telephone contacts, face-to-face street outreach, community engagement,[64] or assertive outreach after a referral is made by a clinician or caseworker. These efforts often occur within or in collaboration with programs for intimate partner violence, homelessness, or HIV/AIDS.[65-68] One study showed that 41 percent of referrals to treatment among substance-using individuals enrolled in a homelessness outreach project successfully resulted in treatment enrollment.[69] This is notable and promising, but additional research is needed to validate that outreach efforts geared at identifying individuals who need treatment are successful at increasing substance use treatment enrollment and subsequent outcomes.

Educational campaigns are also a common strategy for reducing harms associated with substance use. Such campaigns have historically been targeted toward substance-using individuals, giving them information and guidance on risks associated with sharing medications or needles, how to access low or no-cost treatment services, and how to prevent a drug overdose death.[59,61] Other education campaigns target the overall public to improve general understanding about addiction, community health and safety risks, and how to access available treatment services.[70-72] Two examples are SAMHSA's *National Recovery Month*, which seeks to increase awareness and understanding of mental and substance use issues, and the *Anyone.Anytime.* campaign in New Hampshire, which was implemented statewide to educate the public and professionals about addiction, emergency overdose medication, and accessibility to support services for those with opioid use disorders. The National Highway Traffic Safety Administration's (NHTSA's) annual *Drive Sober or Get Pulled Over* campaign is another example, aimed at reducing drunk driving and preventing alcohol-impaired fatalities.

Needle/Syringe Exchange Programs

Drugs such as heroin and other opioids, cocaine, and methamphetamine are commonly used by injection, and this route of administration has been a major source of infectious disease transmission including HIV, Hepatitis B, Hepatitis C, and other blood-borne diseases. Data from the CDC reveal that even though HIV among people who inject drugs is declining, it is still a significant problem: 7 percent (3,096) of the 47,352 newly diagnosed cases of HIV infection in the United States in 2013 were attributable to injection drug use, and another 3 percent (1,270) involved male-to-male sexual contact combined with injection drug use.[73,74] Nearly 20,000 people died from Hepatitis C in 2014, and 3.5 million are living with Hepatitis C. New cases of Hepatitis C infection increased 250 percent between 2010 and 2014, and occur primarily among young White people who inject drugs.[75]

Because of these data, providing sterile needles and syringes to people who inject drugs has become an important strategy for reducing disease transmission. The goal of needle/syringe exchange programs is to minimize infection transmission risks by giving individuals who inject drugs sterile equipment and other support services at little or no cost.[76] Additional services from these programs often include HIV/AIDS counseling and testing; strategies and education for preventing sexually transmitted infections, including condom use and use of medications before or after exposure to HIV to reduce the risk of becoming infected (pre-exposure prophylaxis [PrEP] or post-exposure prophylaxis [PEP]); and other health care services. Needle/syringe exchange programs also attempt to encourage individuals to engage in substance use disorder treatment.[77]

Evaluation studies have clearly shown that needle/syringe exchange programs are effective in reducing HIV transmission and do not increase rates of community drug use.[78] However, most of the research has not examined the impact of these programs on Hepatitis C transmission, therefore currently available data are insufficient to address this question.[79]

Naloxone

Opioid overdose incidents and deaths, either from prescription pain relievers or heroin, are a serious threat to public health in the United States. Overdose deaths from opioid pain relievers and heroin have risen dramatically in the past 14 years,[80] from 5,990 in 1999 to 29,467 in 2014, and most were preventable. Rates of opioid overdose deaths are particularly high among individuals with an opioid use disorder who have recently stopped their use as a result of detoxification or incarceration. As a result, their tolerance for the drug is reduced, making them more vulnerable to an overdose. Those who mix opioids with alcohol, benzodiazepines, or other drugs also have a high risk of overdose.[59]

Opioid overdose does not occur immediately after a person has taken the drug. Rather, the effects develop gradually as the drug depresses a person's breathing and heart rate. This eventually leads to coma and death if the overdose is not treated. This gradual progress means that there is typically a 1- to 3-hour window of opportunity after a user has taken the drug in which bystanders can take action to prevent the user's death.[59]

Naloxone is an opioid antagonist medication approved by the FDA to reverse opioid overdose in injectable and nasal spray forms. It works by displacing opioids from receptors in the brain, thereby blocking their effects on breathing and heart rate.

The rising number of deaths from opioid overdose has led to increasing public health efforts to make naloxone available to at-risk individuals and their families, as well as to emergency medical technicians, police officers, and other first responders, or through community-based opioid overdose prevention programs. Although regulations vary by state, some states have passed laws expanding access to naloxone without a patient-specific prescription in some localities.[81,82] Additionally, some schools across the country are stocking naloxone for use by trained nurses.

Interventions that distribute take-home doses of naloxone along with education and training for those actively using opioids and their peers and family members, have the potential to help decrease overdose-related deaths.[83,84] Current evidence from nonrandomized studies also suggests that family, friends, and other community members who are properly trained can and will administer naloxone appropriately during an overdose incident.[85] And, despite concern that access to naloxone might increase the prevalence or frequency of opioid use, research demonstrates that neither of these problems has occurred.[86]

FDA Approval of Naloxone Nasal Spray

Naloxone, a safe medication that can quickly restore normal breathing to a person in danger of dying from an opioid overdose, is already carried by emergency medical personnel and other first responders. But by the time an overdosing person is reached and treated, it is often too late to save them. To solve this problem, several experimental Overdose Education and Naloxone Distribution (OEND) programs have given naloxone directly to opioid users, their friends or loved ones, and other potential bystanders, along with brief training on how to use this medication. These programs have been shown to be an effective, as well as cost-effective, way of saving lives.

Until recently, only injectable forms of naloxone were approved by the FDA. However, in November 2015, the FDA approved a user-friendly intranasal formulation of naloxone that matches the injectable version in terms of how much of the medication gets into the body and how rapidly. According to the CDC, more than 74 Americans die each day from an overdose involving prescription pain relievers or heroin. To reverse these trends, it is important to do everything possible to ensure that emergency personnel, as well as at-risk opioid users and their loved ones, have access to lifesaving medications like naloxone.

Acute Stabilization and Withdrawal Management

Withdrawal management, often called "detoxification," includes interventions aimed at managing the physical and emotional symptoms that occur after a person stops using a substance. Withdrawal symptoms vary in intensity and duration based on the substance(s) used, the duration and amount of use, and the overall health of the individual. Some substances, such as alcohol, opioids, sedatives, and tranquilizers, produce significant physical withdrawal effects, while other substances, such as marijuana, stimulants, and caffeine, produce primarily emotional and cognitive withdrawal symptoms. Most periods of withdrawal are relatively short (3 to 5 days) and are managed with medications combined with vitamins, exercise, and sleep. One important exception is withdrawal from alcohol and sedatives/tranquilizers, especially if the latter are combined with heavy alcohol use. Rapid or unmanaged withdrawal from these substances can be protracted and can produce seizures and other health complications.[56]

Withdrawal management is highly effective in preventing immediate and serious medical consequences associated with discontinuing substance use,[56] but by itself it is not an effective treatment for any substance use disorder. It is best considered stabilization: The patient is assisted through a period of acute detoxification and withdrawal to being medically stable and substance-free. Stabilization includes preparing the individual for treatment and involving the individual's family and other significant people in the person's life, as appropriate, to support the person's treatment process. Stabilization is considered a first step toward recovery, much like acute management of a diabetic coma or a hypertensive stroke is simply the first step toward managing the underlying illness of diabetes or high blood pressure. Similarly, acute stabilization and withdrawal management are most effective when following evidence-based standards of care.[87]

Unfortunately, many individuals who receive withdrawal management do not become engaged in treatment. Studies have found that half to three quarters of individuals with substance use disorders who receive withdrawal management services do not enter treatment.[88] One common result of not engaging in continuing care is rapid readmission to a detoxification center, an emergency department, or a hospital. For example, 27 percent of people who received detoxification services not followed by continuing care were readmitted within 1 year to public detoxification services in Delaware, Oklahoma, and Washington.[89] Beginning substance use disorder treatment within 14 days of discharge from withdrawal management, however, has been shown to reduce readmission rates.[90]

One of the most serious consequences when individuals do not begin continuing care after withdrawal management is overdose. Because withdrawal management reduces much of an individual's acquired tolerance, those who attempt to re-use their former substance in the same amount or frequency can experience physical problems. Individuals with opioid use disorders may be left particularly vulnerable to overdose and even death. It is critically important for health care providers to be prepared to properly assess the nature and severity of their patients' clinical problems following withdrawal so that they can facilitate engagement into the appropriate intensity of treatment.[56]

Principles of Effective Treatment and Treatment Planning

Principles and Goals of Treatment

Treatment can occur in a variety of settings but most treatment for substance use disorders has traditionally been provided in specialty substance use disorder treatment programs. For this reason, the majority of research has been performed within these specialty settings.[91] The following sections describe what is known from this research about the processes, stages of, and outcomes from traditional substance use disorder treatment programs.

The National Institute on Drug Abuse (NIDA) has detailed the evidence-based principles of effective treatment for adults and adolescents with substance use disorders that apply regardless of the particular setting of care or type of substance use disorder treatment program (Table 4.2).[85,92]

TREATMENT

Table 4.2: Principles of Effective Treatment for Substance Use Disorders

Principles of Effective Treatment for Adults	Principles of Effective Treatment for Adolescents
1. Addiction is a complex but treatable disease that affects brain function and behavior.	1. Adolescent substance use needs to be identified and addressed as soon as possible.
2. No single treatment is appropriate for everyone.	2. Adolescents can benefit from a drug abuse intervention even if they are not addicted to a drug.
3. Treatment needs to be readily available.	
4. Effective treatment attends to multiple needs of the individual, not just his or her drug abuse.	3. Routine annual medical visits are an opportunity to ask adolescents about drug use.
5. Remaining in treatment for an adequate period of time is critical.	4. Legal interventions and sanctions or family pressure may play an important role in getting adolescents to enter, stay in, and complete treatment.
6. Behavioral therapies—including individual, family, or group counseling-- are the most commonly used forms of drug abuse treatment.	5. Substance use disorder treatment should be tailored to the unique needs of the adolescent.
7. Medications are an important element of treatment for many patients, especially when combined with counseling and other behavioral therapies.	6. Treatment should address the needs of the whole person, rather than just focusing on his or her drug use.
8. An individual's treatment and services plan must be assessed continually and modified as necessary to ensure that it meets his or her changing needs.	7. Behavioral therapies are effective in addressing adolescent drug use.
	8. Families and the community are important aspects of treatment.
9. Many drug-addicted individuals also have other mental disorders.	9. Effectively treating substance use disorders in adolescents requires also identifying and treating any other mental health conditions they may have.
10. Medically assisted detoxification is only the first stage of addiction treatment and by itself does little to change long-term drug abuse.	10. Sensitive issues such as violence and child abuse or risk of suicide should be identified and addressed.
11. Treatment does not need to be voluntary to be effective.	11. It is important to monitor drug use during treatment.
12. Drug use during treatment must be monitored continuously, as lapses during treatment do occur.	12. Staying in treatment for an adequate period of time and continuity of care afterward are important.
13. Treatment programs should test patients for the presence of HIV/AIDS, Hepatitis B and C, tuberculosis, and other infectious diseases, provide risk-reduction counseling, and link patients to treatment if necessary.	13. Testing adolescents for sexually transmitted diseases like HIV, as well as Hepatitis B and C, is an important part of drug treatment.

Source: National Institute on Drug Abuse, (2012)[85] and (2014).[92]

The goals of substance use disorder treatment are similar to those of treatments for other serious, often chronic, illnesses: reduce the major symptoms of the illness, improve health and social function, and teach and motivate patients to monitor their condition and manage threats of relapse. Substance use disorder treatment can be provided in inpatient or outpatient settings, depending on the needs of the patient, and typically incorporates a combination of behavioral therapies, medications, and RSS. However, unlike treatments for most other medical illnesses, substance use disorder treatment has traditionally been provided in programs (both residential and outpatient) outside of the mainstream health care system. The intensity of the treatment regimens offered can vary substantially across program types. The American Society of Addiction Medicine (ASAM) has categorized these programs into "levels" of care to guide referral based on an individual patient's needs.[93-95]

Despite differences in care delivery and differences in reimbursement, substance use disorder treatments have approximately the same rates of positive outcomes as treatment for other chronic illnesses. Relapse rates for substance use disorders (40 to 60 percent) are comparable to those for chronic diseases, such as diabetes (20 to 50 percent), hypertension (50 to 70 percent), and asthma (50 to 70 percent).[12]

The general process of treatment planning and delivery for individuals with severe substance use disorders is described below, along with an explanation of the evidence-based therapies, medications, and RSS shown to be effective in treatment.

> **KEY CONCEPT**
>
> **Treatment** varies depending on substance(s) used, severity of substance use disorder, comorbidities, and the individual's preferences.
>
> Treatment typically includes medications and counseling as well as other social supports such as linkage to community recovery groups depending on an individual patient's needs and level of existing family and social support.

Treatment Planning

Assessment and Diagnosis

Among the first steps involved in substance use disorder treatment are assessment and diagnosis. The diagnosis of substance use disorders is based primarily on the results of a clinical interview. Several assessment instruments are available to help structure and elicit the information required to diagnose substance use disorders. The diagnosis of a substance use disorder is made by a trained professional based on 11 symptoms defined in the Fifth Edition of the *Diagnostic and Statistical Manual of Mental Disorders* (DSM-5). These symptoms, which are generally related to loss of control over substance use,[96] are presented in Table 1.5[2] in Chapter 1. The number of diagnostic symptoms present defines the severity of the disorder, ranging from mild to severe (i.e., fewer than 2 symptoms = no disorder; 2 to 3 symptoms = mild disorder; 4 to 5 symptoms = moderate disorder; 6 or more symptoms = severe disorder).[97]

> **FOR MORE ON THIS TOPIC**
>
> See Chapter 1 - *Introduction and Overview.*

Conducting a clinical assessment is essential to understanding the nature and severity of the patient's health and social problems that may have led to or resulted from the substance use. This assessment is important in determining the intensity of care that will be recommended and the composition of the treatment plan.[91] Several validated assessment tools can provide information about an individual's substance use disorder. Table 4.3 gives a brief overview of some of the tools that are available.

TREATMENT

Table 4.3: Detailed Information on Substance Use Disorder Assessment Tools

Addiction Severity Index (ASI)[98]	Substance Abuse Module (SAM)[99]	Global Appraisal of Individual Needs (GAIN)[299]	Psychiatric Research Interview for Substance and Mental Disorders (PRISM)[100]
• Semi-structured interview. • Addresses seven potential problem areas in substance using individuals: medical status, employment and support, drug use, alcohol use, legal status, family/social status, and psychiatric status. • Provides an overview of problems related to substance, rather than focusing on any single area. • Used extensively for treatment planning and outcome evaluation. • A shorter, self-report version of the ASI called the ASI-Lite is also available.	• Expanded and more detailed version of the substance use section of the Composite International Diagnostic Interview (CIDI). • Designed to assess mental disorders as defined by the *Diagnositic and Statistical Manual of Mental Disorders, Fourth Edition* (DSM-IV). • Contains four diagnostic sections on tobacco, alcohol, drugs, and caffeine. • Includes questions about when symptoms began and how recent they are, withdrawal symptoms, and the physical, social and psychological consequences of each substance assessed. • Assesses the respondent's impairment and treatment seeking. • Can assess substance use disorders quickly and accurately in the clinical setting.	• Series of measures (screener, standardized biopsychosocial intake assessment battery, follow-up assessment battery) which integrate research and clinical assessment. • Contains 99 scales and subscales, that are designed to measure the recency, breadth, and frequency of problems and service utilization related to substance use (including diagnosis and course, treatment motivation, and relapse potential), physical health, risk/protective involvement, mental health, environment and vocational situation. • Can assess change over time.	• Semi-structured, clinician-administered interview. • Measures the major DSM-IV diagnoses of alcohol, drug, and psychiatric disorders. • Provides clear guidelines for differentiating between the effects of intoxication and withdrawal, substance-induced disorders, and primary disorders.

Individualized Treatment Planning

After a formal assessment, the information is discussed with the patient to jointly develop a personalized treatment plan designed to address the patient's needs.[91,101] The treatment plan and goals should be person-centered and include strength-based approaches, or ones that draw upon an individual's strengths, resources, potential, and ability to recover, to keep the patient engaged in care. Individualized treatment plans should consider age, gender identity, race and ethnicity, language, health literacy, religion/spirituality, sexual orientation, culture, trauma history, and co-occurring physical and mental health problems. Such considerations are critical for understanding the individual and for tailoring the treatment to his or her specific needs. This increases the likelihood of successful treatment engagement and retention, and research shows that those who participate more fully in treatment typically have better outcomes.[102] Throughout treatment, individuals should be periodically reassessed to determine response to treatment and to make any needed adjustments to the treatment plan.

Maintaining Treatment Engagement and Retention

Treatment plans should be personalized and include engagement and retention strategies to promote participation, motivation, and adherence to the plan.[47] Research has found that individuals who received proactive engagement services such as direct outreach and a specific follow-up plan are more likely to remain engaged in services throughout the treatment process.[47,103,104]

Treatment providers can improve engagement and retention in programs by building a strong therapeutic alliance with the patient, effectively using evidence-based motivational strategies, acknowledging the patient's individual barriers, making reminder phone calls, and creating a positive environment.[105] Further, providers who can recommend and/or provide a broad range of RSS, such as child care, housing, and transportation, can improve retention in treatment.[106]

Engaging, effective treatment also involves culturally competent care. For example, treatment programs that provide gender-specific and gender-responsive care are more likely to enhance women's treatment outcomes.[107] Tailoring treatment to involve family and community is particularly effective for certain groups. For example, American Indians or Alaska Natives may require specific elements in their treatment plan that respond to their unique cultural experiences and to intergenerational and historical trauma and trauma from violent encounters.[108] Language and literacy (including health literacy) may also affect how a person responds to the treatment environment.[109-112] Race and ethnicity, sexual orientation, gender identity, and economic status can play significant roles in treatment initiation, engagement, and completion.[107,113,114]

Substance use disorder treatment programs also have an obligation to prepare for disasters within their communities that can affect the availability of services. A disaster can disrupt a program's ability to provide treatment services or an individual's ability to maintain treatment. Individuals in recovery, for example, may relapse due to sudden discontinuation of services or stress when having to cope with effects of a disaster. Individuals receiving MAT could be at risk of serious withdrawal symptoms if medications are stopped abruptly. Others may face challenges without their treatment program's support.[115] Therefore, planning for disasters and other large scale emergencies is critical to prevent or reduce the impact of interruptions in treatment services.

Treatment Setting and the Continuum of Care

As indicated above, the treatment of addiction is delivered in predominantly freestanding programs that differ in their setting (hospital, residential, or outpatient); in the frequency of care delivery (daily sessions to monthly visits); in the range of treatment components offered; and in the planned duration of care. In general, as patients progress in treatment and begin to meet the goals of their individualized treatment plan, they transfer from clinical management in residential or intensive outpatient programs to less clinically intensive outpatient programs that promote patient self-management.

A typical progression for someone who has a severe substance use disorder might start with 3 to 7 days in a medically managed withdrawal program, followed by a 1- to 3-month period of intensive rehabilitative care in a residential treatment program, followed by continuing care, first in an intensive outpatient program (2 to 5 days per week for a few months) and later in a traditional outpatient program that meets 1 to 2 times per month. For many patients whose current living situations are not conducive to recovery, outpatient services should be provided in conjunction with recovery-supportive housing.

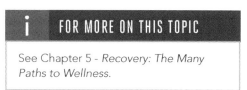

See Chapter 5 - *Recovery: The Many Paths to Wellness.*

In general, patients with serious substance use disorders are recommended to stay engaged for at least 1 year in the treatment process, which may involve participation in three to four different programs or services at reduced levels of intensity, all of which are ideally designed to help the patient prepare for continued self-management after treatment ends.[56,116] This expected trajectory of care explains why efforts to maintain patient motivation and engagement are important. Brief summaries of the major levels of the treatment continuum are discussed below.

Medically monitored and managed inpatient care is an intensive service delivered in an acute, inpatient hospital setting.[18] These programs are typically necessary for individuals who require withdrawal management, primary medical and nursing care, and for those with co-occurring mental and physical health conditions.[18] Treatment is usually provided by an interdisciplinary team of health care professionals, available 24 hours a day, who can address serious mental and physical health needs.[18,91]

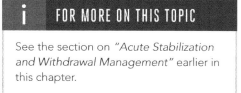

See the section on *"Acute Stabilization and Withdrawal Management"* earlier in this chapter.

Residential services offer organized services, also in a 24-hour setting but outside of a hospital. These programs typically provide support, structure, and an array of evidence-based clinical services.[18] Such programs are appropriate for physically and emotionally stabilized individuals who may not have a living situation that supports recovery, may have a history of relapse, or have co-occurring physical and/or mental illnesses.

Partial hospitalization and intensive outpatient services range from counseling and education to clinically intensive programming.[18] Partial hospitalization programs are used as a step-down treatment option after completing residential treatment and are usually available 6 to 8 hours a day during the work week.[18] These services are considered to be approximately as intensive but less restrictive than residential programs[91] and are appropriate for patients living in an environment that supports recovery but who need structure to avoid relapse.

Outpatient services provide both group and individual behavioral interventions and medications when appropriate.[91] These components of care can be offered during the day, before or after work or school, or in the evenings and weekends. Typically, outpatient programs are appropriate as the initial level of care for individuals with a mild to moderate substance use disorder or as continuing care after completing more intensive treatment.[18] Outpatient programs are also suitable for individuals with co-occurring mental health conditions.

Evidence-based Treatment: Components of Care

Regardless of the substance for which the individual seeks treatment or the setting or level of care, all substance use disorder treatment programs are expected to offer an individualized set of evidence-based clinical components. These components are clinical practices that research has shown to be effective in reducing substance use and improving health and functioning. These include behavioral therapies, medications, and RSS. Treatment programs that offer more of these evidence-based components have the greatest likelihood of producing better outcomes.

> **Evidence-Based Practices**
>
> Research continues to identify new effective components of care. SAMHSA manages the *National Registry of Evidence-based Programs and Practices* (NREPP) that was developed to inform the public and to guide individual choices about treatment.

Medications and Medication-Assisted Treatment

Five medications, approved by the FDA, have been developed to treat alcohol and opioid use disorders. Currently, no approved medications are available to treat marijuana, amphetamine, or cocaine use disorders.[117] Table 4.4 lists these medications and they are discussed individually in the text that follows.

Table 4.4: Pharmacotherapies Used to Treat Alcohol and Opioid Use Disorders

Medication	Use	Dosage Form	DEA Schedule*	Application
Buprenorphine-Naloxone	Opioid use disorder	Sublingual film**:[118] 2mg/0.5mg, 4mg/1mg, 8mg/2mg, and 12mg/3mg Sublingual tablet: 1.4mg/0.36mg, 2mg/0.5mg, 2.9mg/0.71mg, 5.7mg/1.4mg, 8mg/2mg, 8.6mg/2.1mg, 11.4mg/2.9mg Buccal film: 2.1mg/0.3mg, 4.2mg/0.7mg, 6.3mg/1mg	CIII	Used for detoxification or maintenance of abstinence for individuals aged 16 or older. Physicians who wish to prescribe buprenorphine, must obtain a waiver from SAMHSA and be issued an additional registration number by the U.S. Drug Enforcement Administration (DEA).
Buprenorphine Hydrochloride	Opioid use disorder	Sublingual tablet: 2mg, 4mg, 8mg, and 12mg	CIII	This formulation is indicated for treatment of opioid dependence and is preferred for induction. However, it is considered the preferred formulation for pregnant patients, patients with hepatic impairment, and patients with sensitivity to naloxone. It is also used for initiating treatment in patients transferring from methadone, in preference to products containing naloxone, because of the risk of precipitating withdrawal in these patients.

TREATMENT

Medication	Use	Dosage Form	DEA Schedule*	Application
		Probuphine® implants: 80mgx4 implants for a total of 320mg		For those already stable on low to moderate dose buprenorphine. The administration of the implant dosage form requires specific training and must be surgically inserted and removed.
Methadone	Opioid use disorder	Tablet: 5mg, 10mg Tablet for suspension: 40mg Oral concentrate: 10mg/mL Oral solution: 5mg/5mL, 10mg/5mL Injection: 10mg/mL	CII	Methadone used for the treatment of opioid addiction in detoxification or maintenance programs shall be dispensed only by Opioid Treatment Programs (OTPs) certified by SAMHSA and approved by the designated state authority. Under federal regulations it can be used in persons under age 18 at the discretion of an OTP physician.[119]
Naltrexone	Opioid use disorder; alcohol use disorder	Tablets: 25mg, 50mg, and 100mg Extended-release injectable suspension: 380mg/vial	Not Scheduled under the Controlled Substances Act	Provided by prescription; naltrexone blocks opioid receptors, reduces cravings, and diminishes the rewarding effects of alcohol and opioids. Extended-release injectable naltrexone is recommended to prevent relapse to opioids or alcohol. The prescriber need not be a physician, but must be licensed and authorized to prescribe by the state.
Acamprosate	Alcohol use disorder	Delayed-release tablet: 333mg	Not Scheduled under the Controlled Substances Act	Provided by prescription; acamprosate is used in the maintenance of alcohol abstinence. The prescriber need not be a physician, but must be licensed and authorized to prescribe by the state.
Disulfiram	Alcohol use disorder	Tablet: 250mg, 500mg	Not Scheduled under the Controlled Substances Act	When taken in combination with alcohol, disulfiram causes severe physical reactions, including nausea, flushing, and heart palpitations. The knowledge that such a reaction is likely if alcohol is consumed acts as a deterrent to drinking.

Notes: *For more information about the DEA Schedule and classification of specific drugs, see Appendix D - Important Facts about Alcohol and Drugs.

**This dosage form may be used via sublingual or buccal routes of administration; sublingual means placed under the tongue, buccal means applied to the buccal area (in the cheek).

Source: Adapted from Lee et al., (2015).[120]

Like all other FDA-approved medications, those listed in Table 4.4 demonstrate "well-supported" experimental evidence of safety and effectiveness[120] for improving outcomes for individuals with alcohol and opioid use disorders.[117] At the same time, all of these medications have side effects; two (methadone and buprenorphine) have the potential to be misused, and methadone (and to a lesser extent buprenorphine) has the potential for overdose. For these reasons, only appropriately trained health care professionals should decide whether medication is needed as part of treatment, how the medication is provided in the context of other clinical services, and under what conditions the medication should be withdrawn or terminated.

The combination of behavioral interventions and medications to treat substance use disorders is commonly referred to as MAT.[121] MAT is a highly effective treatment option for individuals with alcohol and opioid use disorders. Studies have repeatedly demonstrated the efficacy of MAT at reducing illicit drug use and overdose deaths,[122,123] improving retention in treatment,[124] and reducing HIV transmission.[122]

Some medications used to treat opioid use disorders can be used to manage withdrawal and as maintenance treatment to reduce craving, lessen withdrawal symptoms, and maintain recovery.[56] These medications are used to help a patient function comfortably without illicit opioids or alcohol while balance is gradually restored to the brain circuits that have been altered by prolonged substance use.

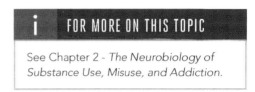

FOR MORE ON THIS TOPIC

See Chapter 2 - *The Neurobiology of Substance Use, Misuse, and Addiction.*

Prescribed in this fashion, medications for substance use disorders are in some ways like insulin for patients with diabetes. Insulin reduces symptoms by normalizing glucose metabolism, but it is part of a broader disease control strategy that also employs diet change, education on healthy living, and self-monitoring. Whether treating diabetes or a substance use disorder, medications are best employed as part of a broader treatment plan involving behavioral health therapies and RSS, as well as regular monitoring.

State agencies that oversee substance use disorder treatment programs use a variety of strategies to promote implementation of MAT, including education and training, financial incentives (e.g., linking funding to the provision of MAT), policy mandates, and support for infrastructure development.[5] Nevertheless, multiple factors create barriers to widespread use of MAT. These include provider, public, and client attitudes and beliefs about MAT; lack of an appropriate infrastructure for providing medications; need for staff training and development; and legislation, policies, and regulations that limit MAT implementation.[5]

Medication-Assisted Treatment for Opioid Use Disorders

MAT for patients with a chronic opioid use disorder must be delivered for an adequate duration in order to be effective. Patients who receive MAT for fewer than 90 days have not shown improved outcomes.[125] One study suggested that individuals who receive MAT for fewer than 3 years are more likely to relapse than those who are in treatment for 3 or more years.[126] Three medications are commonly used to treat opioid use disorders: methadone, buprenorphine, and naltrexone.

TREATMENT

Methadone is a synthetic opioid agonist that has been used to treat the symptoms of withdrawal from heroin and other opioids.[127] More than 40 years of research support the use of methadone as an effective treatment for opioid use disorder.[121,128,129] It is also used in the treatment of patients with chronic, severe pain[130] as a therapeutic alternative to morphine sulfate and other opioid analgesics.[131] Any licensed physician can prescribe methadone for the treatment of pain, but methadone may only be dispensed for treatment of an opioid use disorder within licensed methadone treatment programs.

> **KEY TERMS**
>
> **Agonist.** A chemical substance that binds to and activates certain receptors on cells, causing a biological response. Fentanyl and methadone are examples of opioid receptor agonists.

Long-term methadone maintenance treatment for opioid use disorders has been shown to be more effective than short-term withdrawal management,[132] and it has demonstrated improved outcomes for individuals (including pregnant women and their infants) with opioid use disorders.[133] Studies have also indicated that methadone reduces deaths, HIV risk behaviors, and criminal behavior associated with opioid drug seeking.[134,135]

The use of methadone to treat opioid use disorders has much in common with treatments for other substance use disorders and other chronic illnesses. However, it has one significant structural and cultural difference. Under regulations dating back to the early 1970s, the federal government created special methadone programs for adults with opioid use disorders. Originally referred to as "methadone treatment programs," these treatment facilities were created to provide special management of the medical and legal issues associated with the use of this potent, long-acting opioid.

The use of opioid agonist medications to treat opioid use disorders has always had its critics. Many people, including some policymakers, authorities in the criminal justice system, and treatment providers, have viewed maintenance treatments as "substituting one substance for another"[85] and have adhered instead to an abstinence-only philosophy that avoids the use of medications, especially those that activate opioid receptors. Such views are not scientifically supported; the research clearly demonstrates that MAT leads to better treatment outcomes compared to behavioral treatments alone. Moreover, withholding medications greatly increases the risk of relapse to illicit opioid use and overdose death. Decades of research have shown that the benefits of MAT greatly outweigh the risks associated with diversion.

> **KEY TERMS**
>
> **Drug diversion.** A medical and legal concept involving the transfer of any legally prescribed controlled substance from the person for whom it was prescribed to another person for any illicit use.

Today, methadone treatment programs, now called Opioid Treatment Programs (OTPs), must be certified by SAMHSA and registered by the U.S. Drug Enforcement Administration (DEA). OTPs are predominantly outpatient programs (approximately 95 percent) that provide pharmacotherapy in combination with behavioral therapies and other RSS.[136] OTPs incorporate principles of harm reduction and benefit both program participants and the community[137] by reducing opioid use, mortality, crime associated with opioid use disorders, and infectious disease transmission. Buprenorphine and naltrexone may also be provided in OTPs.[61]

Individuals receiving medication for opioid use disorders in an OTP must initially take their doses daily under observation.[138,139] After a period of orientation, patients are typically started at a dose of 20 to 30 mg and gradually increased to 80 mg or more per day, until craving and opioid misuse are significantly reduced. During this period, all dosing occurs at the OTP, but following stabilization and initially positive results, the stabilized patient may be given a "take-home" supply of his or her dose to self-administer per the federal opioid treatment standard regulations 42 CFR 8.12(i).

Buprenorphine is available as a sublingual tablet and a sublingual or buccal film. In addition, in May 2016, an implantable formulation of buprenorphine was approved by the FDA. For individuals who are already on a stable low to moderate dose of buprenorphine, the implant delivers a constant low dose of buprenorphine for 6 months. Buprenorphine is associated with improved outcomes compared to placebo for individuals (including pregnant women and their infants) with opioid use disorders,[140] and it is effective in reducing illegal opioid use.[129]

Buprenorphine is a partial opioid agonist, meaning that it binds to and activates opioid receptors but with less intensity than full agonists. As a result, there is an upper limit to how much euphoria, pain relief, or respiratory depression buprenorphine can produce.[56,141] However, buprenorphine still may result in overdose if used with tranquilizers and/or alcohol, and some diversion has been reported, although studies suggest most diverted buprenorphine is used therapeutically (e.g., to control cravings), not to get high.[142-144]

Clinical experience and research protocols indicate that buprenorphine initiation and stabilization during the induction period is an important part of successful treatment for individuals with opioid use disorder.[145] Buprenorphine can be prescribed alone or as a combination medication that includes naloxone, an opioid antagonist medication.[145] If this combined medication is taken as prescribed, the naloxone has no appreciable effects. However, if the combined medication is injected, the naloxone component can precipitate an opioid withdrawal syndrome, and in this way serves as a deterrent to misuse by injection.[145]

Buprenorphine may be prescribed by physicians who have met the statutory requirements for a waiver in accordance with the Controlled Substances Act (21 U.S.C. 823(g)(2)(D)(iii)).[146] However, physicians using the waiver are limited in the number of patients they can treat with this medication. This patient limit does not apply to OTPs that dispense buprenorphine on site because the OTP operating in this capacity is doing so under 21 U.S.C. 823(g)(1) and 42 CFR Part 8, and not under 21 U.S.C. 823(g)(2)(B).

When they first receive their waiver, physicians can provide buprenorphine treatment for only up to 30 individuals. After the first year they can request to treat up to 100.[147] However, lack of physician availability to prescribe buprenorphine has been a significant limitation on access to this effective medication. Although approximately 435,000 primary care physicians practice medicine in the United States,[148] only slightly more than 30,000 have a buprenorphine waiver,[149] and only about half of those are actually treating opioid use disorders.[150] To address this limitation and narrow the treatment gap, a final rule was published on July 8, 2016, expanding access to MAT by allowing eligible practitioners to request approval to treat up to 275 patients.[147]

Additionally, on July 22, 2016, the Comprehensive Addiction and Recovery Act (CARA) was signed into law. CARA temporarily expands eligibility to prescribe buprenorphine-based drugs for MAT for substance use disorders to qualifying nurse practitioners and physician assistants through October 1, 2021.

> **FOR MORE ON THIS TOPIC**
>
> See the section on *"Comprehensive Addiction and Recovery Act (CARA)"* in Chapter 6 - Health Care Systems and Substance Use Disorders.

Naltrexone is an opioid antagonist that binds to opioid receptors and blocks their activation; it produces no opioid-like effects and is not abusable. It prevents other opioids from binding to opioid receptors so that they have little to no effect. It also interrupts the effects of any opioids in a person's system, precipitating an opioid withdrawal syndrome in opioid-dependent patients, so it can be administered only after a complete detoxification from opioids. There is also no withdrawal from naltrexone when the patient stops taking it. Naltrexone may be appropriate for people who have been successfully treated with buprenorphine or methadone who wish to discontinue use but still be protected from relapse; people who prefer not to take an opioid agonist; people who have completed detoxifications and/or rehabilitation or are being released from incarceration and expect to return to an environment where drugs may be used and wish to avoid relapse; and adolescents or young adults with opioid dependence.[151]

Because naltrexone is not a controlled substance, it can be prescribed or administered by any physician, nurse practitioner, or physician assistant with prescribing authority. Naltrexone comes in two formulations: oral and extended-release injectable. Oral naltrexone can be effective for those individuals who are highly motivated and/or supported with observed daily dosing. Extended-release injectable naltrexone, which is administered on a monthly basis, addresses the poor compliance associated with oral naltrexone since it provides extended protection from relapse and reduces cravings for 30 days.[152,153]

Medication-Assisted Treatment for Alcohol Use Disorders

A number of factors should be weighed in determining the need for medication when treating an individual for an alcohol use disorder, such as the patient's motivation for treatment, potential for relapse, and severity of co-existing conditions.[120] Three FDA-approved medications are currently available to treat alcohol use disorder: disulfiram, naltrexone, and acamprosate.[117] None of these medications carries a risk of misuse or addiction, and thus none is a DEA-scheduled substance. Each has a distinct effectiveness and side effect profile. Prescribing health care professionals should be familiar with these side effects and take them into consideration before prescribing.[154] Providers can obtain additional information from materials produced by the National Institute on Alcohol Abuse and Alcoholism (NIAAA) and SAMHSA.[155,156]

Research studies on the efficacy of medications to treat alcohol use disorders have demonstrated that most patients show benefit, although individual response can be difficult to predict.[154,157] MAT interventions for alcohol use disorders can be provided in both non-specialty and specialty care settings and are most beneficial when combined with behavioral interventions and brief support.[154]

Disulfiram is a medication that inhibits normal breakdown of acetaldehyde which is produced by the metabolism of alcohol, thus rapidly increasing acetaldehyde in the blood which produces an aversive response. Thus, once disulfiram is taken by mouth, any alcohol consumed results in rapid buildup of acetaldehyde and a negative reaction or sickness results. The intensity of this reaction is dependent on the dose of disulfiram and the amount of alcohol consumed.[158] Effects from a disulfiram-alcohol reaction include warmth and flushing of the skin, increased heart rate, palpitations, a drop in blood pressure, nausea and/or vomiting, sweating, dizziness, and headache.[159] In this way, disulfiram essentially punishes alcohol consumption and indirectly rewards abstinence.[117]

Disulfiram was the first medication approved by the FDA to treat alcohol use disorder and its efficacy has been widely studied.[160] Most studies have demonstrated that disulfiram, when given under supervision, is more effective than placebo in treating alcohol use disorders.[154] A major limitation of disulfiram is adherence, which is typically poor, thereby reducing the medication's effectiveness. Disulfiram is most effective when its use is supervised or observed, which has been found to increase compliance.[154,159] Negotiating with the patient to have a spouse or significant other provide supervision offers both the incentive to take the medication and the documentation that the medication is being taken.[161] The best candidates for disulfiram are patients with motivation for treatment and a desire to be abstinent. Thus, an individual who wants to reduce, but not stop, drinking is *not* a candidate for disulfiram. Disulfiram should also be avoided in individuals with advanced liver disease.[162]

Naltrexone is the opioid antagonist described above that is used to treat opioid use disorder. Because it blocks some opioid receptors, naltrexone counteracts some of the pleasurable aspects of drinking.[154,159] Unlike disulfiram, naltrexone does not interact with alcohol to produce a severe reaction.[163] As noted before, naltrexone comes in two formulations: oral and extended-release injectable.

Many studies have examined the effectiveness of naltrexone in treating alcohol use disorders.[154] Several research reviews have found that it reduces the risk of heavy drinking in patients who are abstinent for at least several days at the time treatment begins.[154,160] However, as with disulfiram, medication compliance can be a problem with the oral formulation. Adherence to taking the medication increases under conditions where it is administered and observed by a trusted family member or when the extended-release injectable, which requires only a single monthly injection, is used.[164] Naltrexone should not be prescribed to patients with acute hepatitis, renal failure, or liver failure.[162]

Acamprosate is a medication that normalizes the alcohol-related neurochemical changes in the brain glutamate systems and thereby reduces the symptoms of craving that can prompt a relapse to pathological drinking.[117] Acamprosate has been found to be an effective medication when used concurrently with behavioral interventions and, as with other medications for alcohol use disorders, works best in motivated patients.[117,165] Reviews show that acamprosate is effective in reducing relapse[166] and effective when used to maintain abstinence from alcohol.[167]

TREATMENT

Behavioral Therapies

Behavioral therapies can be provided in individual, group, and/or family sessions in virtually all treatment settings.[47,56] These structured therapies help patients recognize the impact of their behaviors – such as those dealing with stress or interacting in interpersonal relationships – on their substance use and ability to function in a healthy, safe, and productive manner. These therapies also teach and motivate patients in how to change their behaviors as a way to control their substance use disorders.[56]

For evidence-based behavioral therapies to be delivered appropriately, they must be provided by qualified, trained providers. Despite this, many counselors and therapists working in substance use disorder treatment programs have not been trained to provide evidence-based behavioral therapies, and general group counseling remains the major form of behavioral intervention available in most treatment programs.[168] Unfortunately, despite decades of research, it cannot be concluded that general group counseling is reliably effective in reducing substance use or related problems.[169,170]

The following sections describe behavioral therapies that have been shown to be effective in treating substance use disorders. These therapies have been studied extensively, have a well-supported evidence base indicating their effectiveness, and have been broadly applied across many types of substance use disorders and across ages, sexes, and racial and ethnic groups.

Individual counseling is delivered in structured sessions to help patients reduce substance use and improve function by developing effective coping strategies and life skills.[85,171] Individual counseling has been extensively studied in many specialty care settings but rarely within non-specialty settings. Most studies support the use of individual counseling as an effective intervention for individuals with substance use disorders.[117,169] As indicated above, group counseling is a standard part of most substance use disorder treatments, but should primarily be used only in conjunction with individual counseling[171] or other forms of individual therapy.[85]

Cognitive-Behavioral Therapy

The theoretical foundation for Cognitive-Behavioral Therapy (CBT) is that substance use disorders develop, in part, as a result of maladaptive behavior patterns and dysfunctional thoughts.[117] CBT treatments thus involve techniques to modify such behaviors and improve coping skills by emphasizing the identification and modification of dysfunctional thinking.[117] CBT is a short-term approach, usually involving 12 to 24 weekly individual sessions. These sessions typically explore the positive and negative consequences of substance use, and they use self-monitoring as a mechanism to recognize cravings and other situations that may lead the individual to relapse. They also help the individual develop coping strategies.[85]

CBT may be the most researched and evaluated of all the therapies for substance use disorders.[172,173] Research suggests that self-monitoring and craving-recognition skills can be learned during CBT and that those skills continue to be employed by the individual after treatment has concluded.[85] CBT interventions have been found to be quite effective, and outcomes are enhanced when CBT is combined with other behavioral and/or pharmacologic components of care.[174]

Research has shown that CBT is also an effective treatment for individuals with co-occurring mental disorders. Individuals with a substance use disorder and co-occurring mental disorder who received CBT had significantly improved outcomes on various measures of substance use and mental health symptoms as compared to those who did not receive CBT.[101,175,176]

Contingency Management

Behavior change involves learning new behaviors and changing old behaviors. Positive rewards or incentives for these changes can aid this process. Contingency management, which involves giving tangible rewards to individuals to support positive behavior change,[85] has been found to be effective in treating substance use disorders.[177] In this therapy, patients receive a voucher with monetary value that can be exchanged for food items, healthy recreational options (e.g., movies), or other sought-after goods or services when they exhibit desired behavior such as drug-free urine tests or participation in treatment activities.[85] Clinical studies comparing voucher-based reinforcement to traditional treatment regimens have found that voucher-based reinforcement is associated with longer treatment engagement, longer periods of abstinence, and greater improvements in personal function.[177] These positive findings, initially demonstrated with individuals with cocaine use disorders, have been reproduced in individuals with alcohol, opioid, and methamphetamine use disorders.[177]

Contingency management may be combined with other therapies or treatment components. For example, contingency management has been shown to improve outcomes for adults with cocaine dependence when added to CBT.[178] Similarly, contingency management improves outcomes for young adults with marijuana dependence when included with Motivational Enhancement Therapy (described below) and CBT.[179]

Community Reinforcement Approach

Community Reinforcement Approach (CRA) Plus Vouchers is an intensive 24-week outpatient program that uses incentives and reinforcers to reward individuals who reduce their substance use.[85] Individuals are required to attend one to two counseling sessions each week that emphasize improving relations, acquiring skills to minimize substance use, and reconstructing social activities and networks to support recovery.[85] Individuals receiving this treatment are eligible to receive vouchers with monetary value if they provide drug-free urine tests several times per week.[85] Research has demonstrated that CRA Plus Vouchers promotes treatment engagement and facilitates abstinence.[85] Recent studies have also shown improvements in psychosocial functioning and abstinence among individuals who received CRA Plus Vouchers compared to those who received an intervention of standard care only.[180]

CRA without vouchers has been successfully adapted for adolescents. The Adolescent Community Reinforcement Approach (A-CRA) is a similar program targeting 12 to 22 year olds with substance use disorders. A-CRA, which has been implemented in outpatient and residential treatment settings, seeks to increase family, social, and educational and vocational supports to reinforce abstinence and recovery from substance use. The effectiveness of A-CRA has been supported in multiple randomized clinical trials with adolescents from different settings, sexes, and racial groups.[181,182] Studies have found that A-CRA increased long-term abstinence from marijuana and alcohol and decreased frequency of other substance use.[182]

Motivational Enhancement Therapy

Motivational Enhancement Therapy (MET) is a counseling approach that uses motivational interviewing techniques to help individuals resolve any uncertainties they have about stopping their substance use. MET works by promoting empathy, developing patient awareness of the discrepancy between their goals and their unhealthy behavior, avoiding argument and confrontation, addressing resistance, and supporting self-efficacy[46] to encourage motivation and change.[85,183] The therapist supports the patient in executing the behaviors necessary for change and monitors progress toward patient-expressed goals.

MET has been shown to be an effective treatment in a range of populations and has demonstrated favorable outcomes such as reducing substance use and improving treatment engagement.[169] As with other therapies reviewed, MET is often used concurrently with other behavioral interventions.[184] However, the results of MET are mixed for people who use drugs such as heroin, cocaine, and nicotine, and for adolescents.[185,186] The combination of MET and CBT has shown favorable results for adolescents for multiple substances.[181]

The Matrix Model

The Matrix Model is a structured, multi-component behavioral treatment that consists of evidence-based practices, including relapse prevention, family therapy, group therapy, drug education, and self-help, delivered in a sequential and clinically coordinated manner.[85] The model consists of 16 weeks of group sessions held three times per week, which combine CBT, family education, social support, individual counseling, and urine drug testing.[187]

Several randomized controlled trials over the past 20 years have demonstrated that the Matrix Model is effective at reducing substance misuse and associated risky behaviors.[85] For example, one study demonstrated the model's effectiveness in producing sustained reductions in sexual risk behaviors among individuals who use methamphetamines, thus decreasing their risk of getting or transmitting HIV.[188] The Matrix Model has also been adapted to focus more on relationships, parenting, body image, and sexuality in order to improve women's retention in treatment and facilitate recovery.[189]

Twelve-Step Facilitation Therapy

Twelve-Step Facilitation (TSF), an individual therapy typically delivered in 12 weekly sessions, is designed to prepare individuals to understand, accept, and become engaged in Alcoholics Anonymous (AA), Narcotics Anonymous (NA), or similar 12-step programs.[190,191] As discussed in the next chapter, 12-step programs and other mutual-aid groups are not themselves medical treatments but fall under the category of RSS. Well-supported evidence shows that TSF interventions are effective in a variety of ways:

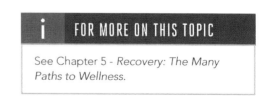

FOR MORE ON THIS TOPIC

See Chapter 5 - *Recovery: The Many Paths to Wellness.*

- As a stand-alone intervention;[192-194]
- When integrated with other treatments, such as CBT;[190]
- As a distinct component of a multi-treatment package;[191] and
- As a modular appendage to treatment.[195]

Some substance use disorder treatment programs that employ TSF also typically encourage AA or NA participation through group counseling.[123] However, TSF is quite different from generic group counseling, not only because it is an individual therapy, but also because it involves a systematic set of sequential sessions focused on three key ideas:[85]

- *Acceptance* - realizing that their substance use is part of a disorder, that life has become unmanageable because of alcohol or drugs, that willpower alone will not overcome the problem, and that abstinence is the best alternative;
- *Surrender* - giving oneself to a higher power, accepting the fellowship and support structure of other recovering individuals, and following the recovery activities laid out by a 12-step program; and
- *Active involvement in a 12-step program.*

> **KEY TERMS**
>
> **12-Step Program.** A group providing mutual support and fellowship for people recovering from addictive behaviors. The first 12-step program was Alcoholics Anonymous (AA), founded in 1935; an array of 12-step groups following a similar model have since emerged and are the most widely used mutual aid groups and steps for maintaining recovery from alcohol and drug use disorders. It is not a form of treatment, and it is not to be confused with the treatment modality called TSF.

TSF has been effective in reducing alcohol use during the first month of treatment for individuals with alcohol use disorders, but these effects disappeared rapidly following treatment completion.[196] In one study, alcohol-dependent women were randomly assigned to TSF, CBT, or a standard counseling group. The women who received TSF and CBT over 12 weeks both had better outcomes on perceived social support from friends and on social functioning than those in the counseling group, and the differences between those receiving TSF and CBT were minimal.[197]

In another study, a randomized controlled trial compared a CBT treatment program alone to the same treatment combined with TSF. TSF in addition to CBT increased AA involvement and days of abstinence over a 12-month follow-up period as compared to CBT alone.[190] Statistical analysis showed the benefits of the TSF stemmed from its ability to increase AA participation in the period after treatment ended. Further, another randomized controlled trial of outpatients with severe alcohol use disorder evaluated a treatment that aimed to change people's social networks away from heavy drinkers and toward non-drinking individuals, including AA members.[194] Those receiving the social network enhancement treatment had 20 percent more abstinent days and greater AA participation at 2-year follow-up than did patients assigned to receive standard case management. Again, AA participation and the number of abstinent friends in the social network were found to account for the treatment's effectiveness.[194]

Project MATCH, the largest study of alcohol use disorder treatment ever conducted, found that TSF increased rates of continuous abstinence and sustained remission at the same rates as two other evidenced-based treatments—CBT and MET. All three treatments reduced the quantity and frequency of alcohol use immediately after treatment. Further, relative to the CBT and MET treatment conditions, significantly more of the patients receiving TSF treatment maintained continuous abstinence in the year following treatment.[193] The same pattern of results was also evident at follow-up 3 years later.[198] Like the other studies discussed, data analysis showed that the effectiveness of the TSF treatment was based on its differential ability to increase post-treatment participation in AA.[196]

The first clinical trial of TSF for patients in treatment for stimulant use disorder was recently completed. Individuals randomized to TSF had higher rates of attending groups such as Crystal Meth Anonymous and higher rates of abstinence at follow-up as well.[199]

Given the common group and social orientation and the similar therapeutic factors operating across different mutual aid groups,[200-202] participation in mutual aid groups other than AA might confer similar benefits at analogous levels of attendance.[203,204] Yet systematic efforts to facilitate entry into non-12-step mutual aid groups have rarely been studied.[204] One exception is a clinical trial evaluating SMART Recovery, a cognitive-behavioral, evidence-based mutual aid group. Patients in treatment for "heavy drinking" were randomly assigned to receive face-to-face SMART Recovery meetings or to an on-line Web meeting. Both groups showed approximately equal rates of post-treatment participation in SMART Recovery and in abstinence.[205]

Family Therapies

Mainstream health care has long acknowledged the benefits of engaging family and social supports to improve treatment adherence and to promote behavioral changes needed to effectively treat many chronic illnesses.[206] This is also true for patients with substance use disorders. Studies of various family therapies have demonstrated positive findings for both adults and adolescents.[85] Family therapies engage partners and/or parents and children to help the individual achieve positive outcomes based on behavior change. Several evidence-based family therapies have been evaluated.

Family behavior therapy (FBT) is a therapeutic approach used for both adolescents and adults that addresses not only substance use but other issues the family may also be experiencing, such as mental disorders and family conflict.[85] FBT includes up to 20 treatment sessions that focus on developing skills and setting behavioral goals. Basic necessities are reviewed and inventoried with the client, and the family pursues resolution strategies and addresses activities of daily living, including violence prevention and HIV/AIDS prevention.[207]

Family therapies used specifically for treating substance use disorders in adolescents include Multi-Systemic Therapy (MST), Multi-Dimensional Family Therapy (MDFT), Brief Strategic Family Therapy (BSFT), and Functional Family Therapy (FFT).[85] Most of these therapies consist of sessions that include the adolescent and at least one other family member, although MDFT uses a combination of both individual and family sessions.[85] These interventions use different approaches, ranging from addressing antisocial behaviors (MST) and unfavorable influences (MDFT) on adolescents to identifying patterns of negative behaviors and interactions within the family (BSFT and FFT).[85]

Perhaps the most widely studied and applied family therapy has been Behavioral Couples Therapy (BCT). A cardinal feature of BCT is the "daily sobriety contract" between the affected patient and his/her spouse in which the patient states his or her intent not to drink or use drugs, and the spouse expresses support for the patient's efforts to stay abstinent. BCT also teaches communication and non-substance-associated positive activities for couples. Findings show that BCT produces more abstinence and better functioning relationships than typical individual-based treatment and that it also reduces social costs and intimate partner violence.[208]

Well-supported evidence demonstrates the effectiveness of substance use disorder therapies that engage the spouse or partner and the family in reducing substance use and/or misuse problems and addressing other issues, such as poor communication, neglect, conflict, and intimate partner violence. In a recent review of controlled studies with alcohol-dependent patients, marital and family therapy, and particularly behavioral couples therapy, was significantly more effective than individual treatments at inducing and sustaining abstinence; improving relationship functioning and reducing intimate partner violence; and reducing emotional problems of children.[209,210] Similar findings have been shown with patients having opioid and cocaine use disorders[208,210] and with gay and lesbian families.[210]

Tobacco Use Cessation Efforts in Substance Use Disorder Treatment Programs

People with mental and/or substance use disorders account for 40 percent of all cigarettes smoked in the United States.[211] Many substance use disorder treatment facilities and programs have adopted tobacco-free policies and tobacco cessation programs. Research has shown that incorporating tobacco cessation programs into substance use disorder treatment does not jeopardize treatment outcomes[212] and is associated with a 25 percent increase in the likelihood of maintaining long-term abstinence from alcohol and drug misuse.[213]

Recovery Support Services

Recovery support services (RSS), provided by both substance use disorder treatment programs and community organizations, help to engage and support individuals in treatment, and provide ongoing support after treatment. These supportive services are typically delivered by trained case managers, recovery coaches, and/or peers.

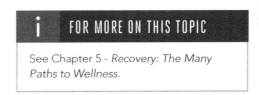

FOR MORE ON THIS TOPIC

See Chapter 5 - *Recovery: The Many Paths to Wellness.*

Specific supports include help with navigating systems of care, removing barriers to recovery, staying engaged in the recovery process, and providing a social context for individuals to engage in community living without substance use.[214] RSS can be effective in promoting healthy lifestyle techniques to increase resilience skills, reduce the risk of relapse, and help those affected by substance use disorders achieve and maintain recovery.[56]

Individuals who participate in substance use disorder treatment and RSS typically have better long-term recovery outcomes than individuals who receive either alone. Further, active recovery and social supports, both during and following treatment, are important in maintaining recovery.[214] This has also been demonstrated for adolescents; the combination of behavioral treatments with assertive continuing care has yielded positive results for this age group, beyond treatment alone.[215]

Emerging Treatment Technologies

Technological advancements are changing not only the face of health care generally, but also the treatment of substance use disorders. In this regard, approximately 20 percent of substance use disorder treatment programs have adopted electronic health record (EHR) systems. With the growing adoption of EHRs, individuals and their providers can more easily access and share treatment records to improve coordination of care.[216] In turn, information sharing through EHRs can lead to improved quality and efficiency of service delivery, reduced treatment gaps, and increased cost savings to health systems.

The use of telehealth to deliver health care, provide health information or education, and monitor the effects of care, has also rapidly increased.[217] Telehealth can be facilitated through a variety of media, including smartphones, the Internet, videoconferencing, wireless communication, and streaming media. It offers alternative, cost-effective care options for individuals living in rural or remote areas or when physically travelling to a health care facility poses significant challenges.

> **KEY TERMS**
>
> **Telehealth.** The use of digital technologies such as EHRs, mobile applications, telemedicine, and web-based tools to support the delivery of health care, health-related education, or other health-related services and functions.[1]
>
> **Telemedicine.** Two-way, real-time interactive communication between a patient and a physician or other health care professional at a distant site. Telemedicine is a subcategory of *telehealth*. Telemedicine refers specifically to remote clinical services, whereas telehealth can include remote non-clinical services such as provider training, administrative meetings, and continuing medical education, and patient-focused technologies, in addition to clinical services.

Technology-based interventions offer many potential advantages. They can increase access to care in underserved areas and settings; free up time so that service providers can care for more clients; provide alternative care options for individuals hesitant to seek in-person treatment; increase the chances that interventions will be delivered as they were designed and intended to be delivered; and decrease costs.[218-222] Further, studies show that most individuals already have access to the necessary tools to engage in technology-based care; about 92 percent of United States adults own a cell phone[223] and 85 percent use the Internet.[224]

Research on the effectiveness of technology-assisted care within substance use disorder treatment focuses on three main applications: (1) technology as an add-on to enhance standard care; (2) technology as a substitute for a portion of standard care; and (3) technology as a replacement for standard care.[221] The current evidence base of technology-based interventions for substance use disorder treatment is limited, though it is growing.[221,225-227] For this reason, these technologies can only be considered "promising" at this time. Table 4.5 shows the state of evidence supporting innovative technology-assisted interventions, several of which are discussed in the Electronic Treatment Interventions and Electronic Clinical and Recovery Support Tools sections.

Table 4.5: Examples of Technology-Assisted Interventions

Intervention	Intervention Overview	Sample (at pretest) /Ethnicity/ Setting Design	Summary/Results	Source
Addiction–Comprehensive Health Enhancement Support System (A-CHESS)	Smartphone-based application offering monitoring, information, communication, and support services.	N = 349 individuals with alcohol dependence entering treatment at residential programs Varied settings, multiethnic RCT	At 4-, 8- and 12-month follow-up, intervention group reported significantly fewer risky drinking days (1.39 vs. 2.75 days on average) and a higher likelihood of consistent abstinence (51.9% vs. 39.6%) as compared to the control group.	Gustafson et al., (2014)[228]
CBT4CBT	Six-module computer-based cognitive behavioral therapy training.	N = 101 cocaine-dependent individuals maintained on methadone Urban, multiethnic RCT	After completing an 8-week program, participants who received the intervention were significantly more likely to attain 3 or more consecutive weeks of abstinence from cocaine than were participants who did not receive the program (36% vs.17%). 6-month follow-up data indicated continued improvement for intervention group.	Carroll et al., (2014)[229]
HealthCall	60 days of patient automated telephone interactive voice response (IVR) calls to self-monitor alcohol- and other health-related behaviors as adjunct to motivational interviewing.	N = 258 HIV-positive individuals reporting alcohol misuse Urban HIV primary care clinic, multiethnic RCT	After 60 days, members of intervention group with alcohol dependence reported significantly fewer drinks per drinking day as compared to control group (3.55 vs. 6.07). Lower rates of drinks per drinking day among intervention group maintained at 12-month follow-up.	Hasin et al., (2013)[230]
Reduce Your Use	Self-guided web-based treatment program for cannabis use disorder based on cognitive, motivational, and behavioral principles.	N = 225 individuals looking to reduce or cease cannabis use Varied settings RCT	After 6 weeks, the intervention group reported significantly fewer days of cannabis use in the past month, significantly lower past-month quantity of cannabis use, and significantly fewer symptoms of cannabis abuse compared to the control group. Similar results at 3-month follow-up.	Rooke et al., (2013)[231]

Intervention	Intervention Overview	Sample (at pretest) /Ethnicity/ Setting Design	Summary/Results	Source
Self-Help for Alcohol and other Drug Use and Depression (SHADE)	Nine sessions of computer-delivered motivational interviewing and cognitive behavior therapy with brief therapist assistance.	N = 274 individuals with comorbid depression and alcohol/cannabis misuse Community-based, Australia RCT	At 3-month follow-up, the intervention group that received computer-delivered care achieved 4 times the reduction in alcohol consumption compared to the control group, and 2.5 times the reduction of the group who received therapist-delivered care.	Kay-Lambkin et al., (2011)[232]
Therapeutic Education System (TES)	62 computer-interactive modules teaching skills for achieving and maintaining abstinence, as well as prize-based motivational incentives based on abstinence and treatment adherence.	N = 507 adult men and women Outpatient addiction treatment programs RCT	Compared to the control group, those receiving TES reduced dropout from treatment (Hazard Ratio=0.72) and increased abstinence (Odds Ratio=1.62).	Cambell et al., (2015)[233]

Note: RCT = randomized controlled trial.

Electronic Assessments and Early Intervention

Several studies have been conducted on technology-assisted screening, assessment, and brief intervention for substance use disorders. Many of these studies focus on Internet-based assessments and brief interventions for at-risk, college-age populations. Examples of evaluated tools include the *Check Your Drinking* screener,[234] electronic alcohol screening and brief intervention (*e-SBI*),[235] *Drinker's Check-up*,[236] *Alcohol electronic Check-Up to Go* (*e-CHUG,*)[237] and *Marijuana eCHECKUP TO GO*.[238] Other studies assessed interventions that can be implemented in general health care settings, including *Project QUIT*, a brief intervention in a primary care setting that also includes follow-up coaching calls for individuals who have been identified through screening as engaging in risky drug use,[50] and use of kiosks in emergency departments to screen for alcohol and drug use.[239] In the latter study, patients in the emergency department were found to be significantly more likely to disclose their substance use at a kiosk compared to a health care professional or other interviewer. Other studies focus on telephone-based assessments and brief interventions related to alcohol and drug use, including *DIAL*,[240] and a telephone-based monitoring and brief counseling intervention.[241] Preliminary evidence shows that Web- and telephone-based assessments and brief interventions are superior to no treatment in reducing substance use, and often result in similar or improved outcomes when compared to alternative brief intervention options.[236,241-247]

Electronic Treatment Interventions

A larger pool of research studies has assessed the effectiveness of substance use disorder treatment approaches (largely outpatient) that incorporate Web- and telephone-based technology. These interventions focus on a wider range of substances, including alcohol (e.g., *Drinking Less*,[248] *HealthCall*[230]), opioids (e.g., *Therapeutic Education System*,[226] *CBT4CBT*[229]), and marijuana (e.g., *Reduce Your Use*,[231] *SHADE*[232]), and target various subpopulations, including veterans and individuals with co-occurring disorders and other chronic illnesses.[230,232,249]

Many of these technology-enhanced treatment interventions are Web-based versions of evidence-based, in-person treatment components such as CBT and MET. Early research suggests the value of applying Web-based treatment approaches for moderate levels of substance misuse and for individuals who may not otherwise seek face-to-face treatment.[221,250] Among studies evaluating Web-based intervention support as an add-on to standard in-person treatment, preliminary evidence shows reduced substance use, better retention, and higher motivation to change among the intervention group.[229,233,251,252] One study explored replacing traditional in-person CBT with a Web-based version and found at least equivalent outcomes among the intervention group, indicating great potential for these Web-based interventions to broaden the dissemination of evidence-based treatments.[232]

Recent studies of telephone-based interventions as adjuncts to or replacements for standard care interventions showed similarly promising results. For example, one study explored the effect of adding daily self-monitoring calls to an interactive voice response technology system with personalized feedback and compared it to standard motivational enhancement practice. Study results showed that those who received the intervention reduced the number of drinks they had on the days they did drink.[230]

Electronic Clinical and Recovery Support Tools

Several studies have examined the application of technology-assisted tools to RSS. In general, Web- and telephone-based recovery support tools focus on providing remote support to individuals following substance use disorder treatment. Examples of e-recovery support tools include: *A-CHESS*, a smartphone application that provides monitoring, information, communication, and support services to patients, including ways for individuals and counselors to stay in contact;[228] and *MORE*, a Web-based recovery support program that delivers assessments, clinical content, and access to recovery coaching support online.[253] Preliminary evidence shows that technology-assisted recovery support approaches may be effective in helping individuals to maintain their recovery.[221,228,253] In 2014, a study found that OTP participants receiving ongoing counseling services through Web-based videoconferencing technology experienced comparable rates of decreased drug use and program attendance as did individuals receiving in-person care.[227]

Considerations for Specific Populations

Culturally Competent Care

A variety of treatment approaches have been developed to address the needs of individuals with substance use disorders. However, disparities exist in the outcomes and effectiveness of substance use treatment for different populations.[109,254] Research has shown that treatment needs can differ across various populations,[255,256] suggesting that treatment interventions should be individually tailored and incorporate culturally competent and linguistically appropriate practices relevant to specific populations and subpopulation groups.[257]

Racial and Ethnic Groups

A study examining a culturally sensitive substance use disorder intervention program targeted at Hispanic or Latino and Black or African American adolescents called *Alcohol Treatment Targeting Adolescents in Need (ATTAIN)* found significant reductions in alcohol and marijuana use for all racial and ethnic groups.[258] Cultural factors, including discrimination, acculturation, ethnic pride, and cultural mistrust, were associated with the pre-intervention levels of alcohol and drug use. The study concluded that accounting for these factors when tailoring a substance use disorder intervention is critical to meeting the needs of the community it is aiming to serve.

Many of the interventions developed for substance use disorder treatment services in general have been evaluated in populations that included Black or African American patients, and many of these interventions are as effective for Black or African American patients as they are for White patients.[259,260] Some motivational interventions that are aligned with the cultural values of the population have been found to reduce substance use among Blacks or African Americans.[27,257]

Dialectical Behavior Therapy (DBT) is an evidence-based therapy that teaches a skill called mindfulness. Multiple research studies have noted that mindfulness, an attentional exercise originally developed in Buddhist cultures, is potentially useful in helping people gain mastery over substance cravings.[261] A study examining patients in a substance use disorder residential treatment center that incorporated DBT with specific cultural, traditional, and spiritual practices for American Indian or Alaska Native adolescents found that 96 percent of the adolescents in their sample either "recovered" or "improved."[262] Treatment included all aspects of comprehensive DBT and included consultation with tribal leaders from the governing body and a medicine man/spiritual counselor from a local tribe.

Asian patients tend to enter treatment with less severe substance misuse problems than do members of other racial or ethnic groups,[263] place less value on substance use disorder treatment, and are less likely to use such services.[264] Studies on Asians and Native Hawaiians and Pacific Islanders have identified culturally specific barriers and facilitators to entering and completing substance use treatment (e.g., family, peers, shame, and involvement in the criminal justice system).[265] Assessing patient experience of shame is an important step when providing substance use disorder treatment to Asian patients because shame and humiliation can be significant barriers to treatment engagement for this population.[266]

Combining Evidence-based Care with Traditional, Spiritual, and Cultural Beliefs

Agency or Organization:

Desert Visions Youth Wellness Center (Desert Visions), Indian Health Service, Sacaton, Arizona

Purpose:

Desert Visions is a federally-operated adolescent residential center whose purpose is to provide substance use and behavioral health treatment to American Indians and Alaska Natives. Desert Visions offers a multi-disciplinary treatment that includes bio-psychosocial, health, education, and cultural activities. Desert Visions uses Dialectical Behavior Therapy (DBT) as the treatment modality, and clients are taught to use the DBT skills to improve their quality of life.

> *"The results demonstrated by the outcome data far exceeded expectations. DBT has dramatically improved the care of adolescents at our facilities. A serendipitous benefit has been the enhancement of the relationship with the multiplicity of referral sources. Our tribal partners have commented positively on the integration of DBT with those traditional, cultural, and spiritual practices that are common to the many tribal nations."*
>
> – Rear Admiral Vincent Berkley, USPHS, Retired Medical Director, Youth Treatment Centers of Arizona and Nevada

Goals:

- Provide holistic care and treatment for the physical, spiritual, and emotional needs of American Indian and Alaska Native adolescents.
- Provide superior outcomes in treating substance use/co-occurring disorders.
- Utilize the DBT skill of mindfulness to allow for the introduction of cultural, spiritual, and traditional practices into treatment while still maintaining fidelity to this evidence-based approach. In essence, the goal of using DBT is to combine the best of "Western-Based" interventions with traditional American Indian/Alaska Native interventions.

Outcomes:

A 3-year program/statistical review of outcome data found that of 229 patients who were enrolled in the treatment program:

- 201 met the criteria for clinically significant change, (i.e., "recovered" or "reliable change" or "improved") and 10 showed no change.
- None of the youth in treatment deteriorated during the treatment period.
- The findings represent a first investigation of the use of DBT within American Indian and Alaska Native populations.

Lesbian, Gay, Bisexual, and Transgender Populations

Lesbian, gay, bisexual, and transgender (LGBT) populations often enter treatment with more severe substance misuse problems,[267] have a greater likelihood of experiencing a substance use disorder in their lifetime, and initiate alcohol consumption earlier than heterosexual clients;[268] thus, developing effective treatment programs that address the specific needs of these populations is critical. For example, the 2013 *National Health Interview Survey*, conducted by the U.S. Census Bureau, found that a higher percentage of LGBT adults, aged 18 to 64, had five or more drinks on one day in the past year compared to heterosexual adults.[269] Research has also shown that LGB adolescents report higher rates of substance use compared to heterosexual youth; on average substance use among LGB youth was 190 percent higher than for heterosexual youth, 340 percent higher for bisexual youth, and 400 percent higher for lesbians and bisexual females.[270] Treatment programs with specialized groups for gay and bisexual clients have shown better outcomes for men compared to gay and bisexual men in non-specialized programs.[113] According to one analysis, a significant minority of the nation's substance use disorder treatment agencies indicated that they offer treatment services tailored to LGBT populations, although only a small portion (7.4 percent) offered a service that they could identify as an LGBT-specialized service.[271]

Research has shown that treatment providers should be knowledgeable about sexuality, sexual orientation, and unique aspects of LGBT developmental and social experiences.[272] For example, factors such as transphobia or homophobia (both internal and societal), violence, family issues, and social isolation, among other problems, may need to be addressed within the substance use disorder treatment environment for transgender people.[273] It is also important to consider the types of treatment that have been shown effective with the LGBT population. Motivational interviewing, social support therapy, contingency management, and CBT have all demonstrated effectiveness specifically for gay or bisexual men with a substance use disorder.[272]

Veterans

Being a veteran or an active member of the military is a unique way of life that involves experiences and sacrifices by the service member and the member's family. Military service members, veterans, and their families have needs unlike other individuals that require culturally competent approaches to treatment and services. Veterans report high rates of substance misuse; between 2004 and 2006, 7.1 percent of all veterans met the criteria for a substance use disorder.[274] Studies of female veterans have shown that between 4 and 37 percent of veterans reported alcohol misuse, 7 to 25 percent reported binge drinking, and between 3 and 16 percent reported substance use disorders.[275] Much of the literature on substance use in the military examines the relationship between post-traumatic stress disorder (PTSD) and alcohol and drug use. For example, a large study examined improvement in substance use outcomes among 12,270 veterans who were diagnosed with PTSD and a substance use disorder and treated in specialized intensive veterans' treatment programs. The study found that treatment in longer-term programs, with prescribed psychiatric medication and planned participation in program reunions for post-discharge support, were all associated with improved outcomes.[276] Reductions in substance use were also associated with improvements in PTSD symptoms and violent behavior. The findings suggested that intensive treatment combined with proper discharge planning for veterans with severe PTSD and a substance use disorder may result in better outcomes than traditional substance use disorder treatment. A study among homeless veterans with a diagnosis of a substance use disorder as well as a mental disorder found that those who took part in a low-intensity wrap-around intervention showed improvements in a number of substance use, mental health, and behavioral health outcomes from the beginning of the study to follow-up 12 months later.[277]

Criminal Justice Populations

It has been estimated that half of the United States prison population has an active substance use disorder.[278] Many incarcerated individuals will experience a lower tolerance for substances due to abstinence while in prison; upon release, many will return to dangerous use levels, not realizing their tolerance is diminished.[279] This is particularly important as it raises the risk of opioid overdose deaths after release from incarceration; one study found that 14.8 percent of all former prisoner deaths from 1999 to 2009 were related to opioids.[280] There is typically insufficient pre-release counseling and post-release follow-up provided to this population to reduce these risks.[281]

In a randomized controlled trial of methadone maintenance for prisoners, participants were randomly assigned to counseling with passive referral to methadone maintenance treatment (MMT) after release, counseling with transfer to MMT, or counseling with pre-release MMT. Prisoners who received counseling and MMT in prison prior to release and continued with community-based MMT after release were significantly less likely to use opioids and engage in criminal activity post-release.[282] Increased access to opioid agonist maintenance may positively impact the needs of substance use disorders among incarcerated individuals.[283]

Another randomized trial assigned some participants to extended-release naltrexone treatment and others to usual treatment, consisting of brief counseling and referrals to community treatment programs. Those who received extended-release naltrexone had a lower rate of relapse (43 percent vs. 64 percent), and a higher rate of opioid-negative urine samples (74 percent vs. 56 percent), and the average time between treatment and relapse was found to be longer—10.5 weeks, compared with 5.0 weeks for those who received usual treatment. Importantly, positive effects diminished after treatment with extended-release naltrexone was discontinued.[284]

Drug Courts

Drug courts are a diverse group of specialized programs that focus on adult or juvenile offenders, as well as parents under child protective supervision who have substance use-related disorders.[285] Drug courts provide treatment and other services, overseen by a judge, in lieu of being processed through the traditional justice system. By 2015, more than 3,400 drug courts were in operation across the United States.[285] An estimated 55,000 defendants per year participate in adult drug courts,[286,287] with each court serving a caseload of approximately 50 individuals each year.[288] These interventions seek to harness the coercive power of the criminal justice system to persuade drug-involved offenders to cease their problematic drug use.

Existing research, including randomized controlled trials, have found positive effects of drug courts, including high rates of treatment completion and reduced rates of recidivism, incarceration, and subsequent drug use.[288-291] Reviews of these evaluations have concluded that the average effect of adult drug court participation is analogous to a drop in recidivism from 50 percent to 38 percent, and that this effect lasts up to 3 years.[289] Evaluations of driving under the influence (DUI) drug courts generally find similar reductions as adult drug courts and substantially smaller effects than are found in juvenile drug courts.[292] Larger reductions in recidivism were found in adult drug courts that had high graduation rates and that accepted only nonviolent offenders, suggesting that this intervention may be more effective among that segment of the substance-using population.

Despite the rapid expansion of drug courts, the number of defendants who pass through such programs remains a small proportion of the more than 1 million offenders with substance use disorders who pass through the United States criminal justice system each year. Capacity constraints provide the most important limitation.[286]

Drug court programs require random drug tests and other monitoring measures. Required abstinence involves making sanctions certain and immediate. *Hawaii's Opportunity Probation with Enforcement* (*HOPE*) program has implemented coerced abstinence for the entire probation population. Promising results of a randomized trial have sparked interest in broader replication.[293] Observed recidivism rates were dramatically lower than for the prior probation population, and the treatment group was incarcerated for roughly half as many days as the control group. Interventions such as *HOPE* do not necessarily involve substance use disorder treatment; this reflects the reality that many drug-involved offenders do not meet the criteria for substance use disorders. For many individuals, regular monitoring, alongside the adverse consequences of a failed urine test, provide powerful motivation to abstain.[294]

A further example is the *24/7 Sobriety Project* (24/7), a South Dakota innovative program to supervise individuals who were arrested in connection with alcohol-related offenses. It addresses problem drinking by imposing close monitoring, followed by swift, certain, yet modest sanctions when there is evidence of renewed alcohol use. Under 24/7, problem drinkers rearrested for DUI and selected other alcohol-related violations were subject to intensive monitoring and sanctions. As a condition of bail, participants were required to take morning and evening breathalyzer tests or wear continuous alcohol-monitoring bracelets. Between 2005 and 2010, 24/7 participants were ordered to take approximately 3.7 million breathalyzer tests, and achieved a pass rate of approximately 99.3 percent.[295] A RAND Corporation program evaluation found that 24/7 tangibly improved public safety in counties where the program was implemented at scale.[295] In counties where the number of 24/7 participants reached one-quarter of DUI arrests, the intervention was associated with a significant reduction in repeat DUI and intimate partner violence arrests. Similar results have been replicated in Montana.[296]

Recommendations for Research

Although the field of treatment for substance use disorders has made substantial progress, additional types of research are needed. Research involving early interventions and various components of treatment must move from rigorously controlled trials to natural delivery settings and a broader mix of patient types. Because rigorously controlled trials must focus on specific diagnoses and carefully characterized patient types, it is often the case that the samples used in these trials are not representative of the real-world populations who need treatment. For example, many opioid medication trials involve "opioid-only" populations, whereas in practice most patients with opioid use disorders also have alcohol, marijuana, and/or cocaine use disorders. Rigorously controlled trials are necessary to establish efficacy, but interventions that seem to be effective in these studies too often cannot be implemented in real-world settings because of a lack of workforce training, inadequate insurance coverage, and an inability to adequately engage the intended patient population.

As has been documented in several chapters within this *Report*, the great majority of patients with substance use disorders do not receive any form of treatment. Nonetheless, many of these individuals do access primary or general medical care in community clinics or school settings and research is needed to determine the availability and efficacy of treatment in these settings and to identify ways in which access to treatment in these settings could be improved. The current failure to acknowledge and address substance use disorders in these settings has reduced the quality and increased the costs of health care. Moreover, access and referral to specialty substance use disorder care from primary care settings is neither easy nor quick. Better integration between primary care and specialty care and additional treatment options within primary care are needed. Primary care physicians need to be better prepared to identify, assist, and refer patients, when appropriate. If treatment is delivered in primary care, it should be practical for delivery within these settings and attractive, engaging, accessible and affordable for affected patients.

Buprenorphine or naloxone treatment for opioid misuse should also be available in emergency departments.[297] Here, the goals of treatment would be the reduction of substance use combined with better engagement in and adherence to treatment for any associated medical illness. Therefore, treatment research outside of traditional substance use disorder treatment programs is needed.

As of June 2016, four states, plus the District of Columbia, have legalized recreational marijuana, and many more have permitted medical marijuana use. The impact of the changes on levels of marijuana and other drug and alcohol use, simultaneous use, and related problems such as motor vehicle crashes and deaths, overdoses, hospitalizations, and poor school and work performance, must be evaluated closely. Accurate and practical marijuana screening and early intervention procedures for use in general and primary care settings are needed. Not only must it be determined which assessment tools are appropriate for the various populations that use marijuana, but also which treatments are generalizable from research to practice, especially in primary care and general mental health care settings.

Current research suggests that it is useful to educate and train first responders, peers, and family members of those who use opioids to use naloxone to prevent and reverse potential overdose-related deaths. However, more research is needed to identify strategies to encourage the subsequent engagement of those who have recovered from overdose into appropriate treatment. In this work, it will be important to consider contextual factors such as age, gender identity, race and ethnicity, sexual orientation, economic status, community resources, faith beliefs, co-occurring mental or physical illness, and many other personal issues that can work against the appropriateness and ultimately the usefulness of a treatment strategy.

Opioid agonist therapies are effective in stabilizing the lives of individuals with severe opioid use disorders. However, many important clinical and social questions remain about whether, when, and how to discontinue medications and related services. This is an important question for many other areas of medicine where maintenance medications are continued without significant change and often without attention to other areas of clinical progress.

At the same time, it is clear from many studies over the decades that detoxification following an arbitrary maintenance time period (e.g., 90 days, 180 days), or performed without continuing supports, is rarely effective in disengaging patients from opioid use disorders and may lead to relapse and overdose. Thus, more research is needed to explore if, when, and how patients can be transitioned from MAT to non-medication status within the context of "personalized medicine," to provide both patients and clinical staff appropriate therapeutic guidance.

Regarding personalized medicine, research is needed on how to implement multidisciplinary, collaborative, and patient-centered care for persons with opioid use disorders and chronic pain, in a manner effectively treating both diseases together with any psychiatric comorbidities that may undermine recovery. Precision medicine research is also needed on how to individually tailor such interventions to optimize care management for patient groups in which there is overlap between pain-related psychological distress and stress-related opioid misuse.[298]

References

1. HealthIT.gov. (2014). What is telehealth? How is telehealth different from telemedicine? Retrieved from https://www.healthit.gov/providers-professionals/faqs/what-telehealth-how-telehealth-different-telemedicine. Accessed on June 17, 2016.

2. Medina, J. (2015). Symptoms of substance use disorders (Revised for DSM-5). Retrieved from http://psychcentral.com/disorders/revised-alcoholsubstance-use-disorder/. Accessed on March 9, 2016.

3. Substance Abuse and Mental Health Services Administration. (2015). Behavioral health treatments and services. Retrieved from http://www.samhsa.gov/treatment. Accessed on January 25, 2016.

4. Evashwick, C. (1988). Creating the continuum of care. *Health Matrix, 7*(1), 30-39.

5. Rieckmann, T., Kovas, A. E., & Rutkowski, B. A. (2010). Adoption of medications in substance abuse treatment: Priorities and strategies of single state authorities. *Journal of Psychoactive Drugs, 42*(Suppl 6), 227-238.

6. Udo, T., Vasquez, E., & Shaw, B. A. (2015). A lifetime history of alcohol use disorder increases risk for chronic medical conditions after stable remission. *Drug and Alcohol Dependence, 157*, 68-74.

7. Kline-Simon, A. H., Weisner, C., & Sterling, S. (2016). Point prevalence of co-occurring behavioral health conditions and associated chronic disease burden among adolescents. *Journal of the American Academy of Child & Adolescent Psychiatry, 55*(5), 408-414.

8. Puddy, R. W., & Wilkins, N. (2011). *Understanding evidence Part 1: Best available research evidence. A guide to the continuum of evidence of effectiveness.* Atlanta, GA: Centers for Disease Control and Prevention.

9. Compton, W. M., Thomas, Y. F., Stinson, F. S., & Grant, B. F. (2007). Prevalence, correlates, disability, and comorbidity of DSM-IV drug abuse and dependence in the United States: Results from the national epidemiologic survey on alcohol and related conditions. *Archives of General Psychiatry, 64*(5), 566-576.

10. Hasin, D. S., Stinson, F. S., Ogburn, E., & Grant, B. F. (2007). Prevalence, correlates, disability, and comorbidity of DSM-IV alcohol abuse and dependence in the United States: Results from the National Epidemiologic Survey on Alcohol and Related Conditions. *Archives of General Psychiatry, 64*(7), 830-842.

11. Ettner, S. L., Huang, D., Evans, E., Ash, D. R., Hardy, M., Jourabchi, M., & Hser, Y. I. (2006). Benefit-cost in the California treatment outcome project: Does substance abuse treatment "pay for itself"? *Health Services Research, 41*(1), 192-213.

12. McLellan, A. T., Lewis, D. C., O'Brien, C. P., & Kleber, H. D. (2000). Drug dependence, a chronic medical illness: Implications for treatment, insurance, and outcomes evaluation. *JAMA, 284*(13), 1689-1695.

13. Pasareanu, A. R., Opsal, A., Vederhus, J., Kristensen, Ø., & Clausen, T. (2015). Quality of life improved following in-patient substance use disorder treatment. *Health and Quality of Life Outcomes, 13*(35).

14. Garner, B. R., Scott, C. K., Dennis, M. L., & Funk, R. R. (2014). The relationship between recovery and health-related quality of life. *Journal of Substance Abuse Treatment, 47*(4), 293-298.

15. Tracy, E. M., Laudet, A. B., Min, M. O., Kim, H., Brown, S., Jun, M. K., & Singer, L. (2012). Prospective patterns and correlates of quality of life among women in substance abuse treatment. *Drug and Alcohol Dependence, 124*(3), 242-249.

16. Sobell, M. B., & Sobell, L. C. (2005). Guided self-change model of treatment for substance use disorders. *Journal of Cognitive Psychotherapy, 19*(3), 199-210.

17. Center for Substance Abuse Treatment. (1999). *Brief interventions and brief therapies for substance abuse. Treatment improvement protocol (TIP) series, No. 34.* (HHS Publication No. (SMA) 12-3952). Rockville, MD: Substance Abuse and Mental Health Services Administration.

18. American Society of Addiction Medicine. (2001). *ASAM patient placement criteria for the treatment of substance-related disorders* (2nd ed.). Chevy Chase, MD: American Society of Addiction Medicine, Inc.

19. Center for Behavioral Health Statistics and Quality. (2016). *Results from the 2015 National Survey on Drug Use and Health: Detailed tables.* Rockville, MD: Substance Abuse and Mental Health Services Administration.

20. Agerwala, S. M., & McCance-Katz, E. F. (2012). Integrating screening, brief intervention, and referral to treatment (SBIRT) into clinical practice settings: A brief review. *Journal of Psychoactive Drugs, 44*(4), 307-317.

21. Manuel, J. K., Satre, D. D., Tsoh, J., Moreno-John, G., Ramos, J. S., McCance-Katz, E. F., & Satterfield, J. M. (2015). Adapting screening, brief intervention, and referral to treatment for alcohol and drugs to culturally diverse clinical populations. *Journal of Addiction Medicine, 9*(5), 343-351.

22. Harris, S. K., & Knight, J. R. (2014). Putting the screen in screening: Technology-based alcohol screening and brief interventions in medical settings. *Alcohol Research: Current Reviews, 36*(1), 63-79.

23. Benningfield, M. M., Riggs, P., & Stephan, S. H. (2015). The role of schools in substance use prevention and intervention. *Child and Adolescent Psychiatric Clinics of North America, 24*(2), 291-303.

24. O'Donnell, A., Anderson, P., Newbury-Birch, D., Schulte, B., Schmidt, C., Reimer, J., & Kaner, E. (2014). The impact of brief alcohol interventions in primary healthcare: A systematic review of reviews. *Alcohol and Alcoholism, 49*(1), 66-78.

25. Schmidt, C. S., Schulte, B., Seo, H. N., Kuhn, S., A, O. D., Kriston, L., . . . Reimer, J. (2016). Meta-analysis on the effectiveness of alcohol screening with brief interventions for patients in emergency care settings. *Addiction, 111*(5), 783-794.

26. Madras, B. K., Compton, W. M., Avula, D., Stegbauer, T., Stein, J. B., & Clark, H. W. (2009). Screening, brief interventions, referral to treatment (SBIRT) for illicit drug and alcohol use at multiple healthcare sites: Comparison at intake and 6 months later. *Drug and Alcohol Dependence, 99*(1), 280-295.

27. Bernstein, J., Bernstein, E., Tassiopoulos, K., Heeren, T., Levenson, S., & Hingson, R. (2005). Brief motivational intervention at a clinic visit reduces cocaine and heroin use. *Drug and Alcohol Dependence, 77*(1), 49-59.

28. Fuster, D., Cheng, D. M., Wang, N., Bernstein, J. A., Palfai, T. P., Alford, D. P., . . . Saitz, R. (2015). Brief intervention for daily marijuana users identified by screening in primary care: A subgroup analysis of the ASPIRE randomized clinical trial. *Substance Abuse*, 1-7.

29. Saitz, R. (2014). Screening and brief intervention for unhealthy drug use: Little or no efficacy. *Frontiers in Psychiatry, 5*(121).

30. Estee, S., He, L., Mancuso, D., & Felver, B. (2006). *Medicaid cost outcomes*. Olympia, WA: Department of Social and Health Services, Research and Data Analysis Division.

31. Levy, S. J., Williams, J. F., & Committee on Substance Use and Prevention. (2016). Substance use screening, brief intervention, and referral to treatment. *Pediatrics, 138*(1).

32. Levy, S. J., & Kokotailo, P. K. (2011). Substance use screening, brief intervention, and referral to treatment for pediatricians. *Pediatrics, 128*(5), e1330-e1340.

33. Coble, Y. D., Estes, E. H., Head, C. A., Karlan, M. S., Kennedy, W. R., Numann, P. J., . . . Strong, J. P. (1993). Confidential health services for adolescents. *JAMA, 269*(11), 1420-1424.

34. Canfield, S. E., & Dahm, P. (2011). Rating the quality of evidence and the strength of recommendations using GRADE. *World Journal of Urology, 29*(3), 311-317.

35. Committee on Health Care for Underserved Women. (2011). At-risk drinking and alcohol dependence: Obstetric and gynecologic implications. *Obstetrics & Gynecology 118*(2 Pt 1), 383-388.

36. Shapiro, B., Coffa, D., & McCance-Katz, E. F. (2013). A primary care approach to substance misuse. *American Family Physician, 88*(2), 113-121.

37. Center for Substance Abuse Treatment. (1999). *Chapter 2—Brief interventions in substance abuse treatment*. In, Brief interventions and brief therapies for substance abuse. Treatment improvement protocol (TIP) series, No. 34. (HHS Publication No. (SMA) 12-3952.). Rockville, MD: Substance Abuse and Mental Health Services Administration.

38. McNeely, J., Cleland, C. M., Strauss, S. M., Palamar, J. J., Rotrosen, J., & Saitz, R. (2015). Validation of self-administered single-item screening questions (SISQs) for unhealthy alcohol and drug use in primary care patients. *Journal of General Internal Medicine, 30*(12), 1757-1764.

39. McNeely, J., Strauss, S. M., Saitz, R., Cleland, C. M., Palamar, J. J., Rotrosen, J., & Gourevitch, M. N. (2015). A brief patient self-administered substance use screening tool for primary care: Two-site validation study of the Substance Use Brief Screen (SUBS). *The American Journal of Medicine, 128*(7), 784.e789-784.e719.

40. Clark, D. B., Martin, C. S., Chung, T., Gordon, A. J., Fiorentino, L., Tootell, M., & Rubio, D. M. (2016). Screening for underage drinking and *Diagnostic and Statistical Manual of Mental Disorders, 5th Edition* alcohol use disorder in rural primary care practice. *The Journal of Pediatrics, 173*, 214-220.

41. Smith, P. C., Schmidt, S. M., Allensworth-Davies, D., & Saitz, R. (2009). Primary care validation of a single-question alcohol screening test. *Journal of General Internal Medicine, 24*(7), 783-788.

42. Levy, S., Dedeoglu, F., Gaffin, J. M., Garvey, K. C., Harstad, E., MacGinnitie, A., . . . Wisk, L. E. (2016). A screening tool for assessing alcohol use risk among medically vulnerable youth. *PLoS One, 11*(5).

43. National Institute on Drug Abuse. (2015). Chart of evidence-based screening tools for adults and adolescents. Retrieved from https://www.drugabuse.gov/nidamed-medical-health-professionals/tool-resources-your-practice/screening-assessment-drug-testing-resources/chart-evidence-based-screening-tools-adults. Accessed on March 9, 2016.

44. Miller, W. R., & Rollnick, S. (2012). *Motivational interviewing: Helping people change* (3rd ed.). New York, NY: Guilford Press.

45. Lundahl, B., Moleni, T., Burke, B. L., Butters, R., Tollefson, D., Butler, C., & Rollnick, S. (2013). Motivational interviewing in medical care settings: A systematic review and meta-analysis of randomized controlled trials. *Patient Education and Counseling, 93*(2), 157-168.

46. Center for Substance Abuse Treatment. (1999). *Chapter 3—Motivational interviewing as a counseling style.* In, Enhancing motivation for change in substance abuse treatment. Treatment improvement protocol (TIP) series, No. 35. (HHS Publication No. (SMA) 13-4212). Rockville, MD: Substance Abuse and Mental Health Services Administration.

47. National Quality Forum. (2005). *Evidence-based treatment practices for substance use disorders: Workshop proceedings.* (NQFWP-06-05). Washington, DC: National Quality Forum.

48. Roy-Byrne, P., Bumgardner, K., Krupski, A., Dunn, C., Ries, R., Donovan, D., . . . Graves, M. C. (2014). Brief intervention for problem drug use in safety-net primary care settings: A randomized clinical trial. *JAMA, 312*(5), 492-501.

49. Saitz, R., Palfai, T. P., Cheng, D. M., Alford, D. P., Bernstein, J. A., Lloyd-Travaglini, C. A., . . . Samet, J. H. (2014). Screening and brief intervention for drug use in primary care: The ASPIRE randomized clinical trial. *JAMA, 312*(5), 502-513.

50. Gelberg, L., Andersen, R. M., Afifi, A. A., Leake, B. D., Arangua, L., Vahidi, M., . . . Fleming, M. F. (2015). Project QUIT (Quit Using Drugs Intervention Trial): A randomized controlled trial of a primary care-based multi-component brief intervention to reduce risky drug use. *Addiction, 110*(11), 1777-1790.

51. Yuma-Guerrero, P. J., Lawson, K. A., Velasquez, M. M., von Sternberg, K., Maxson, T., & Garcia, N. (2012). Screening, brief intervention, and referral for alcohol use in adolescents: A systematic review. *Pediatrics, 130*(1), 115-122.

52. Mitchell, S. G., Gryczynski, J., O'Grady, K. E., & Schwartz, R. P. (2013). SBIRT for adolescent drug and alcohol use: Current status and future directions. *Journal of Substance Abuse Treatment 44*(5), 463-472.

53. Sterling, S., Kline-Simon, A. H., Satre, D. D., Jones, A., Mertens, J., Wong, A., & Weisner, C. (2015). Implementation of screening, brief intervention, and referral to treatment for adolescents in pediatric primary care: A cluster randomized trial. *JAMA Pediatrics, 169*(11).

54. Ozechowski, T. J., Becker, S. J., & Hogue, A. (2016). SBIRT-A: Adapting SBIRT to maximize developmental fit for adolescents in primary care. *Journal of Substance Abuse Treatment, 62,* 28-37.

55. Satre, D. D., Campbell, C. I., Gordon, N. P., & Weisner, C. (2010). Ethnic disparities in accessing treatment for depression and substance use disorders in an integrated health plan. *The International Journal of Psychiatry in Medicine, 40*(1), 57-76.

56. Center for Health Information and Analysis. (2015). *Access to substance use disorder treatment in Massachusetts.* (15-112-CHIA-01). Boston, MA: Center for Health Information and Analysis, Commonwealth of Massachusetts.

57. DeFlavio, J. R., Rolin, S. A., Nordstrom, B. R., & Kazal, L. A., Jr. (2015). Analysis of barriers to adoption of buprenorphine maintenance therapy by family physicians. *Rural Remote Health, 15*(3019), 1-11.

58. Quest, T. L., Merrill, J. O., Roll, J., Saxon, A. J., & Rosenblatt, R. A. (2012). Buprenorphine therapy for opioid addiction in rural Washington: The experience of the early adopters. *Journal of Opioid Management, 8*(1), 29-38.

59. Hawk, K. F., Vaca, F. E., & D'Onofrio, G. (2015). Reducing fatal opioid overdose: Prevention, treatment and harm reduction strategies. *The Yale Journal of Biology and Medicine, 88*(3), 235-245.

60. Ritter, A., & Cameron, J. (2006). A review of the efficacy and effectiveness of harm reduction strategies for alcohol, tobacco and illicit drugs. *Drug and Alcohol Review, 25*(6), 611-624.

61. Hunt, N., Ashton, M., Lenton, S., Mitcheson, L., Nelles, B., & Stimson, G. (2003). A review of the evidence-base for harm reduction approaches to drug use. Retrieved from http://www.forward-thinking-on-drugs.org/review2-print.html. Accessed on June 20, 2016.

62. Wheeler, E., Davidson, P. J., Jones, T. S., & Irwin, K. S. (2012). Community-based opioid overdose prevention programs providing naloxone—United States, 2010. *MMWR, 61*(6), 101-105.

63. Marlatt, G. A., Larimer, M. E., & Witkiewitz, K. (2011). *Harm reduction: Pragmatic strategies for managing high-risk behaviors.* New York, NY: Guilford Press.

64. Gottheil, E., Sterling, R. C., & Weinstein, S. P. (1997). Outreach engagement efforts: Are they worth the effort? *The American Journal of Drug and Alcohol Abuse, 23*(1), 61-66.

65. Center for Substance Abuse Treatment. (2009). *Substance abuse treatment: Addressing the specific needs of women. Treatment improvement protocol (TIP) series, No. 51.* (HHS Publication No. (SMA) 15-4426). Rockville, MD: Substance Abuse and Mental Health Services Administration.

66. Reback, C. J., & Fletcher, J. B. (2014). HIV prevalence, substance use, and sexual risk behaviors among transgender women recruited through outreach. *AIDS and Behavior, 18*(7), 1359-1367.

67. Carmona, J., Slesnick, N., Guo, X., Murnan, A., & Brakenhoff, B. (2015). Predictors of outreach meetings among substance using homeless youth. *Community Mental Health Journal*, 1-10.

68. Tobias, C., Cunningham, W. E., Cunningham, C. O., & Pounds, M. B. (2007). Making the connection: The importance of engagement and retention in HIV medical care. *AIDS Patient Care and STDs, 21*(S1), S-3-S-8.

69. Fisk, D., Rakfeldt, J., & McCormack, E. (2006). Assertive outreach: An effective strategy for engaging homeless persons with substance use disorders into treatment. *The American Journal of Drug and Alcohol Abuse, 32*(3), 479-486.

70. Bowman, S., Engelman, A., Koziol, J., Mahoney, L., Maxwell, C., & Mckenzie, M. (2014). The Rhode Island community responds to opioid overdose deaths. *Rhode Island Medical Journal, 97*(10), 34-37.

71. Substance Abuse and Mental Health Administration. (n.d.). National Recovery Month. Retrieved from http://www.recoverymonth.gov/. Accessed on June 20, 2016.

72. National Safety Council. (2015). *Prescription drug community action kit: Public education and media.* Washington, DC: National Safety Council.

73. Centers for Disease Control and Prevention. (2015). HIV and injection drug use in the United States. Retrieved from http://www.cdc.gov/hiv/risk/idu.html. Accessed on April 6, 2016.

74. Centers for Disease Control and Prevention. (2014). *HIV surveillance report, 2014.* (Vol 26). Atlanta, GA: Centers for Disease Control and Prevention. Retrieved from http://www.cdc.gov/hiv/pdf/library/reports/surveillance/cdc-hiv-surveillance-report-us.pdf. Accessed on April 6, 2016.

75. Centers for Disease Control and Prevention. (2016). Surveillance for viral hepatitis – United States, 2014. Retrieved from https://www.cdc.gov/hepatitis/statistics/2014surveillance/index.htm. Accessed on July 28, 2016.

76. Ingram, M. (2014). *The impact of syringe and needle exchange programs on drug use rates in the United States.* (Master's thesis). Georgetown University, Washington, DC. Retrieved from https://repository.library.georgetown.edu/bitstream/handle/10822/709897/Ingram_georgetown_0076M_12592.pdf?sequence=1. Accessed on April 12, 2016.

77. Rich, J. D., & Adashi, E. Y. (2015). Ideological anachronism involving needle and syringe exchange programs: Lessons from the Indiana HIV outbreak. *JAMA, 314*(1), 23-24.

78. Aspinall, E. J., Nambiar, D., Goldberg, D. J., Hickman, M., Weir, A., Van Velzen, E., . . . Hutchinson, S. J. (2014). Are needle and syringe programmes associated with a reduction in HIV transmission among people who inject drugs: A systematic review and meta-analysis. *International Journal of Epidemiology, 43*(1), 235-248.

79. Palmateer, N., Kimber, J., Hickman, M., Hutchinson, S., Rhodes, T., & Goldberg, D. (2010). Evidence for the effectiveness of sterile injecting equipment provision in preventing hepatitis C and human immunodeficiency virus transmission among injecting drug users: A review of reviews. *Addiction, 105*(5), 844-859.

80. National Institute on Drug Abuse. (2015). Overdose death rates. Retrieved from http://www.drugabuse.gov/related-topics/trends-statistics/overdose-death-rates. Accessed on January 25, 2016.

81. Cowan, K. (2016). CVS pharmacies in NY to sell naloxone without prescription. Retrieved from http://cnycentral.com/news/local/cvs-pharmacies-in-ny-to-sell-naloxone-without-prescription. Accessed on April 11, 2016.

82. StopOverdose.org. (n.d.). Naloxone (Narcan®): Frequently asked questions. Retrieved from http://stopoverdose.org/faq.htm. Accessed on January 25, 2016.

83. European Monitoring Centre for Drugs and Drug Addiction. (2015). *Preventing fatal overdoses: A systematic review of the effectiveness of take-home naloxone.* Luxembourg: EMCDDA Papers, Publications Office of the European Union.

84. Walley, A. Y., Xuan, Z., Hackman, H. H., Quinn, E., Doe-Simkins, M., Sorensen-Alawad, A., . . . Ozonoff, A. (2013). Opioid overdose rates and implementation of overdose education and nasal naloxone distribution in Massachusetts: Interrupted time series analysis. *BMJ, 346*(f174).

85. National Institute on Drug Abuse. (2012). *Principles of drug addiction treatment: A research-based guide.* (NIH Publication No. 12–4180). Rockville, MD: National Institutes of Health, U.S. Department of Health and Human Services.

86. Kim, D., Irwin, K. S., & Khoshnood, K. (2009). Expanded access to naloxone: Options for critical response to the epidemic of opioid overdose mortality. *The American Journal of Public Health, 99*(3), 402-407.

87. American Society of Addiction Medicine. (2014). *The ASAM standards of care for the addiction specialist physician.* Chevy Chase, MD: American Society of Addiction Medicine.

88. Mark, T. L., Dilonardo, J. D., Chalk, M., & Coffey, R. M. (2002). Trends in inpatient detoxification services, 1992-1997. *Journal of Substance Abuse Treatment, 23*(4), 253-260.

89. Mark, T. L., Vandivort-Warren, R., & Montejano, L. B. (2006). Factors affecting detoxification readmission: Analysis of public sector data from three states. *Journal of Substance Abuse Treatment 31*(4), 439-445.

90. Lee, M. T., Horgan, C. M., Garnick, D. W., Acevedo, A., Panas, L., Ritter, G. A., . . . Reynolds, M. (2014). A performance measure for continuity of care after detoxification: Relationship with outcomes. *Journal of Substance Abuse Treatment, 47*(2), 130-139.

91. Millette, S. (2013). *Treatment for substance use disorders – The continuum of care*. National Partnership on Alcohol Misuse and Crime.

92. National Institute on Drug Abuse. (2014). *Principles of adolescent substance use disorder treatment: A research-based guide*. (NIH Publication No. 14-7953). Rockville, MD: National Institutes of Health, U.S. Department of Health and Human Services.

93. Gastfriend, D. R., & Mee-Lee, D. (2004). The ASAM patient placement criteria: Context, concepts and continuing development. *Journal of Addictive Diseases 22*(Suppl 1), 1-8.

94. Stallvik, M., Gastfriend, D. R., & Nordahl, H. M. (2015). Matching patients with substance use disorder to optimal level of care with the ASAM criteria software. *Journal of Substance Use, 20*(6), 389-398.

95. The American Society of Addiction Medicine (ASAM). (n.d.). Continuum: The ASAM criteria decision engine. Retrieved from http://asamcontinuum.org/. Accessed on April 4, 2016.

96. Substance Abuse and Mental Health Services Administration. (2014). *Trauma-informed care in behavioral health services. Treatment Improvement Protocol (TIP) Series, No. 57*. (HHS Publication No. (SMA) 13-4801). Rockville, MD: Substance Abuse and Mental Health Services Administration.

97. American Psychiatric Association. (2013). *Diagnostic and statistical manual of mental disorders (DSM-5)* (5th ed.). Arlington, VA: American Psychiatric Publishing.

98. McLellan, A. T., Luborsky, L., O'Brien, C. P., & Woody, G. E. (n.d.). An improved diagnostic instrument for substance abuse patients: The Addiction Severity Index. *Journal of Nervous & Mental Diseases*(168), 26-33.

99. Cottler, L. B. (2000). *Composite international diagnostic interview—Substance Abuse Module (SAM)*. St. Louis, MO: Washington University School of Medicine, Department of Psychiatry. Retrieved from http://pubs.niaaa.nih.gov/publications/AssessingAlcohol/InstrumentPDFs/65_SAM.pdf. Accessed on July 27, 2016.

100. Hasin, D., & Samet, S. (n.d.). *Psychiatric Research Interview for Substance and Mental Disorders (PRISM)*. New York, NY: New York State Psychiatric Institute. Retrieved from http://pubs.niaaa.nih.gov/publications/AssessingAlcohol/InstrumentPDFs/52_PRISM.pdf. Accessed on January 27, 2016.

101. Kelly, T. M., Daley, D. C., & Douaihy, A. B. (2012). Treatment of substance abusing patients with comorbid psychiatric disorders. *Addictive Behaviors, 37*(1), 11-24.

102. Center for Substance Abuse Treatment. (2006). Chapter 10. Addressing diverse populations in intensive outpatient treatment. *Clinical issues in intensive outpatient treatment. Treatment improvement protocol (TIP) series, No. 47*. Rockville, MD: Substance Abuse and Mental Health Services Administration.

103. Prendergast, M. L., Messina, N. P., Hall, E. A., & Warda, U. S. (2011). The relative effectiveness of women-only and mixed-gender treatment for substance-abusing women. *Journal of Substance Abuse Treatment, 40*(4), 336-348.

104. Messina, N., Grella, C. E., Cartier, J., & Torres, S. (2010). A randomized experimental study of gender-responsive substance abuse treatment for women in prison. *Journal of Substance Abuse Treatment, 38*(2), 97-107.

105. Wisdom, J. P., Pollock, M. N., & Hopping-Winn, A. (2011). *Service engagement and retention for women with substance use disorders*. Berkeley, CA: National Abandoned Infants Assistance Resource Center, University of California, Berkeley.

106. Sheedy, C. K., & Whitter, M. (2009). *Guiding principles and elements of recovery-oriented systems of care: What do we know from the research?* (HHS Publication No. (SMA) 09-4439). Rockville, MD: Center for Substance Abuse Treatment, Substance Abuse and Mental Health Services Administration.

107. Greenfield, S. F., & Grella, C. E. (2009). What is "women-focused" treatment for substance use disorders? *Psychiatric Services, 60*(7), 880-882.

108. Coyhis, D., & Simonelli, R. (2008). The Native American healing experience. *Substance Use & Misuse, 43*(12-13), 1927-1949.

109. Guerrero, E. G., Marsh, J. C., Duan, L., Oh, C., Perron, B., & Lee, B. (2013). Disparities in completion of substance abuse treatment between and within racial and ethnic groups. *Health Services Research, 48*(4), 1450-1467.

110. Guerrero, E. G., Marsh, J. C., Khachikian, T., Amaro, H., & Vega, W. A. (2013). Disparities in Latino substance use, service use, and treatment: Implications for culturally and evidence-based interventions under health care reform. *Drug and Alcohol Dependence, 133*(3), 805-813.

111. Jones, J. H., Treiber, L. A., & Jones, M. C. (2014). Intervening at the intersection of medication adherence and health literacy. *The Journal for Nurse Practitioners, 10*(8), 527-534.

112. Alegría, M., Alvarez, K., Ishikawa, R. Z., DiMarzio, K., & McPeck, S. (2016). Removing obstacles to eliminating racial and ethnic disparities in behavioral health care. *Health Affairs, 35*(6), 991-999.

113. Senreich, E. (2010). Are specialized LGBT program components helpful for gay and bisexual men in substance abuse treatment? *Substance Use & Misuse, 45*(7-8), 1077-1096.

114. Saloner, B., & Le Cook, B. (2013). Blacks and Hispanics are less likely than whites to complete addiction treatment, largely due to socioeconomic factors. *Health Affairs, 32*(1), 135-145.

115. Substance Abuse and Mental Health Services Administration. (2013). *Disaster planning handbook for behavioral health treatment programs. Technical Assistance Publication (TAP) Series, No. 34.* (HHS Publication No. (SMA) 13-4779). Rockville, MD: Substance Abuse and Mental Health Services Administration.

116. National Institute on Drug Abuse. (2016). DrugFacts: Treatment approaches for drug addiction. Retrieved from http://www.drugabuse.gov/publications/drugfacts/treatment-approaches-drug-addiction. Accessed on January 25, 2016.

117. Kleber, H. D., Weiss, R. D., Anton, R. F., George, T. P., Greenfield, S. F., Kosten, T. R., . . . Smith Connery, H. (2006). *Practice guideline for the treatment of patients with substance use disorders*. Arlington, VA: American Psychiatric Association.

118. Food and Drug Administration. (2015). Suboxone®: Highlights of prescribing information Retrieved from http://www.accessdata.fda.gov/drugsatfda_docs/label/2015/022410s020s022lbl.pdf. Accessed on July 8, 2016.

119. Substance Abuse and Mental Health Services Administration. (2015). *Federal Guidelines for Opioid Treatment Programs*. (HHS Publication No. (SMA) PEP15-FEDGUIDEOTP). Rockville, MD: Substance Abuse and Mental Health Services Administration.

120. Lee, J., Kresina, T. F., Campopiano, M., Lubran, R., & Clark, H. W. (2015). Use of pharmacotherapies in the treatment of alcohol use disorders and opioid dependence in primary care. *BioMed Research International, 2015*.

121. Bonhomme, J., Shim, R. S., Gooden, R., Tyus, D., & Rust, G. (2012). Opioid addiction and abuse in primary care practice: a comparison of methadone and buprenorphine as treatment options. *Journal of the National Medical Association, 104*(7-8), 342-350.

122. Kresina, T. F., Melinda, C., Lee, J., Ahadpour, M., & Robert, L. (2015). Reducing mortality of people who use opioids through medication assisted treatment for opioid dependence. *Journal of HIV & Retro Virus, 1*(1).

123. Schwartz, R. P., Gryczynski, J., O'Grady, K. E., Sharfstein, J. M., Warren, G., Olsen, Y., . . . Jaffe, J. H. (2013). Opioid agonist treatments and heroin overdose deaths in Baltimore, Maryland, 1995-2009. *American Journal of Public Health, 103*(5), 917-922.

124. Mattick, R. P., Breen, C., Kimber, J., & Davoli, M. (2014). Buprenorphine maintenance versus placebo or methadone maintenance for opioid dependence. *Cochrane Database of Systematic Reviews, 2*.

125. National Consensus Development Panel on Effective Medical Treatment of Opiate Addiction. (1998). Effective medical treatment of opiate addiction. *JAMA, 280*(22), 1936-1943.

126. Joseph, H., Stancliff, S., & Langrod, J. (2000). Methadone maintenance treatment (MMT): A review of historical and clinical issues. *Mount Sinai Journal of Medicine, 67*(5-6), 347-364.

127. Kreek, M. J., Borg, L., Ducat, E., & Ray, B. (2010). Pharmacotherapy in the treatment of addiction: Methadone. *Journal of Addictive Diseases, 29*(2), 200-216.

128. Perkins, M. E., & Bloch, H. I. (1970). Survey of a methadone maintenance treatment program. *American Journal of Psychiatry, 126*(10), 1389-1396.

129. Fiellin, D. A., Friedland, G. H., & Gourevitch, M. N. (2006). Opioid dependence: Rationale for and efficacy of existing and new treatments. *Clinical Infectious Diseases, 43*(Suppl 4), S173-S177.

130. Anderson, I. B., & Kearney, T. E. (2000). Use of methadone. *Western Journal of Medicine, 172*(1), 43-46.

131. Säwe, J., Hansen, J., Ginman, C., Hartvig, P., Jakobsson, P., Nilsson, M., . . . Anggård, E. (1981). Patient-controlled dose regimen of methadone for chronic cancer pain. *BMJ, 282*(6266), 771-773.

132. Sees, K. L., Delucchi, K. L., Masson, C., Rosen, A., Clark, H. W., Robillard, H., . . . Hall, S. M. (2000). Methadone maintenance vs 180-day psychosocially enriched detoxification for treatment of opioid dependence: A randomized controlled trial. *JAMA, 283*(10), 1303-1310.

133. Fullerton, C. A., Kim, M., Thomas, C. P., Lyman, D. R., Montejano, L. B., Dougherty, R. H., . . . Delphin-Rittmon, M. E. (2014). Medication-assisted treatment with methadone: Assessing the evidence. *Psychiatric Services, 65*(2), 146-157.

134. Connock, M., Juarez-Garcia, A., Jowett, S., Frew, E., Liu, Z., Taylor, R. J., . . . Taylor, R. S. (2007). Methadone and buprenorphine for the management of opioid dependence: A systematic review and economic evaluation. *Health Technology Assessment, 11*(9), 1-171.

135. Stotts, A. L., Dodrill, C. L., & Kosten, T. R. (2009). Opioid dependence treatment: Options in pharmacotherapy. *Expert Opinion on Pharmacotherapy, 10*(11), 1727-1740.

136. Substance Abuse and Mental Health Services Administration. (2014). *National Survey of Substance Abuse Treatment Services (N-SSATS): 2013. Data on substance abuse treatment facilities.* (BHSIS Series S-73, HHS Publication No. (SMA) 14-4890). Rockville, MD: Substance Abuse and Mental Health Services Administration.

137. Stancliff, S., Joseph, H., Fong, C., Furst, T., Comer, S. D., & Roux, P. (2012). Opioid maintenance treatment as a harm reduction tool for opioid-dependent individuals in New York City: The need to expand access to buprenorphine/naloxone in marginalized populations. *Journal of Addictive Diseases, 31*(3), 278-287.

138. Volkow, N. D., Frieden, T. R., Hyde, P. S., & Cha, S. S. (2014). Medication-assisted therapies—tackling the opioid-overdose epidemic. *New England Journal of Medicine, 370*(22), 2063-2066.

139. Center for Substance Abuse Treatment. (2005). *Medication-assisted treatment for opioid addiction in opioid treatment programs. Treatment Improvement Protocol (TIP) Series, No. 43.* (HHS Publication No. (SMA) 12-4214). Rockville, MD: Substance Abuse and Mental Health Services Administration.

140. Thomas, C. P., Fullerton, C. A., Kim, M., Montejano, L., Lyman, D. R., Dougherty, R. H., . . . Delphin-Rittmon, M. E. (2014). Medication-assisted treatment with buprenorphine: Assessing the evidence. *Psychiatric Services, 65*(2), 158-170.

141. Pathan, H., & Williams, J. (2012). Basic opioid pharmacology: An update. *British Journal of Pain, 6*(1), 11-16.

142. Schuman-Olivier, Z., Albanese, M., Nelson, S. E., Roland, L., Puopolo, F., Klinker, L., & Shaffer, H. J. (2010). Self-treatment: Illicit buprenorphine use by opioid-dependent treatment seekers. *Journal of Substance Abuse Treatment, 39*(1), 41-50.

143. Cicero, T. J., Ellis, M. S., Surratt, H. L., & Kurtz, S. P. (2014). Factors contributing to the rise of buprenorphine misuse: 2008 - 2013. *Drug and Alcohol Dependence, 142,* 98-104.

144. Monico, L. B., Mitchell, S. G., Gryczynski, J., Schwartz, R. P., O'Grady, K. E., Olsen, Y. K., & Jaffe, J. H. (2015). Prior experience with non-prescribed buprenorphine: Role in treatment entry and retention. *Journal of Substance Abuse Treatment, 57,* 57-62.

145. Jacobs, P., Ang, A., Hillhouse, M. P., Saxon, A. J., Nielsen, S., Wakim, P. G., . . . Blaine, J. D. (2015). Treatment outcomes in opioid dependent patients with different buprenorphine/naloxone induction dosing patterns and trajectories. *The American Journal on Addictions, 24*(7), 667-675.

146. Center for Substance Abuse Treatment. (2004). *Clinical guidelines for the use of buprenorphine in the treatment of opioid addiction. Treatment improvement protocol (TIP) series, No. 40.* Rockville, MD: Substance Abuse and Mental Health Services Administration.

147. Medication assisted treatment for opioid use disorders; 81 Fed. Reg. 44712 (July 8, 2016) (to be codified at 42 C.F.R. pt 8).

148. The Henry J. Kaiser Family Foundation. (2015). Primary care physicians by field. Retrieved from http://kff.org/other/state-indicator/primary-care-physicians-by-field/. Accessed on July 27, 2016.

149. Stein, B. D., Pacula, R. L., Gordon, A. J., Burns, R. M., Leslie, D. L., Sorbero, M. J., . . . Dick, A. W. (2015). Where is buprenorphine dispensed to treat opioid use disorders? The role of private offices, opioid treatment programs, and substance abuse treatment facilities in urban and rural counties. *Milbank Quarterly, 93*(3), 561-583.

150. Sigmon, S. C. (2015). The untapped potential of office-based buprenorphine treatment. *JAMA Psychiatry, 72*(4), 395-396.

151. Substance Abuse and Mental Health Services Administration. (2009). *The facts about naltrexone for treatment of opioid addiction.* (HHS Publication No. (SMA) 15-4444). Rockville, MD: Substance Abuse and Mental Health Services Administration.

152. Substance Abuse and Mental Health Services Administration. (2012). An introduction to extended-release injectable naltrexone for the treatment of people with opioid dependence. *SAMHSA Advisory, 11*(1).

153. Substance Abuse and Mental Health Services Administration. (2015). *Clinical use of extended-release injectable naltrexone in the treatment of opioid use disorder: A brief guide.* (HHS Publication No. (SMA) 14-4892R). Rockville, MD: Substance Abuse and Mental Health Services Administration.

154. Miller, P. M., Book, S. W., & Stewart, S. H. (2011). Medical treatment of alcohol dependence: A systematic review. *The International Journal of Psychiatry in Medicine, 42*(3), 227-266.

155. National Institute on Alcohol Abuse and Alcoholism. (2005). Helping patients who drink too much: A clinician's guide. Retrieved from http://pubs.niaaa.nih.gov/publications/Practitioner/CliniciansGuide2005/clinicians_guide.htm. Accessed on March 20, 2015.

156. Substance Abuse and Mental Health Services Administration, & National Institute on Alcohol Abuse and Alcoholism. (2015). *Medication for the treatment of alcohol use disorder: A brief guide.* (HHS Publication No. (SMA) 15-4907). Rockville, MD: Substance Abuse and Mental Health Services Administration.

157. Lin, S. K. (2014). Pharmacological means of reducing human drug dependence: A selective and narrative review of the clinical literature. *The British Journal of Clinical Pharmacology, 77*(2), 242-252.

158. National Council on Alcoholism and Drug Dependence. (n.d.). *NCADD's consumer guide to medication-assisted recovery.* New York, NY: National Council on Alcohol and Drug Dependence, Inc.

159. Kufahl, P. R., Watterson, L. R., & Olive, M. F. (2014). The development of acamprosate as a treatment against alcohol relapse. *Expert Opinion on Drug Discovery, 9*(11), 1355-1369.

160. Zindel, L. R., & Kranzler, H. R. (2014). Pharmacotherapy of alcohol use disorders: Seventy-five years of progress. *Journal of Studies on Alcohol and Drugs, 75*(Suppl 17), 79-88.

161. Chick, J., Gough, K., Falkowski, W., Kershaw, P., Hore, B., Mehta, B., . . . Torley, D. (1992). Disulfiram treatment of alcoholism. *The British Journal of Psychiatry, 161*(1), 84-89.

162. Vuittonet, C. L., Halse, M., Leggio, L., Fricchione, S. B., Brickley, M., Haass-Koffler, C. L., . . . Kenna, G. A. (2014). Pharmacotherapy for alcoholic patients with alcoholic liver disease. *American Journal of Health-System Pharmacy, 71*(15), 1265-1276.

163. alcoholrehab.com. (n.d.). Naltrexone and alcohol rehab. Retrieved from http://alcoholrehab.com/drug-addiction-treatment/opiate-antagonist-naltrexone-alcohol-rehab/. Accessed on January 25, 2016.

164. Mannelli, P., Peindl, K., Masand, P. S., & Patkar, A. A. (2007). Long-acting injectable naltrexone for the treatment of alcohol dependence. *Expert Review of Neurotherapeutics, 7*(10), 1265-1277.

165. Rösner, S., Hackl-Herrwerth, A., Leucht, S., Lehert, P., Vecchi, S., & Soyka, M. (2010). Acamprosate for alcohol dependence. *The Cochrane Database of Systematic Reviews,* (9).

166. Jonas, D. E., Amick, H. R., Feltner, C., et al., Bobashev, G., Thomas, K., . . . Garbutt, J. C. (2014). Pharmacotherapy for adults with alcohol use disorders in outpatient settings: A systematic review and meta-analysis. *JAMA, 311*(18), 1889-1900.

167. Maisel, N. C., Blodgett, J. C., Wilbourne, P. L., Humphreys, K., & Finney, J. W. (2013). Meta-analysis of naltrexone and acamprosate for treating alcohol use disorders: When are these medications most helpful? *Addiction, 108*(2), 275-293.

168. Substance Abuse and Mental Health Services Administration. (2013). *Report to Congress on the nation's substance abuse and mental health workforce issues*. Rockville, MD: Substance Abuse and Mental Health Services Administration.

169. McGovern, M. P. (2003). Evidence-based practices for substance use disorders. *Psychiatric Clinics of North America, 26*(4), 991-1010.

170. Center for Substance Abuse Treatment. (2005). *Substance abuse treatment: Group therapy. Treatment improvement protocol (TIP) series, No. 41*. Rockville, MD: Substance Abuse and Mental Health Services Administration.

171. Wandersman, A., Imm, P., Chinman, M., & Kaftarian, S. (2000). Getting to outcomes: A results-based approach to accountability. *Evaluation and Program Planning, 23*(3), 389-395.

172. Morgenstern, J., Blanchard, K. A., Morgan, T. J., Labouvie, E., & Hayaki, J. (2001). Testing the effectiveness of cognitive-behavioral treatment for substance abuse in a community setting: Within treatment and posttreatment findings. *Journal of Consulting and Clinical Psychology, 69*(6), 1007-1017.

173. Carroll, K. M., & Onken, L. S. (2005). Behavioral therapies for drug abuse. *Journal of the American Psychiatric Association, 162*(8), 1452-1460.

174. McHugh, R. K., Hearon, B. A., & Otto, M. W. (2010). Cognitive-behavioral therapy for substance use disorders. *Psychiatric Clinics of North America, 33*(3), 511-525.

175. Gregory, V. L. (2011). Cognitive-behavioral therapy for comorbid bipolar and substance use disorders: A systematic review of controlled trials. *Mental Health and Substance Use, 4*(4), 302-313.

176. Quello, S. B., Brady, K. T., & Sonne, S. C. (2005). Mood disorders and substance use disorder: A complex comorbidity. *Science & Practice Perspectives, 3*(1), 13-21.

177. Higgins, S. T., Heil, S. H., & Sigmon, S. C. (2013). Voucher-based contingency management in the treatment of substance use disorders. In G. J. Madden, W. V. Dube, T. D. Hackenberg, G. P. Hanley, & K. A. Lattal (Eds.), *APA handbook of behavior analysis, Vol. 2: Translating principles into practice*. (pp. 481-500). Washington, DC, US: American Psychological Association.

178. Carroll, K. M., Nich, C., Petry, N. M., Eagan, D. A., Shi, J. M., & Ball, S. A. (2016). A randomized factorial trial of disulfiram and contingency management to enhance cognitive behavioral therapy for cocaine dependence. *Drug and Alcohol Dependence, 160*, 135-142.

179. Carroll, K. M., Easton, C. J., Nich, C., Hunkele, K. A., Neavins, T. M., Sinha, R., ... Rounsaville, B. J. (2006). The use of contingency management and motivational/skills-building therapy to treat young adults with marijuana dependence. *Journal of Consulting and Clinical Psychology, 74*(5), 955-966.

180. Secades-Villa, R., Garcia-Rodriguez, O., Garcia-Fernandez, G., Sanchez-Hervas, E., Fernandez-Hermida, J. R., & Higgins, S. T. (2011). Community reinforcement approach plus vouchers among cocaine-dependent outpatients: Twelve-month outcomes. *Psychology of Addictive Behaviors, 25*(1), 174-179.

181. Dennis, M., Godley, S. H., Diamond, G., Tims, F. M., Babor, T., Donaldson, J., ... Webb, C. (2004). The Cannabis Youth Treatment (CYT) Study: Main findings from two randomized trials. *Journal of Substance Abuse Treatment, 27*(3), 197-213.

182. Slesnick, N., Prestopnik, J. L., Meyers, R. J., & Glassman, M. (2007). Treatment outcome for street-living, homeless youth. *Addictive Behaviors, 32*(6), 1237-1251.

183. Burlew, A. K., Montgomery, L., Kosinski, A. S., & Forcehimes, A. A. (2013). Does treatment readiness enhance the response of African American substance users to motivational enhancement therapy? *Psychology of Addictive Behaviors, 27*(3), 744-753.

184. Miles, L. A. (2015). Motivational enhancement therapy: Treatment for substance abuse & more. Retrieved from http://psychcentral.com/blog/archives/2013/07/12/motivational-enhancement-therapy-treatment-for-substance-abuse-more/. Accessed on April 4, 2016.

185. Tevyaw, T. O. L., & Monti, P. M. (2004). Motivational enhancement and other brief interventions for adolescent substance abuse: Foundations, applications and evaluations. *Addiction, 99*(s2), 63-75.

186. Helstrom, A., Hutchison, K., & Bryan, A. (2007). Motivational enhancement therapy for high-risk adolescent smokers. *Addictive Behaviors, 32*(10), 2404-2410.

187. Rawson, R. A., Gonzales, R., Pearce, V., Ang, A., Marinelli-Casey, P., & Brummer, J. (2008). Methamphetamine dependence and HIV risk behavior. *Journal of Substance Abuse Treatment, 35*(3), 279-284.

188. Shoptaw, S., & Reback, C. J. (2007). Methamphetamine use and infectious disease-related behaviors in men who have sex with men: Implications for interventions. *Addiction, 102*(Suppl 1), 130-135.

189. Substance Abuse and Mental Health Services Administration. (2012). *Using matrix with women clients: A supplement to the matrix intensive outpatient treatment for people with stimulant use disorders.* (HHS Pub. No. (SMA) 12-4698). Rockville, MD: Substance Abuse and Mental Health Services Administration.

190. Walitzer, K. S., Dermen, K. H., & Barrick, C. (2009). Facilitating involvement in Alcoholics Anonymous during out-patient treatment: A randomized clinical trial. *Addiction, 104*(3), 391-401.

191. Kaskutas, L. A., Subbaraman, M. S., Witbrodt, J., & Zemore, S. E. (2009). Effectiveness of making Alcoholics Anonymous easier: A group format 12-step facilitation approach. *Journal of Substance Abuse Treatment, 37*(3), 228-239.

192. Crits-Christoph, P., Siqueland, L., Blaine, J., Frank, A., Luborsky, L., Onken, L. S., . . . Beck, A. T. (1999). Psychosocial treatments for cocaine dependence: National Institute on Drug Abuse Collaborative Cocaine Treatment Study. *Archives of General Psychiatry, 56*(6), 493-502.

193. Allen, J. P., Mattson, M. E., Miller, W. R., Tonigan, J. S., Connors, G. J., Rychtarik, R. G., . . . Litt, M. (1997). Matching alcoholism treatments to client heterogeneity: Project MATCH posttreatment drinking outcomes. *Journal of Studies on Alcohol, 58*(1), 7-29.

194. Litt, M. D., Kadden, R. M., Kabela-Cormier, E., & Petry, N. M. (2009). Changing network support for drinking: Network support project 2-year follow-up. *Journal of Consulting and Clinical Psychology, 77*(2), 229-242.

195. Timko, C., & DeBenedetti, A. (2007). A randomized controlled trial of intensive referral to 12-step self-help groups: One-year outcomes. *Drug and Alcohol Dependence, 90*(2), 270-279.

196. Longabaugh, R., Wirtz, P. W., Zweben, A., & Stout, R. L. (1998). Network support for drinking, Alcoholics Anonymous and long-term matching effects. *Addiction, 93*(9), 1313-1333.

197. Thevos, A. K., Thomas, S. E., & Randall, C. L. (2001). Social support in alcohol dependence and social phobia: Treatment comparisons. *Research on Social Work Practice, 11*(4), 458-472.

198. Cooney, N. L., Babor, T. F., DiClemente, C. C., & Del Boca, F. K. (2003). Clinical and scientific implications of Project MATCH. In T. F. Babor & F. K. D. Boca (Eds.), *Treatment Matching in Alcoholism.* (pp. 222-237). Cambridge, UK: Cambridge University Press.

199. Donovan, D. M., Daley, D. C., Brigham, G. S., Hodgkins, C. C., Perl, H. I., Garrett, S., . . . Zammarelli, L. (2013). Stimulant abuser groups to engage in 12-step (STAGE-12): A multisite trial in the NIDA clinical trials network. *Journal of Substance Abuse Treatment, 44*(1), 103-114.

200. Yalom, I. D., & Leszcz, M. (2005). *Theory and practice of group psychotherapy* (5 ed.). New York, NY: Basic Books.

201. Humphreys, K. (2004). Tale telling in an alcohol mutual help organization. *New Directions in Alcohol Studies, 29,* 33-44.

202. Labbe, A. K., Slaymaker, V., & Kelly, J. F. (2014). Toward enhancing 12-step facilitation among young people: A systematic qualitative investigation of young adults' 12-step experiences. *Substance Abuse, 35*(4), 399-407.

203. Kelly, J. F., Magill, M., & Stout, R. L. (2009). How do people recover from alcohol dependence? A systematic review of the research on mechanisms of behavior change in Alcoholics Anonymous. *Addiction Research & Theory, 17*(3), 236-259.

204. White, W. L., Kelly, J. F., & Roth, J. D. (2012). New addiction-recovery support institutions: Mobilizing support beyond professional addiction treatment and recovery mutual aid. *Journal of Groups in Addiction & Recovery, 7*(2-4), 297-317.

205. Hester, R. K., Lenberg, K. L., Campbell, W., & Delaney, H. D. (2013). Overcoming addictions, a web-based application, and SMART recovery, an online and in-person mutual help group for problem drinkers, Part 1: Three-month outcomes of a randomized controlled trial. *Journal of Medical Internet Research, 15*(7), 11-25.

206. Norris, S. L., Nichols, P. J., Caspersen, C. J., Glasgow, R. E., Engelgau, M. M., Jack, L., . . . McCulloch, D. (2002). Increasing diabetes self-management education in community settings: A systematic review. *American Journal of Preventive Medicine, 22*(Suppl 4), 39-66.

207. Donohue, B., Azrin, N., Allen, D. N., Romero, V., Hill, H. H., Tracy, K., . . . Van Hasselt, V. B. (2009). Family behavior therapy for substance abuse and other associated problems: A review of its intervention components and applicability. *Behavior Modification, 33*(5), 495-519.

208. Winters, J., Fals-Stewart, W., O'Farrell, T. J., Birchler, G. R., & Kelley, M. L. (2002). Behavioral couples therapy for female substance-abusing patients: Effects on substance use and relationship adjustment. *Journal of Consulting and Clinical Psychology, 70*(2), 344-355.

209. Stanton, D., & Heath, A. (2004). Family/couples approaches to treatment engagement and therapy. In J. H. Lowinson & P. Ruiz (Eds.), *Substance abuse: A comprehensive textbook.* Philadelphia, PA: Lippincott Williams & Wilkins.

210. O'Farrell, T. J., & Clements, K. (2012). Review of outcome research on marital and family therapy in treatment for alcoholism. *Journal of Marital & Family Therapy, 38*(1), 122-144.

211. Center for Behavioral Health Statistics and Quality. (2013). *The NSDUH Report: Adults with mental illness or substance use disorder account for 40 percent of all cigarettes smoked.* Rockville, MD: Substance Abuse and Mental Health Services Administration.

212. Baca, C. T., & Yahne, C. E. (2009). Smoking cessation during substance abuse treatment: What you need to know. *Journal of Substance Abuse Treatment, 36*(2), 205-219.

213. Prochaska, J. J., Delucchi, K., & Hall, S. M. (2004). A meta-analysis of smoking cessation interventions with individuals in substance abuse treatment or recovery. *Journal of Consulting and Clinical Psychology, 72*(6), 1144-1156.

214. Substance Abuse and Mental Health Administration. (2015). Recovery and recovery support. Retrieved from http://www.samhsa.gov/recovery. Accessed on June 22, 2016.

215. Ruiz, B. S., Korchmaros, J. D., Greene, A., & Hedges, K. (2011). Evidence-based substance abuse treatment for adolescents: Engagement and outcomes. *Practice: Social Work in Action, 23*(4), 215-233.

216. National Council for Community Behavioral Healthcare. (2012). *HIT adoption and readiness for meaningful use in community behavioral health: Report on the 2012 National Council Survey.* Washington, DC: National Council for Community Behavioral Healthcare.

217. Health Resources and Services Administration. (n.d.). What is telehealth? Retrieved from http://www.hrsa.gov/healthit/toolbox/RuralHealthITtoolbox/Telehealth/whatistelehealth.html. Accessed on April 11, 2016.

218. Kiluk, B. D., & Carroll, K. M. (2013). New developments in behavioral treatments for substance use disorders. *Current Psychiatry Reports, 15*(12), 1-14.

219. Olmstead, T. A., Ostrow, C. D., & Carroll, K. M. (2010). Cost-effectiveness of computer-assisted training in cognitive-behavioral therapy as an adjunct to standard care for addiction. *Drug and Alcohol Dependence, 110*(3), 200-207.

220. Marsch, L. A., & Dallery, J. (2012). Advances in the psychosocial treatment of addiction: The role of technology in the delivery of evidence-based psychosocial treatment. *The Psychiatric Clinics of North America, 35*(2), 481-493.

221. Rosa, C., Campbell, A. N. C., Miele, G. M., Brunner, M., & Winstanley, E. L. (2015). Using e-technologies in clinical trials. *Contemporary Clinical Trials, 45*, 41-54.

222. Johnson, K., Isham, A., Shah, D. V., & Gustafson, D. H. (2011). Potential roles for new communication technologies in treatment of addiction. *Current Psychiatry Reports, 13*(5), 390-397.

223. Anderson, M. (2015). Technology device ownership: 2015. Retrieved from http://www.pewinternet.org/2015/10/29/technology-device-ownership-2015. Accessed on June 10, 2016.

224. Anderson, M., & Perrin, A. (2015). 15% of Americans don't use the internet. Who are they? Retrieved from http://www.pewresearch.org/fact-tank/2015/07/28/15-of-americans-dont-use-the-internet-who-are-they/. Accessed on June 10, 2016.

225. Kiluk, B. D., Sugarman, D. E., Nich, C., Gibbons, C. J., Martino, S., Rounsaville, B. J., & Carroll, K. M. (2011). A methodological analysis of randomized clinical trials of computer-assisted therapies for psychiatric disorders: Toward improved standards for an emerging field. *American Journal of Psychiatry, 168*(8), 790-799.

226. Marsch, L. A., Guarino, H., Acosta, M., Aponte-Melendez, Y., Cleland, C., Grabinski, M., . . . Edwards, J. (2014). Web-based behavioral treatment for substance use disorders as a partial replacement of standard methadone maintenance treatment. *Journal of Substance Abuse Treatment, 46*(1), 43-51.

227. King, V. L., Brooner, R. K., Peirce, J. M., Kolodner, K., & Kidorf, M. S. (2014). A randomized trial of Web-based videoconferencing for substance abuse counseling. *Journal of Substance Abuse Treatment, 46*(1), 36-42.

228. Gustafson, D. H., McTavish, F. M., Chih, M. Y., Atwood, A. K., Johnson, R. A., Boyle, M. G., . . . Shah, D. (2014). A smartphone application to support recovery from alcoholism: A randomized clinical trial. *JAMA Psychiatry, 71*(5), 566-572.

229. Carroll, K. M., Kiluk, B. D., Nich, C., Gordon, M. A., Portnoy, G. A., Marino, D. R., & Ball, S. A. (2014). Computer-assisted delivery of cognitive-behavioral therapy: Efficacy and durability of CBT4CBT among cocaine-dependent individuals maintained on methadone. *American Journal of Psychiatry, 171*(4), 436-444.

230. Hasin, D. S., Aharonovich, E., O'Leary, A., Greenstein, E., Pavlicova, M., Arunajadai, S., . . . Johnston, B. (2013). Reducing heavy drinking in HIV primary care: A randomized trial of brief intervention, with and without technological enhancement. *Addiction, 108*(7), 1230-1240.

231. Rooke, S., Copeland, J., Norberg, M., Hine, D., & McCambridge, J. (2013). Effectiveness of a self-guided web-based cannabis treatment program: Randomized controlled trial. *Journal of Medical Internet Research, 15*(2), e26.

232. Kay-Lambkin, F. J., Baker, A. L., Kelly, B., & Lewin, T. J. (2011). Clinician-assisted computerised versus therapist-delivered treatment for depressive and addictive disorders: A randomised controlled trial. *Medical Journal of Australia, 195*(3), S44-S50.

233. Campbell, A. N., Nunes, E. V., Matthews, A. G., Stitzer, M., Miele, G. M., Polsky, D., . . . Ghitza, U. E. (2014). Internet-delivered treatment for substance abuse: A multisite randomized controlled trial. *Journal of the American Psychiatric Association, 171*(6), 683-690.

234. Cunningham, J. A., Wild, T. C., Cordingley, J., Van Mierlo, T., & Humphreys, K. (2009). A randomized controlled trial of an internet-based intervention for alcohol abusers. *Addiction, 104*(12), 2023-2032.

235. Kypri, K., McCambridge, J., Vater, T., Bowe, S. J., Saunders, J. B., Cunningham, J. A., & Horton, N. J. (2013). Web-based alcohol intervention for Māori university students: Double-blind, multi-site randomized controlled trial. *Addiction, 108*(2), 331-338.

236. Hester, R. K., Delaney, H. D., & Campbell, W. (2012). The college drinker's check-up: Outcomes of two randomized clinical trials of a computer-delivered intervention. *Psychology of Addictive Behaviors, 26*(1), 1-12.

237. Walters, S. T., Vader, A. M., & Harris, T. R. (2007). A controlled trial of web-based feedback for heavy drinking college students. *Prevention Science, 8*(1), 83-88.

238. Palfai, T., Tahaney, K., Winter, M., & Saitz, R. (2016). Readiness-to-change as a moderator of a web-based brief intervention for marijuana among students identified by health center screening. *Drug and Alcohol Dependence, 161*, 368-371.

239. Hankin, A., Haley, L., Baugher, A., Colbert, K., & Houry, D. (2015). Kiosk versus in-person screening for alcohol and drug use in the emergency department: patient preferences and disclosure. *Western Journal of Emergency Medicine, 16*(2), 220-228.

240. Mello, M. J., Longabaugh, R., Baird, J., Nirenberg, T., & Woolard, R. (2008). DIAL: A telephone brief intervention for high-risk alcohol use with injured emergency department patients. *Annals of Emergency Medicine, 51*(6), 755-764.

241. McKay, J. R., Lynch, K. G., Shepard, D. S., & Pettinati, H. M. (2005). The effectiveness of telephone-based continuing care for alcohol and cocaine dependence: 24-month outcomes. *Archives of General Psychiatry, 62*(2), 199-207.

242. Bewick, B. M., Trusler, K., Barkham, M., Hill, A. J., Cahill, J., & Mulhern, B. (2008). The effectiveness of web-based interventions designed to decrease alcohol consumption—A systematic review. *Preventive Medicine, 47*(1), 17-26.

243. Carey, K. B., Scott-Sheldon, L. A., Elliott, J. C., Bolles, J. R., & Carey, M. P. (2009). Computer-delivered interventions to reduce college student drinking: A meta-analysis. *Addiction, 104*(11), 1807-1819.

244. Elliott, J. C., Carey, K. B., & Bolles, J. R. (2008). Computer-based interventions for college drinking: A qualitative review. *Addictive Behaviors, 33*(8), 994-1005.

245. Kypri, K., Saunders, J. B., Williams, S. M., McGee, R. O., Langley, J. D., Cashell-Smith, M. L., & Gallagher, S. J. (2004). Web-based screening and brief intervention for hazardous drinking: A double-blind randomized controlled trial. *Addiction, 99*(11), 1410-1417.

246. Neumann, T., Neuner, B., Weiss-Gerlach, E., Tonnesen, H., Gentilello, L. M., Wernecke, K. D., ... Spies, C. D. (2006). The effect of computerized tailored brief advice on at-risk drinking in subcritically injured trauma patients. *Journal of Trauma and Acute Care Surgery, 61*(4), 805-814.

247. Community Preventive Services Task Force. (2012). Preventing excessive alcohol consumption: Electronic screening and brief interventions (e-SBI). Retrieved from http://www.thecommunityguide.org/alcohol/RReSBI.html. Accessed on June 10, 2016.

248. Riper, H., Kramer, J., Conijn, B., Smit, F., Schippers, G., & Cuijpers, P. (2009). Translating effective web-based self-help for problem drinking into the real world. *Alcoholism: Clinical and Experimental Research, 33*(8), 1401-1408.

249. Brief, D. J., Rubin, A., Keane, T. M., Enggasser, J. L., Roy, M., Helmuth, E., ... Rosenbloom, D. (2013). Web intervention for OEF/OIF veterans with problem drinking and PTSD symptoms: A randomized clinical trial. *Journal of Consulting and Clinical Psychology, 81*(5), 890-900.

250. Litvin, E. B., Abrantes, A. M., & Brown, R. A. (2013). Computer and mobile technology-based interventions for substance use disorders: An organizing framework. *Addictive Behaviors, 38*(3), 1747-1756.

251. Moore, B. A., Fazzino, T., Garnet, B., Cutter, C. J., & Barry, D. T. (2011). Computer-based interventions for drug use disorders: A systematic review. *Journal of Substance Abuse Treatment, 40*(3), 215-223.

252. Kiluk, B. D., Nich, C., Babuscio, T., & Carroll, K. M. (2010). Quality vs. quantity: Acquisition of coping skills following computerized cognitive behavioral therapy for substance use disorders. *Addiction 105*(12), 2120-2127.

TREATMENT

253. Klein, A. A., Slaymaker, V. J., Dugosh, K. L., & McKay, J. R. (2012). Computerized continuing care support for alcohol and drug dependence: A preliminary analysis of usage and outcomes. *Journal of Substance Abuse Treatment, 42*(1), 25-34.

254. Davis, T. A., & Ancis, J. (2012). Look to the relationship: A review of African American women substance users' poor treatment retention and working alliance development. *Substance Use & Misuse, 47*(6), 662-672.

255. Substance Abuse and Mental Health Services Administration, & Center for Behavioral Health Statistics and Quality. (2012). *The NSDUH Report: Need for and receipt of substance use treatment among Hispanics.* Rockville, MD: Substance Abuse and Mental Health Services Administration.

256. Substance Abuse and Mental Health Services Administration, & Center for Behavioral Health Statistics and Quality. (2013). *Need for and receipt of substance use treatment among Blacks.* Rockville, MD: Substance Abuse and Mental Health Services Administration.

257. Longshore, D., & Grills, C. (2000). Motivating illegal drug use recovery: Evidence for a culturally congruent intervention. *Journal of Black Psychology, 26*(3), 288-301.

258. Gil, A. G., Wagner, E. F., & Tubman, J. G. (2004). Culturally sensitive substance abuse intervention for Hispanic and African American adolescents: Empirical examples from the Alcohol Treatment Targeting Adolescents in Need (ATTAIN) project. *Addiction, 99*(s2), 140-150.

259. Milligan, C. O., Nich, C., & Carroll, K. M. (2004). Ethnic differences in substance abuse treatment retention, compliance, and outcome from two clinical trials. *Psychiatric Services, 55,* 167-173.

260. Tonigan, J. S. (2003). Project Match treatment participation and outcome by self-reported ethnicity. *Alcoholism: Clinical & Experimental Research, 27*(8), 1340-1344.

261. Witkiewitz, K., Bowen, S., Douglas, H., & Hsu, S. H. (2013). Mindfulness-based relapse prevention for substance craving. *Addictive Behaviors, 38*(2), 1563-1571.

262. Beckstead, D. J., Lambert, M. J., DuBose, A. P., & Linehan, M. (2015). Dialectical behavior therapy with American Indian/Alaska Native adolescents diagnosed with substance use disorders: Combining an evidence based treatment with cultural, traditional, and spiritual beliefs. *Addictive Behaviors, 51,* 84-87.

263. Niv, N., Wong, E. C., & Hser, Y.-I. (2007). Asian Americans in community-based substance abuse treatment: Service needs, utilization, and outcomes. *Journal of Substance Abuse Treatment, 33*(3), 313-319.

264. Yu, J., & Warner, L. A. (2013). Substance abuse treatment readmission patterns of Asian Americans: Comparisons with other ethnic groups. *The American Journal of Drug and Alcohol Abuse, 39*(1), 23-27.

265. Wu, L.-T., & Blazer, D. G. (2015). Substance use disorders and co-morbidities among Asian Americans and Native Hawaiians/Pacific Islanders. *Psychological Medicine, 45*(03), 481-494.

266. Substance Abuse and Mental Health Services Administration, & Center for Behavioral Health Statistics and Quality. (2014). *Improving cultural competence. Treatment Improvement Protocol (TIP) Series, No. 59.* (HHS Publication No. (SMA) 14-4849). Rockville, MD: Substance Abuse and Mental Health Services Administration.

267. Cochran, B. N., & Cauce, A. M. (2006). Characteristics of lesbian, gay, bisexual, and transgender individuals entering substance abuse treatment. *Journal of Substance Abuse Treatment, 30*(2), 135-146.

268. McCabe, S. E., West, B. T., Hughes, T. L., & Boyd, C. J. (2013). Sexual orientation and substance abuse treatment utilization in the United States: Results from a national survey. *Journal of Substance Abuse Treatment, 44*(1), 4-12.

269. Ward, B. W., Dahlhamer, J. M., Galinsky, A. M., & Joestl, S. S. (2014). Sexual orientation and health among US adults: National Health Interview Survey, 2013. *National Health Statistics Reports, 77*, 1-10.

270. Marshal, M. P., Friedman, M. S., Stall, R., King, K. M., Miles, J., Gold, M. A., . . . Morse, J. Q. (2008). Sexual orientation and adolescent substance use: A meta-analysis and methodological review. *Addiction, 103*(4), 546-556.

271. Cochran, B. N., Peavy, K. M., & Robohm, J. S. (2007). Do specialized services exist for LGBT individuals seeking treatment for substance misuse? A study of available treatment programs. *Substance Use & Misuse, 42*(1), 161-176.

272. Green, K. E., & Feinstein, B. A. (2012). Substance use in lesbian, gay, and bisexual populations: An update on empirical research and implications for treatment. *Psychology of Addictive Behaviors, 26*(2), 265-278.

273. Lombardi, E. L., & van Servellen, G. (2000). Building culturally sensitive substance use prevention and treatment programs for transgendered populations. *Journal of Substance Abuse Treatment, 19*(3), 291-296.

274. Substance Abuse and Mental Health Administration. (2014). Veterans and military families. Retrieved from http://www.samhsa.gov/veterans-military-families. Accessed on June 9, 2016.

275. Hoggatt, K. J., Jamison, A. L., Lehavot, K., Cucciare, M. A., Timko, C., & Simpson, T. L. (2015). Alcohol and drug misuse, abuse, and dependence in women veterans. *Epidemiologic Reviews, 37*, 23-37.

276. Coker, K. L., Stefanovics, E., & Rosenheck, R. (2016). Correlates of improvement in substance abuse among dually diagnosed veterans with post-traumatic stress disorder in specialized intensive VA treatment. *Psychological Trauma: Theory, Research, Practice, and Policy, 8*(1), 41-48.

277. Smelson, D. A., Kline, A., Kuhn, J., Rodrigues, S., O'Connor, K., Fisher, W., . . . Kane, V. (2013). A wraparound treatment engagement intervention for homeless veterans with co-occurring disorders. *Psychological Services, 10*(2), 161-167.

278. The Pew Center on the States. (2008). *One in 100: Behind bars in America 2008*. Washington, DC: The Pew Charitable Trusts.

279. Krinsky, C. S., Lathrop, S. L., Brown, P., & Nolte, K. B. (2009). Drugs, detention, and death: A study of the mortality of recently released prisoners. *The American Journal of Forensic Medicine and Pathology, 30*(1), 6-9.

280. Binswanger, I. A., Blatchford, P. J., Mueller, S. R., & Stern, M. F. (2013). Mortality after prison release: Opioid overdose and other causes of death, risk factors, and time trends from 1999 to 2009. *Annals of Internal Medicine, 159*(9), 592-600.

TREATMENT

281. Møller, L. F., Matic, S., van Den Bergh, B. J., Moloney, K., Hayton, P., & Gatherer, A. (2010). Acute drug-related mortality of people recently released from prisons. *Public Health, 124*(11), 637-639.

282. Gordon, M. S., Kinlock, T. W., Schwartz, R. P., & O'Grady, K. E. (2008). A randomized clinical trial of methadone maintenance for prisoners: Findings at 6 months post-release. *Addiction, 103*(8), 1333-1342.

283. Wakeman, S. E., & Rich, J. D. (2015). Addiction treatment within U.S. Correctional facilities: Bridging the gap between current practice and evidence-based care. *Journal of Addictive Diseases, 34*(2-3), 220-225.

284. Lee, J. D., Friedmann, P. D., Kinlock, T. W., Nunes, E. V., Boney, T. Y., Hoskinson, R. A. J., … O'Brien, C. P. (2016). Extended-release naltrexone to prevent opioid relapse in criminal justice offenders. *New England Journal of Medicine, 374*(13), 1232-1242.

285. U.S. Department of Justice Office of Justice Programs. (2015). Drug courts. Retrieved from https://www.ncjrs.gov/pdffiles1/nij/238527.pdf. Accessed on July 10, 2016.

286. Bhati, A. S., Roman, J. K., & Chalfin, A. (2008). *To treat or not to treat: Evidence on the prospects of expanding treatment to drug-involved offenders.* Washington, DC: Urban Institute Justice Policy Center.

287. Wilson, D. B., Mitchell, O., & MacKenzie, D. L. (2013). Drug courts. In G. Bruinsma & D. Weisburd (Eds.), *Encyclopedia of Criminology and Criminal Justice.* (pp. 1170-1178). New York, NY: Springer.

288. Sevigny, E. L., Fuleihan, B. K., & Ferdik, F. V. (2013). Do drug courts reduce the use of incarceration? A meta-analysis. *Journal of Criminal Justice, 41*(6), 416–425.

289. Wilson, D. B., Mitchell, O., & MacKenzie, D. L. (2006). A systematic review of drug court effects on recidivism. *Journal of Experimental Criminology, 2*(4), 459-487.

290. Gottfredson, D. C., Najaka, S. S., Kearley, B. W., & Rocha, C. M. (2006). Long-term effects of participation in the Baltimore City drug treatment court: Results from an experimental study. *Journal of Experimental Criminology, 2*(1), 67-98.

291. Belenko, S., Patapis, P., & French, M. T. (2005). Economic benefits of drug treatment: A critical review of the evidence for policy makers. Retrieved from http://www.fccmh.org/resources/docs/EconomicBenefits_of_Drug_Trx_02.05_.pdf. Accessed on October 14, 2015.

292. Mitchell, O., Wilson, D., Eggers, A., & MacKenzie, D. (2012). Drug courts' effects on criminal offending for juveniles and adults. *Campbell Systematic Reviews, 8*(4).

293. Hawken, A., & Kleiman, M. (2009). Managing drug involved probationers with swift and certain sanctions: Evaluating Hawaii's HOPE. Retrieved from https://www.ncjrs.gov/pdffiles1/nij/grants/229023.pdf. Accessed on October 12, 2015.

294. Pollack, H., Sevigny, E. L., & Reuter, P. (2011). If drug treatment works so well, why are so many drug users in prison? In P. J. Cook, J. Ludwig, & J. McCrary (Eds.), *Controlling Crime: Strategies and Tradeoffs.* (pp. 125 - 160). Chicago, Illinois: University of Chicago Press.

295. Kilmer, B., Nicosia, N., Heaton, P., & Midgette, G. (2013). Efficacy of frequent monitoring with swift, certain, and modest sanctions for violations: Insights from South Dakota's 24/7 sobriety project. *American Journal of Public Health, 103*(1), e37-e43.

296. Midgette, G., & Kilmer, B. (2015). *The effect of Montana's 24/7 sobriety program on DUI re-arrest: Insights from a natural experiment with limited administrative data.* Santa Monica, CA: RAND Corporation.

297. D'Onofrio, G., O'Connor, P. G., Pantalon, M. V., Chawarski, M. C., Busch, S. H., Owens, P. H., ... Fiellin, D. A. (2015). Emergency department–initiated buprenorphine/naloxone treatment for opioid dependence: A randomized clinical trial. *JAMA, 313*(16), 1636-1644.

298. Ghitza, U. E. (2016). Overlapping mechanisms of stress-induced relapse to opioid use disorder and chronic pain: Clinical implications. *Frontiers in Psychiatry, 7*(80).

299. Dennis, M. l., Titus, J. C., White, M. K., Unsicker, J. I., & Hodgkins, D. (2003). *Global appraisal of individual needs Administration guide for the GAIN and related measures.* Bloomington, IL: Chestnut Health Systems.

CHAPTER 5. RECOVERY: THE MANY PATHS TO WELLNESS

Chapter 5 Preview

On October 4, 2015, tens of thousands of people attended the UNITE to Face Addiction rally in Washington, D.C. The event was one of many signs that a new movement is emerging in America: People in recovery, their family members, and other supporters are banding together to decrease the discrimination associated with substance use disorders and spread the message that people do recover. Much of the success of the event hinged on the growing network of recovery community organizations (RCOs) that have proliferated across the country, creating cultures of recovery and advancing recovery-positive attitudes, programs, and prevention strategies. Recovery advocates have created a once-unimagined vocal and visible recovery presence, as living proof that long-term recovery exists in the millions of individuals who have attained degrees of health and wellness, are leading productive lives, and making valuable contributions to society. Meanwhile, policymakers and health care system leaders in the United States and abroad are beginning to embrace recovery as an organizing framework for approaching addiction as a chronic disorder from which individuals can recover, so long as they have access to evidence-based treatments and responsive long-term supports.[1-4]

Despite the growing popularity and importance of "recovery" as a concept, many people wonder what the term really means and why it matters. This chapter answers these questions by first defining the concept of recovery from substance use disorders and then reviewing the research on the methods and procedures used by mutual aid groups and recovery support services (RSS) to foster and sustain recovery.

KEY FINDINGS*

- Recovery from substance use disorders has had several definitions. Although specific elements of these definitions differ, all agree that recovery goes beyond the remission of symptoms to include a positive change in the whole person. In this regard, "abstinence," though often necessary, is not always sufficient to define recovery.
- Remission from substance use disorders—the reduction of key symptoms below the diagnostic threshold—is more common than most people realize. "Supported" scientific evidence indicates that approximately 50 percent of adults who once met diagnostic criteria for a substance use disorder—or about 25 million people—are currently in stable remission (1 year or longer). Even so, remission from a substance use disorder can take several years and multiple episodes of treatment, RSS, and/or mutual aid.
- There are many paths to recovery. People will choose their pathway based on their cultural values, their socioeconomic status, their psychological and behavioral needs, and the nature of their substance use disorder.
- Mutual aid groups and newly emerging recovery support programs and organizations are a key part of the system of continuing care for substance use disorders in the United States. A range of recovery support services have sprung up all over the United States, including in schools, health care systems, housing, and community settings.
- The state of the science is varied in the recovery field.
  - Well-supported scientific evidence demonstrates the effectiveness of 12-step mutual aid groups focused on alcohol and 12-step facilitation interventions.
  - Evidence for the effectiveness of other recovery supports (educational settings, drug-focused mutual aid groups, and recovery housing) is promising.
  - Many other recovery supports have been studied little or not at all.

*The Centers for Disease Control and Prevention (CDC) summarizes strength of evidence as: "Well-supported": when evidence is derived from multiple controlled trials or large-scale population studies; "Supported": when evidence is derived from rigorous but fewer or smaller trials; and "Promising": when evidence is derived from a practical or clinical sense and is widely practiced.[6]

Recovery Definitions, Values, and Controversies

"Recovery" Has Many Meanings

The word "recovery" is used to mean a range of different things.[4,7] For example, members of Alcoholics Anonymous (AA) may say they are "in recovery" or are "recovering alcoholics." Substance use treatment program directors sometimes speak of their "recovery rate," meaning the proportion of patients who have graduated and remained abstinent. Some activists describe themselves as being part of a "recovery movement." One simple way to make sense of these different definitions of recovery is to divide them into those that describe individual people and their experience and those that describe a set of recovery values and beliefs that could be embraced by individuals, organizations, and activist movements.

Recovery as a Term for Individuals

Like any other chronic health condition, substance use disorders can go into remission. Among individuals with substance use disorders, this commonly involves the person stopping substance use, or at least reducing it to a safer level—for example, a student who was binge drinking several nights a week during college but reduced his alcohol consumption to one or two drinks a day after graduation. In general health care, treatments that reduce major disease symptoms to normal or "sub-clinical" levels are said to produce remission, and such treatments are thereby considered effective. However, serious substance use disorders are chronic conditions that can involve cycles of abstinence and relapse, possibly over several years following attempts to change.[4,8-11] Thus, sustaining remission among those seriously affected typically requires a personal program of sustained recovery management.[12]

> **KEY TERMS**
>
> **Remission**. A medical term meaning that major disease symptoms are eliminated or diminished below a pre-determined, harmful level.

For some people with substance use disorders, especially those whose problems are not severe, remission is the end of a chapter in their life that they rarely think about later, if at all. But for others, particularly those with more severe substance use disorders, remission is a component of a broader change in their behavior, outlook, and identity. That change process becomes an ongoing part of how they think about themselves and their experience with substances. Such people describe themselves as being "in recovery."

Various definitions of individual recovery have been offered nationally and internationally.[13-17] Although they differ in some respects, all of these recovery definitions describe personal changes that are well beyond simply stopping substance use. As such, they are conceptually broader than "abstinence" or "remission." For example, the Betty Ford Institute Consensus Panel defined recovery as "a voluntarily maintained lifestyle characterized by sobriety, personal health, and citizenship."[13] Similarly, the Substance Abuse and Mental Health Services Administration (SAMHSA) defines recovery as "a process of change through which individuals improve their health and wellness, live a self-directed life, and strive to reach their full potential."[16]

The specific meaning of recovery can also vary across cultures and communities. Among some American Indians, recovery is inherently understood to involve the entire family[18] and to draw upon cultural and community resources (see, for example, the organization White Bison). On the other hand, European Americans tend to define recovery in more individual terms. Blacks or African Americans are more likely than individuals of other racial backgrounds to see recovery as requiring complete abstinence from alcohol and drugs.[19] Within some communities, recovery is seen as being aligned with a particular religion, yet in other communities such as the AA fellowship, recovery is explicitly not religious but is instead considered spiritual. Still other communities, such as LifeRing Secular Recovery, SMART Recovery, and Secular Organization for Sobriety, view recovery as an entirely secular process.

Adding further to the diversity of concepts and definitions associated with recovery, in recent years the term has been increasingly applied to recovery from mental illness. Studies of people with schizophrenia, some of whom have co-occurring substance use disorders, have found that recovery is often characterized by increased hope and optimism, and greater life satisfaction.[20] This same research revealed that whether someone experienced such benefits was strongly related to their experience with broader recovery benefits, such as improved health, improved finances, and a better social life.[21]

Recovery-Related Values and Beliefs

When people talk about the recovery movement, they often invoke a set of values and beliefs that may be embraced by individuals with substance use disorders, families, treatment professionals, and even entire health care systems. Some examples of these values and beliefs include:[22]

- People who suffer from substance use disorders (recovering or not) have essential worth and dignity.
- The shame and discrimination that prevents many individuals from seeking help must be vigorously combated.
- Recovery can be achieved through diverse pathways and should be celebrated.
- Access to high-quality treatment is a human right, although recovery is more than treatment.
- People in recovery and their families have valuable experiences and encouragement to offer others who are struggling with substance use.

Conceptual Controversies in Recovery

Most people who define themselves as being "in recovery" have experience with 12-step-oriented mutual aid groups such as AA and Narcotics Anonymous (NA), but many others enter recovery through professional treatment services, non-12-step mutual aid groups, or other routes of support, such as family, friends, or faith-based organizations.[7] The diversity in pathways to recovery has sometimes provoked debate about the value of some pathways over others.

For example, people who achieve recovery with the support of medications (e.g., methadone, buprenorphine, disulfiram, acamprosate, naltrexone, or even antidepressants) have sometimes been denounced by those who do not take medications, based on assumptions that using medication is inconsistent with recovery principles or a form of drug substitutions or replacement. Nonetheless, members of the National Alliance for Medication Assisted Recovery or Methadone Anonymous refer to themselves as practicing medication-assisted recovery.[23]

Finally, some people who have had severe substance use disorders in the past but no longer meet criteria for a substance use disorder do not think of themselves as operating from a recovery perspective or consider themselves part of a recovery movement, even if they endorse some or all of the beliefs and values associated with recovery.

Perspectives of Those in Recovery

The most comprehensive study of how people define recovery recruited over 9,000 individuals with previous substance use disorders from a range of recovery pathways. Almost all (98 percent) reported characteristics that met formal medical criteria for a severe substance use disorder and three-quarters labeled themselves as being "in recovery."[7] The study results shed light on how people vary in their understanding of recovery:

- **Abstinence:** 86.0 percent saw abstinence as part of their recovery. The remainder either did not think abstinence was part of recovery in general or felt it was not important for their recovery.[7] Endorsement of abstinence as "essential" was most common among those who were affiliated with 12-step mutual aid groups.[24] This finding was consistent with previous research showing that the great majority of people (about 6 in 7) who have experienced serious substance use disorders consider abstinence essential for recovery.[19]

- **Personal growth:** "Being honest with myself" was endorsed as part of recovery by 98.6 percent of participants.[7] Other almost universally-endorsed elements included "handling negative feelings without using alcohol or drugs" and "being able to enjoy life without alcohol or drugs." Almost all study participants viewed their recovery as a process of growth and development, and about two-thirds saw it as having a spiritual dimension.

- **Service to others:** Engaging in service to others was another prominent component of how study participants defined recovery, perhaps because during periods of heavy substance use, individuals often do damage to others that they later regret. Importantly, service to others has evidence of helping individuals maintain their own recovery.[25,26] A survey of more than 3,000 people in recovery indicated that fulfilling important roles and being civically engaged, such as paying taxes, holding a job, and being a responsible parent and neighbor, became much more common after their substance use ended.[27]

Estimating the Number of People "In Recovery"

How much recovery one sees in the world depends on where one looks. Substance use disorders are highly variable in their course, complexity, severity, and impact on health and well-being. In the general population, many people who once met diagnostic criteria for low-severity, "mild" substance use disorders but who later drink or use drugs without related problems do not define themselves as being in recovery. This reality has two implications:

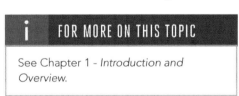

FOR MORE ON THIS TOPIC

See Chapter 1 - Introduction and Overview.

- **First**, the number of people who are in remission from a substance use disorder is, by definition, greater than the number of people who define themselves as being in recovery.

- **Second**, depending on how survey questions are asked and interpreted by respondents, estimates of recovery prevalence may differ substantially. Someone who once met formal criteria for a substance use disorder but no longer does may respond "Yes" to a question asking whether they had "ever had a problem with alcohol or drugs," but may say "No" when asked "Do you consider yourself as being in recovery?"

Perhaps because of this definitional complexity, most clinical outcome studies and community studies of substance use disorders over the years have not included "recovery" as an outcome measure. Instead, abstinence or remission are usually the outcomes that are considered to indicate recovery.[28]

Summarizing data from six large studies, one analysis estimated that the proportion of the United States adult population that is in remission from a substance use disorder of any severity is approximately 10.3 percent (with a range of 5.3 to 15.3 percent).[29] This estimate is consistent with findings from a different national survey, which found that approximately 10 percent, or 1 in 10, of United States adults say, "Yes," when asked, "Did you once have a problem with drugs or alcohol but no longer do?" These percentages translate to roughly 25 million United States adults being in remission.[29] It is not yet known what proportion of adolescents defines themselves as being in recovery.

Despite negative stereotypes of "hopeless addicts," rigorous follow-up studies of treated adult populations, who tend to have the most chronic and severe disorders, show more than 50 percent achieving sustained remission, defined as remission that lasted for at least 1 year.[29] Latest estimates from national epidemiological research using the Fifth Edition of the *Diagnostic and Statistical Manual of Mental Disorders* (DSM-5) criteria for substance use disorder show similar rates of remission.[30,31] Despite these findings, widely held pessimistic views about the chances of remission or recovery from substance use disorders may continue to affect public opinion in part because sustained recovery lasting a year or longer can take several years and multiple episodes of treatment, recovery support, and/or mutual aid services to achieve. By some estimates, it can take as long as 8 or 9 years after a person first seeks formal help to achieve sustained recovery.[32,33]

In studies published since 2000, the rate of sustained remission following substance use disorder treatment among adolescents is roughly 35 percent. This estimate is provisional because most studies used small samples and/or had short follow-up durations.[29] Despite the potentially lower remission rate for adolescents, early detection and intervention can help a young person get to remission faster.[29]

Recovery-oriented Systems of Care

Increasingly, RSS are being organized into a framework for infusing the entire health and social service system with recovery-related beliefs, values, and approaches.[34] This transformation has been described as:

> ...a shift away from crisis-oriented, deficit-focused, and professionally-directed models of care to a vision of care that is directed by people in recovery, emphasizes the reality and hope of long-term recovery, and recognizes the many pathways to healing for people with addiction and mental health challenges.[35]

Recovery-oriented Systems of Care (ROSC) embrace the idea that severe substance use disorders are most effectively addressed through a chronic care management model that includes longer term, outpatient care; recovery housing; and recovery coaching and management checkups.[36] Recovery-oriented systems are designed to be easy to navigate for people seeking help, transparent in their operations, and responsive to the cultural diversity of the communities they serve.[36] Treatment in recovery-oriented systems is offered as one component in a range of other services, including recovery supports. Treatment professionals act in a partnership/consultation role, drawing upon each person's goals and strengths, family supports, and community resources. On a systems level, outcomes from Connecticut's Department of Mental Health and Addiction Services (DMHAS) ROSC initiative have demonstrated a 46 percent increase in individuals served, with 40 percent using outpatient care at lower costs, resulting in a decrease of 25 percent annual cost per client and a 24 percent decrease in overall treatment expenses.[36]

An example of a successful municipal ROSC has been evolving since 2004 in Philadelphia's Department of Behavioral Health and Intellectual disAbility Services (DBHIDS). Three focus areas were aligned to achieve a complete systems transformation in the design and delivery of recovery-oriented services: a change in thinking (concept); a change in behavior (practice); and a change in fiscal, policy, and administrative functions (context). To achieve successful implementation, DBHIDS conducted ongoing activities with a variety of stakeholders including individuals in recovery and their family members, peer and professional providers, administrators and fiscal agents, and agency staff and leadership.[37]

SAMHSA has been instrumental in setting the stage for the emergence of the organized recovery community and its role in the development of ROSC, as well as peer and other RSS. Beginning with the Recovery Community Support Program (RCSP) in 1998, SAMHSA's Center for Substance Abuse Treatment introduced a number of grant initiatives that support recovery, such as Access to Recovery and Targeted Capacity Expansion grants for ROSC and Peer-to-Peer programs. These grants have given states, tribes, and community-based organizations resources and opportunities to create innovative practices and programs that address substance use disorders and promote long-term recovery. Valuable lessons from these grants have been applied to enhance the field, creating movement towards a strong recovery orientation, and highlight the need for rigorous research to identify evidence-based practices for recovery.

In 2010, SAMHSA rolled out Recovery Supports as one of its Strategic Initiatives, highlighting the importance of recovery as a valuable component in the continuum of care. Directly following the establishment of the Recovery Support Strategic Initiative, SAMHSA developed a five-year technical assistance contract to support recovery, known as BRSS-TACS (Bringing Recovery Supports to Scale – Technical Assistance Center Strategy). Through a series of actions and activities, this initiative has served to conceptualize and implement recovery-oriented services and systems across the country; examined the scope and depth of existing and needed recovery supports; supported the growth and quality of the peer workforce; enhanced and extended local, regional, and state recovery initiatives; and supported collaborations and capacity within the recovery movement.

Recovery Supports

Even after a year or 2 of remission is achieved—through treatment or some other route—it can take 4 to 5 more years before the risk of relapse drops below 15 percent, the level of risk that people in the general population have of developing a substance use disorder in their lifetime.[29] As a result, similar to other chronic conditions, a person with a serious substance use disorder often requires ongoing monitoring and management to maintain remission and to provide early re-intervention should the person relapse.[10,32] Recovery support services refer to the collection of community services that can provide emotional and practical support for continuing remission as well as daily structure and rewarding alternatives to substance use.

Just as the development of a substance use disorder involves profound changes in the brain, behavior, and social functioning,[38,39] the process of recovery also involves changes in these and other areas. These changes are typically marked and promoted by acquiring healthy life resources—sometimes called "recovery capital."[14,40-42] These recovery resources include housing, education, employment, and social resources, as well as better overall health and well-being. Recovery support services have been evaluated for effectiveness and are reviewed in the following sections.

Mutual Aid Groups

Mutual aid groups, such as 12-step groups, are perhaps the best known type of RSS, and they share a number of features. The members share a problem or status and they value experiential knowledge—learning from each other's experiences is a central element—and they focus on personal-change goals. The groups are voluntary associations that charge no fees and are self-led by the members.[43]

Mutual aid groups focused on substance use differ from other RSS in important respects. First, they have been in existence longer, having originally been created by American Indians in the 18th century after the introduction of alcohol to North America by Europeans.[44] The best-known mutual aid group today, AA, was founded in 1935. Other more recent RSS innovations and have yet to be studied extensively.[45] Second, mutual aid groups advance specific pathways to recovery, in contrast to the general supports provided by other RSS. They have been studied extensively for problems with alcohol, but not with illicit drugs. For example, an experienced AA member will help new members learn and incorporate AA's specific approach to recovery. In contrast, recovery coaches will support a variety of recovery options and support services, of which AA may be one of many. Third, mutual aid groups have their own self-supporting ecosystem that interacts with, but is fundamentally independent of, other health and social service systems. In contrast, other RSS are often part of formal health and social service systems.

12-Step Mutual Aid Groups

Mutual aid groups such as AA, Women for Sobriety, SMART Recovery, and many others are the historical precursors of RSS.[33,46] Most mutual aid group research has been conducted on AA, because AA is the most widely accessed and best-known form of help for alcohol problems in the United States.[46] Research on AA includes systematic reviews of its effectiveness and randomized controlled trials on AA-oriented interventions that actively link individuals with substance use disorders to mutual aid groups.[47-53] Research suggests that professional treatment programs that facilitate involvement in AA and NA lower health care costs by reducing relapses and need for further treatment.[54,55]

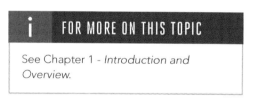

FOR MORE ON THIS TOPIC

See Chapter 1 - *Introduction and Overview*.

Beginning in the 1950s, the AA approach was adapted to illegal drugs by the founders of NA, and in later decades it was adapted to other drugs as well (e.g., Cocaine Anonymous, Marijuana Anonymous, Crystal Meth Anonymous). Alcoholics Anonymous and its derivative programs share two major components: A social fellowship and a 12-step program of action that was formulated based on members' experiences of recovery from severe alcohol use disorders. These 12 steps are ordered in a logical progression, beginning with accepting that one cannot control one's substance use, followed by abstaining from substances permanently, and transforming one's spiritual outlook, character, and relationships with other people.

Members of 12-step mutual aid groups tend to have a history of chronic and severe substance use disorders and participate in 12-step groups to support their long-term recovery. About 50 percent of adults who begin participation in a 12-step program after participating in a treatment program are still attending 3 years later.[56] Rates of continued attendance for individuals who seek AA directly without first going to treatment are also high, with 41.6 percent of those who start going to meetings still attending 9 to 16 years later.[57]

In the years since the Institute of Medicine called for more rigorous research on AA's effects and mechanisms in its 1990 report *Broadening the Base of Treatment for Alcohol Problems*,[58] research has moved from correlational studies with no control groups to carefully conducted randomized controlled trials. The most rigorous of these clinical trials have compared treatments that link patients to 12-step mutual aid groups to the same treatments without the AA linkage. Most of these trials have focused exclusively on AA, but some have involved mutual aid groups for drug use disorder as either an alternative or a supplement to AA.[52,59,60] A substantial body of research indicates AA is an effective recovery resource;[61-65] NA has been studied less extensively than AA, but evidence on its effectiveness is promising.[43]

> **KEY TERMS**
>
> **Clinical trial.** Any research study that prospectively assigns human participants or groups of participants to one or more health-related interventions to evaluate the effects on health outcomes.
>
> **Randomized controlled trial.** A clinical trial of an intervention in which people are randomly assigned either to a group receiving the intervention being studied or to a control group receiving a standard intervention, a placebo (a medicine with no therapeutic effect), or no intervention. At the end of the study, the results from the different groups are compared.

Research studying 12-step mutual aid groups, specifically those focused on alcohol, has shown that participation in the groups promotes an individual's recovery by strengthening recovery-supportive social networks; increasing members' ability to cope with risky social contexts and negative emotions; augmenting motivation to recover; reducing depression, craving, and impulsivity; and enhancing psychological and spiritual well-being.[66-69] Thus, with perhaps the exception of spirituality, many of the same mechanisms of behavior change thought to operate in professional treatments also appear to be important benefits of AA participation.[70]

A strength of 12-step mutual aid group research is that it has included many studies involving people of diverse racial backgrounds, as well as studies focused exclusively on women.[43] For example, American Indian and Alaskan Native groups have adapted AA to incorporate Native spirituality and to allow attendance by entire families. These groups do not limit talking time and incorporate cultural traditions and languages.[71] A culturally appropriate variation of AA[72] includes *The Red Road to Wellbriety*, a Native adaptation of the basic text of AA.[18] Similarly, AA adaptations by Latino immigrants incorporate languages and interaction styles from members' countries of origin.[73,74] Chapters focused on serving Black or African American or gay and lesbian participants also tailor 12-step mutual aid groups to a style that fits the culture of the participants.[46,75] This cultural adaptability, combined with the fact that 12-step groups are easily available, free of charge, and require no paperwork or insurance company documentation to attend, helps explain why these groups are attractive to a remarkably diverse range of people.[76]

Even though mutual aid groups are run by peers, professionals can and should play an important role in helping patients engage and participate. Multiple clinical trials have demonstrated that several clinical procedures are effective in increasing participation in mutual aid groups, and increase the chances for sustained remission and recovery. Health care professionals who help link patients with members of a mutual aid group can significantly increase the likelihood that the patients will attend the group.[50,52,59,77,78] Also, the more time health care professionals spend introducing, explaining, discussing, and encouraging mutual aid group participation during treatment sessions, the more likely the patients will engage, stay involved, and benefit.[47-49,51,53,79-81]

Non-12-step mutual aid group meetings are far less available than are 12-step mutual aid group meetings.[43] This points to a need for more groups aimed at those not comfortable with the 12-step approach,[82] as well as studies assessing their effectiveness.

Al-Anon Family Groups

Friends and family members often suffer when a loved one has a substance use disorder. This may be due to worry about the loved one experiencing accidents, injuries, negative social and legal consequences, diseases, or death, as well as fear of the loved one engaging in destructive behavior, such as stealing, manipulating, or being verbally or physically aggressive. Consequently, a number of mutual aid groups have emerged to provide emotional support to concerned significant others and families and to help them systematically and strategically alter their own unproductive behaviors that have emerged in their efforts to deal with the substance use problems of their affected loved one.

Al-Anon is a mutual aid group commonly sought by families dealing with substance use in a loved one. Like AA, Al-Anon is based on a 12-step philosophy[83] and provides support to concerned family members, affected significant others, and friends through a network of face-to-face and online meetings, whether or not their loved one seeks help and achieves remission or recovery. More than 80 percent of Al-Anon members are women.[84] The principal goal of Al-Anon is to foster emotional stability and "loving detachment" from the loved one rather than coaching members to "get their loved one into treatment or recovery." Al-Anon includes Alateen, which focuses on the specific needs of adolescents affected by a parent's or other family member's substance use.

Clinical trials and other studies of Al-Anon show that participating family members experience reduced depression, anger, and relationship unhappiness, at rates and levels comparable to those of individuals receiving psychological therapies.[85-89] Descriptive research suggests that about half of the newcomers to Al-Anon are still attending 6 months later.[90] Many other family-focused mutual aid groups, such as Nar-Anon, Co-Anon, and Grief Recovery After Substance Passing, have not been researched.

Recovery Coaching

Voluntary and paid recovery coach positions are a new development in the addiction field. Coaches do not provide "treatment" per se, but they often help individuals discharging from treatment to connect to community services while addressing any barriers or problems that may hinder the recovery process.[91] A recovery coach's responsibilities may include providing strategies to maintain abstinence, connecting people to recovery housing and social services, and helping people develop personal skills that maintain recovery.[92] Recovery coaches may or may not be in recovery themselves, but in either case they do not presume that the same path toward recovery will work for everyone they coach. Some community-based recovery organizations offer training programs for recovery coaches,[93] but no national standardized approach to training coaches has been developed. Because of the role that recovery coaches play in linking patients to RSS, they are increasingly becoming a part of formal clinical treatment teams.[94]

Recovery coaching has the potential to become an important part of RSS and the recovery process. A descriptive study of 56 recently homeless veterans with substance use disorder suggested that supplementing psychotherapy with recovery coaching increased length of abstinence at follow-up 6 months later.[95] Recovery coaches may complement, although not replace, professional case management services in the child welfare, criminal justice, and educational systems.[91] One large randomized trial showed that providing recovery coaches to mothers with a substance use disorder who were involved in the child welfare system reduced the likelihood of the mother's child being arrested by 52 percent.[96] Other rigorous studies have found that providing recovery coaches for mothers with substance use disorder reduces subsequent births with prenatal substance exposure[97] and also increases rates of family reunification.[98]

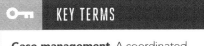

KEY TERMS

Case management. A coordinated approach to delivering general health care, substance use disorder treatment, mental health, and social services. This approach links clients with appropriate services to address specific needs and goals.

Recovery Housing

Recovery-supportive houses provide both a substance-free environment and mutual support from fellow recovering residents. Many residents stay in recovery housing during and/or after outpatient treatment, with self-determined residency lasting for several months to years. Residents often informally share resources with each other, giving advice borne of experience about how to access health care, find employment, manage legal problems, and interact with the social service system. Some recovery houses are connected with affiliates of the National Alliance of Recovery Residences, a non-profit organization that serves 25 regional affiliate organizations that collectively support more than 25,000 persons in recovery across over 2,500 certified recovery residences.

A leading example of recovery-supportive houses is Oxford Houses, which are peer-run, self-sustaining, substance-free residences that host 6 to 10 recovering individuals per house and require that all members maintain abstinence.[99] They encourage, but do not require, participation in 12-step mutual aid groups. A randomized controlled trial found that people with severe substance use disorders who were randomly assigned to live in an Oxford House after substance use disorder treatment were two times more likely to be abstinent and had higher monthly incomes and lower incarceration rates at follow-up 2 years later than similar individuals assigned to receive standard continuing care.[99] Despite high intervention costs, the net cost benefit to the health care and criminal justice systems from the Oxford House assignment relative to standard care was estimated at approximately $29,000 per person over the 2-year follow-up period.[100] Such beneficial effects of recovery housing may be further enhanced for patients with high levels of 12-step mutual aid group participation.[101,102]

Sober living homes are another type of substance-free living environment.[103] Many of these have a house manager or leader and mandate attendance by residents at 12-step mutual aid groups. An 18-month descriptive study found that residents in sober living homes reduced their alcohol and other

PEER RECOVERY COACHES: WHAT THEY ARE AND WHAT THEY ARE NOT

While some RSS described in this chapter can be delivered by people who are not in recovery, peer recovery coaches identify as being in recovery and use their knowledge and lived experience to inform their work. Although research on peer RSS is limited, results so far are promising.[5] The following are some important distinctions regarding peer recovery coaches.

Peer recovery coaches are...

- Individuals in recovery who help others with substance use disorders achieve and maintain recovery using four types of support:
    - Emotional (empathy, caring, concern);
    - Informational (practical knowledge and vocational assistance);
    - Instrumental (concrete assistance to help individuals gain access to health and social services);
    - Affiliational (introductions to healthy social contacts and recreational pursuits).
- Embedded in the community in a variety of settings, including recovery community organizations; community health, mental health, or addiction clinics; sober living homes and recovery residences; and recovery high school and collegiate recovery programs.
- Peer workers in various treatment and recovery contexts including primary care, emergency departments, mental health clinics, criminal justice, child welfare, homeless agencies, and crisis outreach teams.

They are not...

- Substance use disorder treatment counselors. They do not diagnose or provide formal treatment. Rather, they focus on instilling hope and modeling recovery through the personal, lived experience of addiction and recovery.
- Case managers. Case management typically involves professional or patient service delivery models. The terms "peer" and "recovery coach" are used purposely to reflect a mutual, peer-based collaboration to help people achieve sustained recovery.[90]
- AA or NA sponsors. Peer recovery coaches do not espouse any specific recovery pathway or orientation but rather facilitate all pathways to recovery.
- Nationally standardized, with manuals describing their activities. Peer recovery coaches vary around the country. This stems from the newness of this practice and the diversity of the populations that recovery coaches serve. As use of this type of support expands, some national norms of practice and behavior will likely form over time, but with significant flexibility to enable sensitivity to local realities.

drug use as well as increased employment over time.[104,105] However, unlike the clinical trial of Oxford House, this study had no comparison group, and individuals chose whether to reside in sober living homes rather than being randomly assigned to one. Therefore, residence in the sober living home cannot be assumed to have caused the better outcomes observed.

Taken together, these studies provide promising evidence to suggest that recovery-supportive housing can be both cost-effective and effective in supporting recovery.

RECOVERY HOUSING

Agency or Organization:

Oxford House, Inc. - Silver Spring, Maryland

Purpose:

Oxford House, Inc. is a publicly-supported, nonprofit umbrella organization that provides an oversight network connecting Oxford Houses in 43 states and the District of Columbia. Each Oxford House is a self-supporting and democratically-run substance-free residence.

Goals:

- Provide substance-free housing to individuals in recovery as an effective cost-efficient model.
- Ensure that houses are self-governed and run according to Oxford House standards and guidelines.
- Implement infrastructure to oversee existing houses and establish new houses in areas of need.

Outcomes:

- An 87 percent abstinence rate at the end of a 2-year period living in an Oxford House, four to five times greater than typical outcomes following detoxification and treatment.
- Comparisons between a group living in Oxford House and going to AA/NA versus a similar group that only goes to AA/NA show that the group living in an Oxford House had higher and more positive rates of self-efficacy and self-mastery.
- In a comparison study between Oxford House residents and a group that was assigned usual aftercare services, the Oxford House group had significantly lower substance use (31.3 percent vs. 64.8 percent), higher monthly income ($989 vs. $440), and lower incarceration rates (3 percent vs. 9 percent).

> *"Living in an Oxford House reinforced and reestablished a lot of things that I was not able to do or unwilling to do when I was using. Things like paying rent and working. Things like learning how to live without using drugs. Things like becoming a responsible person. Things like developing healthy relationships. While I resided at an Oxford House, I started working for Oxford House, Inc. As a result, I was willing to help open more Oxford Houses, especially for women."*
>
> – Debbie D., former Oxford House resident

Recovery Management

Recovery-oriented care often use long-term recovery management protocols, such as recovery management check-ups (RMCs),[106] and telephone case monitoring.[107,108] These models have only been studied with professionals, but similar protocols are also being used in peer-directed RSS, where they have yet to be formally evaluated.

Recovery Management Check-ups

The RMC model for substance use disorders draws heavily from monitoring and early re-intervention protocols used for other chronic diseases, such as diabetes and hypertension. With the core components of tracking, assessment, linkage, engagement, and retention, patients are monitored quarterly for several years following an initial treatment. If a relapse occurs, the patient is connected with the necessary services and encouraged to remain in treatment. The main assumption is that early detection and treatment of relapse will improve long-term outcomes.[109]

A clinical trial showed that, compared with patients assigned to usual care, individuals receiving RMCs returned to treatment sooner after relapses, had fewer misuse problems, had more days of abstinence, and were less likely to need treatment at follow-up 2 and 4 years later.[106,110] Recovery management check-ups have also been shown to be effective for people who have co-occurring substance use disorders and mental illnesses[111] and for women with substance use disorders who have been released from jail.[112] RMCs are also cost-effective.[113] Although the check-ups add somewhat to annual care costs, a randomized study showed that they produce greater reductions in costs associated with health care and criminal justice.[113]

Telephone Case Monitoring

Telephone case monitoring is another long-term recovery management and monitoring method for maintaining contact with patients without requiring an in-person appointment. It can be provided by professionals or by peers, although only the former approach has been rigorously studied. One example is an extended case monitoring intervention, which consisted of phone calls on a tapering schedule over the course of several years, with contact becoming more frequent when needed, such as when risk of relapse was high. This intervention was designed to optimize the cost-effectiveness of alcohol treatment through long-term engagement with clients beyond the relatively short treatment episodes.[108]

In a randomized clinical trial, patients receiving telephone case monitoring were half as likely as those not receiving it to drink heavily at 3-year follow-up. Case monitoring also reduced the costs of subsequent outpatient treatment by $240 per person at 1-year follow-up, relative to patients who did not receive the telephone monitoring.[114] Another clinical trial compared weekly telephone monitoring plus brief counseling with two other treatments: standard continuing care and individualized relapse prevention. Telephone monitoring produced the highest rates of abstinence from alcohol at follow-up 12 months later.[115] Furthermore, at 24 months, participants who received telephone monitoring continued to have significantly higher rates of total abstinence than those in standard care.[116] Adding telephone monitoring and counseling to intensive outpatient treatment also has been shown to improve alcohol use outcomes in a randomized clinical trial.[117]

Recovery Community Centers

To further distinguish the peer-led services of these centers from professional treatment services, individuals using the center are referred to as "peers" or "members" and center staff hold positions such as "peer leaders" or "recovery mentors."[92,94]

These centers may host mutual aid group meetings and offer recovery coaching, recovery-focused educational and social events; access to resources, including housing, education, and employment; telephone-based recovery services; and additional recovery community education, advocacy, and service events.[33,118] Some recovery community centers are sites in which community members can engage in advocacy to combat negative public attitudes, educate the community, and improve supports for recovery in the community. Many recovery community centers are typically operated by recovery community organizations.[119]

Recovery community centers have yet to be studied in a rigorous fashion; therefore it is not possible to estimate their effectiveness. Evaluation studies currently underway may provide a more conclusive judgment of whether and how recovery community centers benefit their members. Recovery community centers are different from professionally-operated substance use disorder treatment programs because they offer support beyond the clinical setting.

Recovery-based Education

High school and college environments can be difficult for students in recovery because of perceived and actual high levels of substance use among other students, peer pressure to engage in substance use, and widespread availability of alcohol and drugs.[120,121] The emergence of high school and collegiate recovery support programs is an important response to this challenge in that they provide recovery-supportive environments, recovery norms, and peer engagement with other students in recovery.

Recovery High Schools

Recovery high schools help students in recovery focus on academic learning while simultaneously receiving RSS. Such schools support abstinence and student efforts to overcome personal issues that may compromise academic performance or threaten continued recovery.[122] The earliest known program opened in 1979, and the number slowly increased to approximately 35 schools in 15 states by 2015.[123]

A study of 17 recovery high schools found that most had small and rapidly changing enrollments, ranging from 12 to 25 students. Rates of abstinence from "all alcohol and other drugs" increased from 20 percent during the 90 days before enrolling to 56 percent since enrolling. Students' opinions of the schools were positive, with 87 percent reporting overall satisfaction.[124] A study of graduates from one recovery high school found that 39 percent reported no drug or alcohol use in the past 30 days and more than 90 percent had enrolled in college.[125] These results are promising, pointing to the need for more research. A rigorous outcomes study is nearing completion that will give a better idea of the impact of recovery high schools.

Recovery in Colleges

Collegiate recovery support programs vary in number and type of RSS. Most provide some combination of recovery residence halls or recovery-specific wings, counseling services, on-site mutual aid group meetings, and other educational and social supports. These services are provided within an environment that facilitates social role modeling of sobriety and connection among recovering peers. The programs often require participants to demonstrate 3 to 6 months with no use of alcohol and drugs as a requirement for admission. Recovering college peers may help these new students effectively manage the environmental risks present on many college campuses.[126]

Participants in collegiate recovery programs often have significant accompanying mental health problems, such as depression or an eating disorder, in addition to their substance use disorder, which can complicate recovery.[127] Nevertheless, observational data from two model programs suggest that rates of return to use (defined as any use of alcohol or other substance) are only 4 to 13 percent in any given semester.[126,128,129] Further, the academic achievement (grade point average and graduation rates) of students in collegiate recovery support programs is better than that of the rest of the undergraduates at the same institution.[127,128,130] Although these results are promising, more research is needed on these programs[131] to fully evaluate their effectiveness.[126]

Social and Recreational Recovery Infrastructures and Social Media

In keeping with the need to support long-term remission and recovery from substance use disorders, social and recreational entities are emerging that make it easier for people in recovery to enjoy activities and social interaction that do not involve alcohol or drugs. Examples include recovery cafes and clubhouses, recovery sports leagues and other sporting activities, and a variety of recovery-focused creative arts, including music and musicians' organizations, visual arts, and theatre and poetry events.[33] Providing these positive alternatives is intended to support recovery as well as provide access to healthy, enjoyable activities. However, no research has yet examined whether participation in these activities produces a significant benefit beyond what might be obtained from other RSS.

Social media, mobile health applications, and recovery-specific online social networking and support sites are growing platforms for providing both intervention and long-term RSS for individuals with substance use disorders, as well as social interaction, friendship, and humor. These are easily accessible and have wide reach. Although research on the impact of these new tools is limited, studies are beginning to show positive benefits, particularly in preventing relapse and supporting recovery.[132,133] Social media supports appear to be especially helpful for young people in particular.[132]

Specific Populations and Recovery

As mentioned earlier, practice and research in the recovery field are relatively new. This has disadvantages in terms of how much is known from scientific research, but it has a compensating advantage: Most studies have been conducted recently and usually with diverse populations. Indeed, the majority of participants in many of the studies cited in this chapter have included Blacks or African Americans, Hispanics or Latinos, and American Indians or Alaska Natives.

Recovery-oriented policies have also supported diverse populations. For example, SAMHSA's Recovery Community Services Program made advancing recovery in diverse communities a central goal and helped support organizations serving a broad range of ethnic, racial, and sexual minority communities. Further, 12-step fellowships such as AA and NA have a long history of supporting meeting spaces that are specific to women; Lesbian, Gay, Bisexual, and Transgender (LGBT) populations; young people; and other groups, including meetings that are conducted in other languages.

For all these reasons, the research and practice conclusions of this chapter can be assumed to be broadly applicable to a range of populations. However, not every single population has received comparable attention:

- Blacks or African Americans have been well represented in recovery research, including in the studies of ROSC, mutual aid groups, and recovery housing discussed in this chapter.

- American Indians or Alaska Natives have maintained recovery movements for centuries. More recently culturally-specific adaptations of recovery approaches (e.g., *The Red Road to Wellbriety*) have been developed. Hispanic or Latino adaptations of AA have been studied, and ROSC have been studied in areas with significant Hispanic or Latino populations (e.g., Philadelphia).

- Native Hawaiians or Other Pacific Islanders have not been studied by recovery researchers, probably because of their small number (one tenth of one percent of the population). They are a population that should be studied in the future.
- Asian-tailored recovery interventions have not been extensively studied and remain an important focus for future research.
- Research on the effectiveness of various recovery pathways within LGBT communities has been limited in quantity and comparability across studies.

Recommendations for Research

Health and social service providers, funders, policymakers, and most of all people with substance use disorders and their families need better information about the effectiveness of the recovery options reviewed in this chapter. Thus, a key research goal for the future is to understand and evaluate the effectiveness, and cost effectiveness, of the emerging range of mutual aid groups and RSS, particularly peer recovery support services and practices and recovery coaches. Another focus of research is new, culturally specific adaptations of long-existent recovery supports, such as AA and NA, as they evolve to meet the needs of an increasingly diverse membership. Such research could increase public and professional awareness of these potentially cost-effective recovery strategies and resources.

Research is also needed on how health care systems themselves can work best with RSS and the workforce that provides RSS. Professional and formal treatment services and RSS have different roots and represent different cultures historically. Creating a fluid, responsive, and more effective recovery-oriented "system" will require greater sensitivity and understanding of the strengths and benefits of each, including rigorous cross-site evaluations for professional RSS strategies. Research should determine the efficacy of peer supports including peer recovery support services, recovery housing, recovery chronic disease management, high school and collegiate recovery programs, and recovery community centers through rigorous, cross-site evaluations.

Although the professionally-led health and social service system should engage with peer-led service organizations, maintaining the informal, grassroots nature of many RSS may be central to their appeal and quite possibly their effectiveness. Thus, a diverse group of stakeholders in the recovery field should come together to create a strategic research agenda that includes:

- The establishment of recovery outcomes and measures;
- The development of a credible methodology for estimating the prevalence of those in recovery;
- Protocols on initiating, stabilizing, and sustaining long-term recovery; and
- Measuring the value of ROSC.

References

1. Best, D. W., & Lubman, D. I. (2012). The recovery paradigm: A model of hope and change for alcohol and drug addiction. *Australian Family Physician, 41*(8), 593-597.

2. Humphreys, K., & Lembke, A. (2014). Recovery-oriented policy and care systems in the UK and USA. *Drug and Alcohol Review, 33*(1), 13-18.

3. Humphreys, K., & McLellan, A. T. (2010). Brief intervention, treatment, and recovery support services for Americans who have substance use disorders: An overview of policy in the Obama administration. *Psychological Services, 7*(4), 275-284.

4. White, W. L. (2007). The new recovery advocacy movement in America. *Addiction, 102*(5), 696-703.

5. Bassuk, E. L., Hanson, J., Greene, R. N., Richard, M., & Laudet, A. (2016). Peer-delivered recovery support services for addictions in the United States: A systematic review. *Journal of Substance Abuse Treatment 63*, 1-9.

6. Puddy, R. W., & Wilkins, N. (2011). *Understanding evidence Part 1: Best available research evidence. A guide to the continuum of evidence of effectiveness.* Atlanta, GA: Centers for Disease Control and Prevention.

7. Kaskutas, L. A., Borkman, T. J., Laudet, A., Ritter, L. A., Witbrodt, J., Subbaraman, M. S., . . . Bond, J. (2014). Elements that define recovery: The experiential perspective. *Journal of Studies on Alcohol and Drugs, 75*(6), 999-1010.

8. Humphreys, K., & Tucker, J. A. (2002). Toward more responsive and effective intervention systems for alcohol-related problems. *Addiction, 97*(2), 126-132.

9. McLellan, A. T., Lewis, D. C., O'Brien, C. P., & Kleber, H. D. (2000). Drug dependence, a chronic medical illness: Implications for treatment, insurance, and outcomes evaluation. *JAMA, 284*(13), 1689-1695.

10. Kelly, J. F., & White, W. L. (2010). *Addiction recovery management: Theory, research and practice.* New York, NY: Springer Science & Business Media.

11. Simpson, C. A., & Tucker, J. A. (2002). Temporal sequencing of alcohol-related problems, problem recognition, and help-seeking episodes. *Addictive Behaviors, 27*(5), 659-674.

12. White, W. L., Evans, A. C., & Achara-Abrahams, I. (2012). Recovery management service design matrices Retrieved from http://www.williamwhitepapers.com/pr/2012%20Recovery%20Management%20Service%20Design%20Matrices.pdf. Accessed on April 6, 2016.

13. The Betty Ford Institute Consensus Panel. (2007). What is recovery? A working definition from the Betty Ford Institute. *Journal of Substance Abuse Treatment, 33*(3), 221-228.

14. Kelly, J. F., & Hoeppner, B. (2015). A biaxial formulation of the recovery construct. *Addiction Research and Theory, 23*(1), 5-9.

15. The Scottish Government. (2008). *The road to recovery: A new approach to tackling Scotland's drug problem.* (0755956575). Edinburgh, Scotland: The Scottish Government.

16. Substance Abuse and Mental Health Services Administration. (2012). SAMHSA's working definition of recovery: 10 guiding principles of recovery. Rockville, MD: Substance Abuse and Mental Health Services Administration.

17. el-Guebaly, N. (2012). The meanings of recovery from addiction: Evolution and promises. *Journal of Addiction Medicine, 6*(1), 1-9.

18. Coyhis, D., & White, W. (2002b). Addiction and recovery in Native America: Lost history, enduring lessons. *Counselor, 3*(5), 16-20.

19. Laudet, A. B. (2007). What does recovery mean to you? Lessons from the recovery experience for research and practice. *Journal of Substance Abuse Treatment, 33*(3), 243-256.

20. Resnick, S. G., Rosenheck, R. A., & Lehman, A. F. (2004). An exploratory analysis of correlates of recovery. *Psychiatric Services, 55*(5), 540-547.

21. Laudet, A. B. (2011). The case for considering quality of life in addiction research and clinical practice. *Addiction Science & Clinical Practice, 6*(1), 44-55.

22. White, W. (2000). *Toward a new recovery advocacy movement.* Paper presented at the Recovery Community Support Program Conference: "Working Together for Recovery" (April 3-5, 2000), Arlington, VA.

23. White, W. L. (2011). *Narcotics Anonymous and the pharmacotherapeutic treatment of opioid addiction in the United States.* Chicago, IL: Philadelphia Department of Behavioral Health and Intellectual Disability Services & Great Lakes Addiction Technology Transfer Center.

24. Witbrodt, J., Kaskutas, L. A., & Grella, C. E. (2015). How do recovery definitions distinguish recovering individuals? Five typologies. *Drug and Alcohol Dependence, 148,* 109-117.

25. Zemore, S. E., & Kaskutas, L. A. (2008). 12-step involvement and peer helping in day hospital and residential programs. *Substance Use & Misuse, 43*(12-13), 1882-1903.

26. Zemore, S. E., Kaskutas, L. A., & Ammon, L. N. (2004). In 12-step groups, helping helps the helper. *Addiction, 99*(8), 1015-1023.

27. Laudet, A. (2013). *Life in recovery: Report on the survey findings.* Washington, DC: Faces and Voices of Recovery.

28. Berglund, M., Thelander, S., & Jonsson, E. (2003). *Treating alcohol and drug abuse: An evidence based review.* New York, NY: John Wiley & Sons.

29. White, W. L. (2012). *Recovery/remission from substance use disorders: An analysis of reported outcomes in 415 scientific reports, 1868-2011.* Philadelphia, PA: Philadelphia Department of Behavioral Health and Intellectual Disability Services.

30. Grant, B. F., Goldstein, R. B., Saha, T. D., Chou, S. P., Jung, J., Zhang, H., . . . Hasin, D. S. (2015). Epidemiology of DSM-5 alcohol use disorder: Results from the national epidemiologic survey on alcohol and related conditions III. *JAMA Psychiatry, 72*(8), 757-766.

31. Recovery Research Institute. (2016). Estimates of alcohol use disorder in the United States. Retrieved from www.recoveryanswers.org/pressrelease/estimates-of-alcohol-use-disorder-in-the-united-states/. Accessed on April 6, 2016.

32. Dennis, M., & Scott, C. K. (2007). Managing addiction as a chronic condition. *Addiction Science and Clinical Practice, 4*(1), 45-55.

33. White, W. L., Kelly, J. F., & Roth, J. D. (2012). New addiction-recovery support institutions: Mobilizing support beyond professional addiction treatment and recovery mutual aid. *Journal of Groups in Addiction & Recovery, 7*(2-4), 297-317.

34. White, W. (2008). *Recovery management and recovery-oriented systems of care: Scientific rationale and promising practices* (Vol. 6). Pittsburgh, PA: Northeast Addiction Technology Transfer Center.

35. Achara-Abrahams, I., Evans, A. C., & King, J. K. (2011). Recovery-focused behavioral health system transformation: A framework for change and lessons learned from Philadelphia. In J. F. Kelly & W. L. White (Eds.), *Addiction recovery management: Theory, research and practice.* (pp. 187-208). Totowa, NJ: Humana Press.

36. Kirk, T. A. (2010). Connecticut's journey to a statewide recovery-oriented health-care system: Strategies, successes, and challenges. *Addiction recovery management.* (pp. 209-234). New York, NY: Springer.

37. Evans, A. C. (2007). The recovery-focused transformation of an ubran behavioral health care system: An interview with Arthur Evans, PhD. In W. White (Ed.), *Perspectives on systems transformation: How visionary leaders are shifting addiction treatment toward a recovery-oriented system of care.* (pp. 39-58). Chicago, IL: Great Lakes Addiction Technology Transfer Center.

38. Edwards, G. (1982). Cannabis and the question of dependence. *Advisory Council on the Misuse of Drugs. Report of the Expert Group on the Effects of Cannabis Use.* (pp. 34-49). London, UK: Home Office.

39. Edwards, G., & Gross, M. M. (1976). Alcohol dependence: Provisional description of a clinical syndrome. *British Medical Journal Publishing Group, 1*(6017), 1058-1061.

40. Granfield, R., & Cloud, W. (1999). *Coming clean: Overcoming addiction without treatment.* New York, NY: New York University Press.

41. Granfield, R., & Cloud, W. (2004). The elephant that no one sees: Natural recovery among middle-class addicts. In J. Inciardi & K. McElrath (Eds.), *The American drug scene: An anthology.* (4th ed.). Los Angeles, CA: H.W. Roxbury Publishing.

42. Groshkova, T., Best, D., & White, W. (2013). The assessment of recovery capital: Properties and psychometrics of a measure of addiction recovery strengths. *Drug and Alcohol Review, 32*(2), 187-194.

43. Humphreys, K. (2004). *Circles of recovery: Self-help organizations for addictions.* Cambridge, UK: Cambridge University Press.

44. Coyhis, D., & White, W. L. (2002a). Alcohol problems in Native America: Changing paradigms and clinical practices. *Alcoholism Treatment Quarterly, 20*(3-4), 157-165.

45. Laudet, A. B., & Humphreys, K. (2013). Promoting recovery in an evolving policy context: What do we know and what do we need to know about recovery support services? *Journal of Substance Abuse Treatment, 45*(1), 126-133.

46. Humphreys, K. (2004). Tale telling in an alcohol mutual help organization. *New Directions in Alcohol Studies, 29,* 33-44.

47. Allen, J. P., Mattson, M. E., Miller, W. R., Tonigan, J. S., Connors, G. J., Rychtarik, R. G., . . . Litt, M. (1997). Matching alcoholism treatments to client heterogeneity: Project MATCH posttreatment drinking outcomes. *Journal of Studies on Alcohol, 58*(1), 7-29.

48. Kaskutas, L. A., Ye, Y., Greenfield, T. K., Witbrodt, J., & Bond, J. (2008). Epidemiology of Alcoholics Anonymous participation. In M. Galanter & L. A. Kaskutas (Eds.), *Recent developments in alcoholism: Research on Alcoholics Anonymous and spiritual aspects in addiction recovery.* (Vol. 18, pp. 261-282). New York, NY: Springer.

49. Litt, M. D., Kadden, R. M., Kabela-Cormier, E., & Petry, N. (2007). Changing network support for drinking: Initial findings from the network support project. *Journal of Consulting and Clinical Psychology, 75*(4), 542-555.

50. Timko, C., & DeBenedetti, A. (2007). A randomized controlled trial of intensive referral to 12-step self-help groups: One-year outcomes. *Drug and Alcohol Dependence, 90*(2), 270-279.

51. Litt, M. D., Kadden, R. M., Kabela-Cormier, E., & Petry, N. M. (2009). Changing network support for drinking: Network support project 2-year follow-up. *Journal of Consulting and Clinical Psychology, 77*(2), 229-242.

52. Timko, C., DeBenedetti, A., & Billow, R. (2006). Intensive referral to 12-Step self-help groups and 6-month substance use disorder outcomes. *Addiction, 101*(5), 678-688.

53. Walitzer, K. S., Dermen, K. H., & Barrick, C. (2009). Facilitating involvement in Alcoholics Anonymous during out-patient treatment: A randomized clinical trial. *Addiction, 104*(3), 391-401.

54. Humphreys, K., & Moos, R. (2001). Can encouraging substance abuse patients to participate in self-help groups reduce demand for health care? A quasi-experimental study. *Alcoholism: Clinical and Experimental Research, 25*(5), 711-716.

55. Humphreys, K., & Moos, R. H. (2007). Encouraging posttreatment self-help group involvement to reduce demand for continuing care services: Two-year clinical and utilization outcomes. *Alcoholism: Clinical and Experimental Research, 31*(1), 64-68.

56. Kelly, J. F., Stout, R., Zywiak, W., & Schneider, R. (2006). A 3-year study of addiction mutual-help group participation following intensive outpatient treatment. *Alcoholism: Clinical and Experimental Research, 30*(8), 1381-1392.

57. Moos, R. H., & Moos, B. S. (2005). Paths of entry into Alcoholics Anonymous: Consequences for participation and remission. *Alcoholism: Clinical and Experimental Research, 29*(10), 1858-1868.

58. Institute of Medicine Division of Mental Health and Behavioral Medicine. (1990). *Broadening the base of treatment for alcohol problems.* Washington, DC: National Academy of Sciences.

59. Donovan, D. M., Daley, D. C., Brigham, G. S., Hodgkins, C. C., Perl, H. I., Garrett, S., . . . Zammarelli, L. (2013). Stimulant abuser groups to engage in 12-step (STAGE-12): A multisite trial in the NIDA clinical trials network. *Journal of Substance Abuse Treatment, 44*(1), 103-114.

60. Weiss, R. D., Griffin, M. L., Gallop, R. J., Najavits, L. M., Frank, A., Crits-Christoph, P., . . . Luborsky, L. (2005). The effect of 12-step self-help group attendance and participation on drug use outcomes among cocaine-dependent patients. *Drug and Alcohol Dependence, 77*(2), 177-184.

61. Emrick, C. D., Tonigan, J. S., Montgomery, H., & Little, L. (1993). Alcoholics Anonymous: What is currently known? In B. McCrady & W. Miller (Eds.), *Research on Alcoholics Anonymous: Opportunities and alternatives.* (pp. 41-77). New Brunswick, NJ: Rutgers Center of Alcohol Studies.

62. Kelly, J. F., & Yeterian, J. D. (2008). Mutual-help groups. In W. O'Donohue & J. R. Cunningham (Eds.), *Evidence-based adjunctive treatments.* (pp. 61-106). New York, NY: Elsevier.

63. Humphreys, K., Blodgett, J. C., & Wagner, T. H. (2014). Estimating the efficacy of Alcoholics Anonymous without self-selection bias: An instrumental variables re-analysis of randomized clinical trials. *Alcoholism: Clinical and Experimental Research, 38*(11), 2688-2694.

64. Ferri, M., Amato, L., & Davoli, M. (2006). Alcoholics Anonymous and other 12-step programmes for alcohol dependence. *Cochrane Database of Systematic Reviews, 3*(3).

65. Kaskutas, L. A. (2009). Alcoholics Anonymous effectiveness: Faith meets science. *Journal of Addictive Diseases, 28*(2), 145-157.

66. Kelly, J. F., Hoeppner, B., Stout, R. L., & Pagano, M. (2012). Determining the relative importance of the mechanisms of behavior change within Alcoholics Anonymous: A multiple mediator analysis. *Addiction, 107*(2), 289-299.

67. Morgenstern, J., Labouvie, E., McCrady, B. S., Kahler, C. W., & Frey, R. M. (1997). Affiliation with Alcoholics Anonymous after treatment: A study of its therapeutic effects and mechanisms of action. *Journal of Consulting and Clinical Psychology, 65*(5), 768-777.

68. Kelly, J. F., & Yeterian, J. D. (2013). Mutual-help groups for alcohol and other substance use disorders. In B. S. McCrady & E. E. Epstein (Eds.), *Addictions: A comprehensive guidebook.* (2nd ed.). New York, NY: Oxford University Press.

69. Christo, G., & Franey, C. (1995). Drug users' spiritual beliefs, locus of control and the disease concept in relation to Narcotics Anonymous attendance and six-month outcomes. *Drug and Alcohol Dependence, 38*(1), 51-56.

70. Kelly, J. F., Magill, M., & Stout, R. L. (2009). How do people recover from alcohol dependence? A systematic review of the research on mechanisms of behavior change in Alcoholics Anonymous. *Addiction Research & Theory, 17*(3), 236-259.

71. Jilek-Aall, L. (1981). Acculturation, alcoholism and Indian-style Alcoholics Anonymous. *Journal of Studies on Alcohol*(Suppl 9), 143-158.

72. Womack, M. L. (1996). *The Indianization of Alcoholics Anonymous: An examination of Native American recovery movements.* (Master's thesis). University of Arizona Native American Research and Training Center, Tucson, AZ. Accessed

73. Garcia, A., Anderson, B., & Humphreys, K. (2015). Fourth and fifth step groups: A new and growing self-help organization for underserved Latinos with substance use disorders. *Alcoholism Treatment Quarterly, 33*(2), 235-243.

74. Hoffman, F. (1994). Cultural adaptations of Alcoholics Anonymous to serve Hispanic populations. *International Journal of the Addictions, 29*(4), 445-460.

75. Hudson, H. L. (1985). How and why Alcoholics Anonymous works for Blacks. *Alcoholism Treatment Quarterly, 2*(3-4), 11-30.

76. McCrady, B. S., & Miller, W. R. (Eds.). (1993). *Research on Alcoholics Anonymous: Opportunities and alternatives.* New Brunswick, NJ: Rutgers Center of Alcohol Studies.

77. Sisson, R. W., & Mallams, J. H. (1981). The use of systematic encouragement and community access procedures to increase attendance at Alcoholic Anonymous and Al-Anon meetings. *The American Journal of Drug and Alcohol Abuse, 8*(3), 371-376.

78. Manning, V., Best, D., Faulkner, N., Titherington, E., Morinan, A., Keaney, F., . . . Strang, J. (2012). Does active referral by a doctor or 12-Step peer improve 12-Step meeting attendance? Results from a pilot randomised control trial. *Drug and Alcohol Dependence, 126*(1), 131-137.

79. Donovan, D. M., Ingalsbe, M. H., Benbow, J., & Daley, D. C. (2013). 12-step interventions and mutual support programs for substance use disorders: An overview. *Social Work in Public Health, 28*(3-4), 313-332.

80. Kelly, J. F., & Moos, R. (2003). Dropout from 12-step self-help groups: Prevalence, predictors, and counteracting treatment influences. *Journal of Substance Abuse Treatment, 24*(3), 241-250.

81. Crits-Christoph, P., Siqueland, L., Blaine, J., Frank, A., Luborsky, L., Onken, L. S., . . . Beck, A. T. (1999). Psychosocial treatments for cocaine dependence: National Institute on Drug Abuse Collaborative Cocaine Treatment Study. *Archives of General Psychiatry, 56*(6), 493-502.

82. Kelly, J. F., & White, W. L. (2012). Broadening the base of addiction mutual-help organizations. *Journal of Groups in Addiction & Recovery, 7*(2-4), 82-101.

83. Al-Anon Family Groups. (2015). About Al-Anon family group meetings. Retrieved from http://www.al-anon.org/about-group-meetings. Accessed on April 11, 2016.

84. Short, N. A., Cronkite, R., Moos, R., & Timko, C. (2015). Men and women who attend Al-Anon: Gender differences in reasons for attendance, health status and personal functioning, and drinker characteristics. *Substance Use and Misuse, 50*(1), 53-61.

85. O'Farrell, T. J., & Clements, K. (2012). Review of outcome research on marital and family therapy in treatment for alcoholism. *Journal of Marital & Family Therapy, 38*(1), 122-144.

86. O'Farrell, T. J., & Fals-Stewart, W. (2002). Family-involved alcoholism treatment an update. *Recent Developments in Alcoholism.* (Vol. 15, pp. 329-356). New York, NY: Springer.

87. Barber, J. G., & Gilbertson, R. (1996). An experimental study of brief unilateral intervention for the partners of heavy drinkers. *Research on Social Work Practice, 6*(3), 325-336.

88. Miller, W. R., Meyers, R. J., & Tonigan, J. S. (1999). Engaging the unmotivated in treatment for alcohol problems: A comparison of three strategies for intervention through family members. *Journal of Consulting and Clinical Psychology, 67*(5), 688-697.

89. Dittrich, J. E., & Trapold, M. A. (1984). A treatment program for wives of alcoholics: An evaluation. *Bulletin of the Society of Psychologists in Addictive Behaviors, 3*(2), 91-102.

90. Timko, C., Laudet, A., & Moos, R. H. (2014). Newcomers to Al-Anon family groups: Who stays and who drops out? *Addictive Behaviors, 39*(6), 1042-1049.

91. Loveland, D., & Boyle, M. (2005). *Manual for recovery coaching and personal recovery plan development.* Chicago, IL: Illinois Department of Human Services, Department of Alcoholism and Substance Abuse.

92. White, W. (2006). *Sponsor, recovery coach, addiction counselor: The importance of role clarity and role integrity.* Philadelphia, PA: Philadelphia Department of Behavioral Health and Mental Retardation Services.

93. Connecticut Community for Addiction Recovery. (n.d.). Recovery coach academy. Retrieved from http://ccar.us/training-and-products/recovery-coach-academy/. Accessed on April 13, 2016.

94. Center for Substance Abuse Treatment. (2009). *What are peer recovery support services?* (HHS Publication No. (SMA) 09-4454). Rockville, MD: Substance Abuse and Mental Health Services Administration, U.S. Department of Health and Human Services.

95. LePage, J. P., & Garcia-Rea, E. A. (2012). Lifestyle coaching's effect on 6-month follow-up in recently homeless substance dependent veterans: A randomized study. *Psychiatric Rehabilitation Journal, 35*(5), 396-402.

96. Douglas-Siegel, J. A., & Ryan, J. P. (2013). The effect of recovery coaches for substance-involved mothers in child welfare: Impact on juvenile delinquency. *Journal of Substance Abuse Treatment, 45*(4), 381-387.

97. Ryan, J. P., Choi, S., Hong, J. S., Hernandez, P., & Larrison, C. R. (2008). Recovery coaches and substance exposed births: An experiment in child welfare. *Child Abuse & Neglect, 32*(11), 1072-1079.

98. Ryan, J. P., Marsh, J. C., Testa, M. F., & Louderman, R. (2006). Integrating substance abuse treatment and child welfare services: Findings from the Illinois alcohol and other drug abuse waiver demonstration. *Social Work Research, 30*(2), 95-107.

99. Jason, L. A., Olson, B. D., Ferrari, J. R., & Lo Sasso, A. T. (2006). Communal housing settings enhance substance abuse recovery. *American Journal of Public Health, 96*(10), 1727-1729.

100. Lo Sasso, A. T., Byro, E., Jason, L. A., Ferrari, J. R., & Olson, B. (2012). Benefits and costs associated with mutual-help community-based recovery homes: The Oxford House model. *Evaluation and Program Planning, 35*(1), 47-53.

101. Bergman, B. G., Hoeppner, B. B., Nelson, L. M., Slaymaker, V., & Kelly, J. F. (2015). The effects of continuing care on emerging adult outcomes following residential addiction treatment. *Drug and Alcohol Dependence, 153*, 207-214.

102. Groh, D. R., Jason, L. A., Ferrari, J. R., & Davis, M. I. (2009). Oxford House and Alcoholics Anonymous: The impact of two mutual-help models on abstinence. *Journal of Groups in Addiction and Recovery, 4*(1-2), 23-31.

103. Polcin, D. L., & Henderson, D. M. (2008). A clean and sober place to live: Philosophy, structure, and purported therapeutic factors in sober living houses. *Journal of Psychoactive Drugs, 40*(2), 153-159.

104. Polcin, D. L., Korcha, R., Bond, J., & Galloway, G. (2010a). Eighteen-month outcomes for clients receiving combined outpatient treatment and sober living houses. *Journal of Substance Use, 15*(5), 352-366.

105. Polcin, D. L., Korcha, R. A., Bond, J., & Galloway, G. (2010b). Sober living houses for alcohol and drug dependence: 18-month outcomes. *Journal of Substance Abuse Treatment, 38*(4), 356-365.

106. Dennis, M. L., & Scott, C. K. (2012). Four-year outcomes from the early re-intervention (ERI) experiment using recovery management checkups (RMCs). *Drug and Alcohol Dependence, 121*(1-2), 10-17.

107. McKay, J. R., Van Horn, D., Oslin, D. W., Ivey, M., Drapkin, M. L., Coviello, D. M., . . . Lynch, K. G. (2011). Extended telephone-based continuing care for alcohol dependence: 24-month outcomes and subgroup analyses. *Addiction, 106*(10), 1760-1769.

108. Stout, R. L., Rubin, A., Zwick, W., Zywiak, W., & Bellino, L. (1999). Optimizing the cost-effectiveness of alcohol treatment: A rationale for extended case monitoring. *Addictive Behaviors, 24*(1), 17-35.

109. Scott, C. K., & Dennis, M. L. (2003). *Recovery management checkups: An early re-intervention model.* Chicago, IL: Chestnut Health Systems.

110. Dennis, M., Scott, C. K., & Funk, R. (2003). An experimental evaluation of recovery management checkups (RMC) for people with chronic substance use disorders. *Evaluation and Program Planning, 26*(3), 339-352.

111. Rush, B. R., Dennis, M. L., Scott, C. K., Castel, S., & Funk, R. R. (2008). The interaction of co-occurring mental disorders and recovery management checkups on substance abuse treatment participation and recovery. *Evaluation Review, 32*(1), 7-38.

112. Scott, C. K., & Dennis, M. L. (2012). The first 90 days following release from jail: Findings from the Recovery Management Checkups for Women Offenders (RMCWO) experiment. *Drug and Alcohol Dependence, 125*(1-2), 110-118.

113. McCollister, K. E., French, M. T., Freitas, D. M., Dennis, M. L., Scott, C. K., & Funk, R. R. (2013). Cost-effectiveness analysis of recovery management checkups (RMC) for adults with chronic substance use disorders: Evidence from a 4-year randomized trial. *Addiction, 108*(12), 2166-2174.

114. Hilton, M. E., Maisto, S. A., Conigliaro, J., McNiel, M., Kraemer, K., Kelley, M. E., . . . Savetsky, J. (2001). Improving alcoholism treatment across the spectrum of services. *Alcoholism: Clinical and Experimental Research, 25*(1), 128-135.

115. McKay, J. R., Lynch, K. G., Shepard, D. S., Ratichek, S., Morrison, R., Koppenhaver, J., & Pettinati, H. M. (2004). The effectiveness of telephone-based continuing care in the clinical management of alcohol and cocaine use disorders: 12-month outcomes. *Journal of Consulting and Clinical Psychology, 72*(6), 967-979.

116. McKay, J. R., Lynch, K. G., Shepard, D. S., & Pettinati, H. M. (2005). The effectiveness of telephone-based continuing care for alcohol and cocaine dependence: 24-month outcomes. *Archives of General Psychiatry, 62*(2), 199-207.

117. McKay, J. R., Van Horn, D. H., Oslin, D. W., Lynch, K. G., Ivey, M., Ward, K., . . . Coviello, D. M. (2010). A randomized trial of extended telephone-based continuing care for alcohol dependence: Within-treatment substance use outcomes. *Journal of Consulting and Clinical Psychology, 78*(6), 912-923.

118. White, W. L. (2009). *Peer-based addiction recovery support: History, theory, practice, and scientific evaluation.* Chicago, IL: Great Lakes Addiction Technology Transfer Center and Philadelphia Department of Behavioral Health and Mental Retardation Services.

119. Haberle, B. J., Conway, S., Valentine, P., Evans, A. C., White, W. L., & Davidson, L. (2014). The recovery community center: A new model for volunteer peer support to promote recovery. *Journal of Groups in Addiction & Recovery, 9*(3), 257-270.

120. Cleveland, H. H., & Wiebe, R. P. (2003). The moderation of adolescent–to–peer similarity in tobacco and alcohol use by school levels of substance use. *Child Development, 74*(1), 279-291.

121. Spear, S. F., & Skala, S. Y. (1995). Posttreatment services for chemically dependent adolescents. In E. Rahdert & D. Czechowicz (Eds.), *Adolescent drug abuse: Clinical assessment and therapeutic interventions (NIDA Research Monograph 156).* (Vol. 156, pp. 341-364). Rockville, MD: U.S. Department of Health and Human Services, National Institute on Drug Abuse.

122. Finch, A. J., Moberg, D. P., & Krupp, A. L. (2014). Continuing care in high schools: A descriptive study of recovery high school programs. *Journal of Child and Adolescent Substance Abuse, 23*(2), 116-129.

123. Association of Recovery Schools. (n.d.). Accreditation. Retrieved from http://www.recoveryschools.org/accreditation. Accessed on April 11, 2016.

124. Moberg, D. P., & Finch, A. J. (2008). Recovery high schools: A descriptive study of school programs and students. *Journal of Groups in Addiction & Recovery, 2*(2-4), 128-161.

125. Lanham, C. C., & Tirado, J. A. (2011). Lessons in sobriety: An exploratory study of graduate outcomes at a recovery high school. *Journal of Groups in Addiction & Recovery, 6*(3), 245-263.

126. Laudet, A., Harris, K., Kimball, T., Winters, K. C., & Moberg, D. P. (2014). Collegiate recovery communities programs: What do we know and what do we need to know? *Journal of Social Work Practice in the Addictions, 14*(1), 84-100.

127. Laudet, A. B., Harris, K., Kimball, T., Winters, K. C., & Moberg, D. P. (2015). Characteristics of students participating in collegiate recovery programs: A national survey. *Journal of Substance Abuse Treatment, 51*, 38-46.

128. Cleveland, H. H., Harris, K. S., Baker, A. K., Herbert, R., & Dean, L. R. (2007). Characteristics of a collegiate recovery community: Maintaining recovery in an abstinence-hostile environment. *Journal of Substance Abuse Treatment, 33*(1), 13-23.

129. Harris, K. S., Baker, A. K., Kimball, T. G., & Shumway, S. T. (2008). Achieving systems-based sustained recovery: A comprehensive model for collegiate recovery communities. *Journal of Groups in Addiction & Recovery, 2*(2-4), 220-237.

130. Laudet, A. B., & White, W. L. (2008). Recovery capital as prospective predictor of sustained recovery, life satisfaction, and stress among former poly-substance users. *Substance Use and Misuse, 43*(1), 27-54.

131. Dickard, N., Downs, T., & Cavanaugh, D. (2011). *Recovery/relapse prevention in educational settings for youth with substance use & co-occurring mental health disorders: 2010 consultative sessions report.* Washington, DC: U.S. Department of Education, Office of Safe and Drug-Free Schools.

132. Dennis, M. L., Scott, C. K., Funk, R. R., & Nicholson, L. (2015). A pilot study to examine the feasibility and potential effectiveness of using smartphones to provide recovery support for adolescents. *Substance Abuse, 36*(4), 486-492.

133. Elison, S., Humphreys, L., Ward, J., & Davies, G. (2014). A pilot outcomes evaluation for computer assisted therapy for substance misuse—An evaluation of Breaking Free Online. *Journal of Substance Use, 19*(4), 313-318.

CHAPTER 6.
HEALTH CARE SYSTEMS AND SUBSTANCE USE DISORDERS

Chapter 6 Preview

Services for the prevention and treatment of substance misuse and substance use disorders have traditionally been delivered separately from other mental health and general health care services. Because substance misuse has traditionally been seen as a social or criminal problem, prevention services were not typically considered a responsibility of health care systems[i]; and people needing care for substance use disorders have had access to only a limited range of treatment options that were generally not covered by insurance. Effective integration of prevention, treatment, and recovery services across health care systems is key to addressing substance misuse and its consequences and it represents the most promising way to improve access to and quality of treatment. Recent health care reform laws, as well as a wide range of other trends in the health care landscape, are facilitating greater integration to better serve individual and public health, reduce health disparities, and reduce costs to society.

> **KEY TERMS**
>
> **Integration.** The systematic coordination of general and behavioral health care. Integrating services for primary care, mental health, and substance use-related problems together produces the best outcomes and provides the most effective approach for supporting whole-person health and wellness.[3]

This chapter describes the key components of health care systems; historical reasons substance use and its consequences have been addressed separately from other health problems; the key role that health care systems can play in providing prevention, treatment, and recovery support services (RSS) for substance use disorders; and the recent developments that are leading to improved integration of substance use-related care with the rest of medicine. This chapter also describes the challenges to effective integration, as well as promising trends, such as in health information technology (health IT) that will facilitate it. Because these changes are still underway, much

---

i The World Health Organization defines a health care system as (1) all the activities whose primary purpose is to promote, restore, and/or maintain health, and (2) the people, institutions, and resources, arranged together in accordance with established policies, to improve the health of the population they serve.[1] Health care systems may provide a wide range of clinical services, from primary through subspecialty care and be delivered in offices, clinics, and hospitals. They can be run by private, government, non-profit, or for-profit agencies and organizations.

HEALTH CARE SYSTEMS

of the relevant research is still formative and descriptive; information presented in this chapter often derives from reports and descriptive papers.

KEY FINDINGS*

- Well-supported scientific evidence shows that the traditional separation of substance use disorder treatment and mental health services from mainstream health care has created obstacles to successful care coordination. Efforts are needed to support integrating screening, assessments, interventions, use of medications, and care coordination between general health systems and specialty substance use disorder treatment programs or services.

- Supported scientific evidence indicates that closer integration of substance use-related services in mainstream health care systems will have value to both systems. Substance use disorders are medical conditions and their treatment has impacts on and is impacted by other mental and physical health conditions. Integration can help address health disparities, reduce health care costs for both patients and family members, and improve general health outcomes.

- Supported scientific evidence indicates that individuals with substance use disorders often access the health care system for reasons other than their substance use disorder. Many do not seek specialty treatment but they are over-represented in many general health care settings.

- Promising scientific evidence suggests that integrating care for substance use disorders into mainstream health care can increase the quality, effectiveness, and efficiency of health care. Many of the health home and chronic care model practices now used by mainstream health care to manage other diseases could be extended to include the management of substance use disorders.

- Insurance coverage for substance use disorder services is becoming more robust as a result of the Paul Wellstone and Pete Domenici Mental Health Parity and Addiction Equity Act (MHPAEA) and the Affordable Care Act. The Affordable Care Act also requires non-grandfathered individual and small group market plans to cover services to prevent and treat substance use disorders.

- Health care delivery organizations, such as health homes and accountable care organizations (ACOs), are being developed to better integrate care. The roles of existing care delivery organizations, such as community health centers, are also being expanded to meet the demands of integrated care for substance use disorder prevention, treatment, and recovery.

- Use of Health IT is expanding to support greater communication and collaboration among providers, fostering better integrated and collaborative care, while at the same time protecting patient privacy. It also has the potential for expanding access to care, extending the workforce, improving care coordination, reaching individuals who are resistant to engaging in traditional treatment settings, and providing outcomes and recovery monitoring.

- Supported evidence indicates that one fundamental way to address racial and ethnic disparities in health care is to increase the number of people who have health insurance coverage.

- Well-supported evidence shows that the current substance use disorder workforce does not have the capacity to meet the existing need for integrated health care, and the current general health care workforce is undertrained to deal with substance use-related problems. Health care now requires a new, larger, more diverse workforce with the skills to prevent, identify, and treat substance use disorders, providing "personalized care" through integrated care delivery.

*The Centers for Disease Control and Prevention (CDC) summarizes strength of evidence as: "Well-supported": when evidence is derived from multiple controlled trials or large-scale population studies; "Supported": when evidence is derived from rigorous but fewer or smaller trials; and "Promising": when evidence is derived from a practical or clinical sense and is widely practiced.[5]

Key Components of Health Care Systems

In 2015, 20.8 million Americans had a substance use disorder. As discussed in <u>Chapter 1 - Introduction and Overview</u>, these disorders vary in intensity and may respond to different intensities of intervention. Diverse health care systems have many roles to play in addressing our nation's substance misuse and substance use disorder problems, including:

- Screening for substance misuse and substance use disorders;
- Delivering prevention interventions to prevent substance misuse and related health consequences;
- Early intervention to prevent escalation of misuse to a substance use disorder;
- Engaging patients with substance use disorders into treatment;
- Treating substance use disorders of all levels of severity;
- Coordinating care across both health care systems and social services systems including criminal justice, housing and employment support, and child welfare;
- Linking patients to RSS; and
- Long-term monitoring and follow-up.

There is a great diversity of health care systems across the United States, with varying levels of integration across health care settings and wide-ranging workforces that incorporate diverse structural and financing models and leverage different levels of technology.

Health Care Settings

Health care systems are made up of diverse health care organizations ranging from primary care, specialty substance use disorder treatment (including residential and outpatient settings), mental health care, infectious disease clinics, school clinics, community health centers, hospitals, emergency departments, and others.

It is known that most people with substance use disorders do not seek treatment on their own, many because they do not believe they need it or they are not ready for it, and others because they are not aware that treatment exists or how to access it. But individuals with substance use disorders often do access the health care system for other reasons, including acute health problems like illness, injury, or overdose, as well as chronic health conditions such as HIV/AIDS, heart disease, or depression. Thus, screening for substance misuse and substance use disorders in diverse health care settings is the first step to identifying substance use problems and engaging patients in the appropriate level of care.

Mild substance use disorders may respond to brief counseling sessions in primary care, while severe substance use disorders are often chronic conditions requiring substance use disorder treatment like specialty residential or intensive outpatient treatment as well as long-term management through primary care. A wide range of health care settings is needed to effectively meet the diverse needs of patients.

Workforce

Just as a diversity of health care settings is needed to meet the needs of patients, a diversity of health care professionals is also critical. Health care services can be delivered by a wide-range of providers including doctors, nurses, nurse practitioners, psychologists, licensed counselors, care managers, social workers, health educators, peer workers, and others. With limited resources for prevention and treatment, matching patients to the appropriate level of care, delivered by the appropriate level of provider, is crucial for extending those resources to reach the most patients possible.

Structural and Financing Models

A range of promising health care structures and financing models are currently being explored for integrating general health care and substance use disorder treatment within health care systems, as well as integrating the substance use disorder treatment system with the overall health care system. As part of ongoing health reform efforts, both federal and state governments are investing in models and innovations ranging from health homes and ACOs, to managed care and Coordinated Care Organizations (CCOs), to pay-for-performance and shared-savings models. These new models are developing and testing strategies for effectively and sustainably financing high-quality care that integrates behavioral health and general health care.

> **FOR MORE ON THIS TOPIC**
>
> See the sections on *"Health Homes"* and *"Accountable Care Organizations"* later in this chapter.

Technology Integration

Technology can play a key role in supporting these integrated care models. Electronic health records (EHRs), telehealth, health information exchanges (HIE), patient registries, mobile applications, Web-based tools, and other innovative technologies have the potential to extend the reach of the workforce; support quality measurement and improvement initiatives to drive a learning health care system; electronically deliver prevention, treatment, and recovery interventions; efficiently monitor patients; identify population health trends and threats; and engage patients who are hesitant to participate in formal care.

> **KEY TERMS**
>
> **Learning Health Care System.** As described by the Institute of Medicine (IOM), a learning health care system is "designed to generate and apply the best evidence for the collaborative healthcare choices of each patient and provider; to drive the process of discovery as a natural outgrowth of patient care; and to ensure innovation, quality, safety, and value in health care."[4]

The Promise of Integration

When health care is not well integrated and coordinated across systems, too many patients fall through the cracks, leading to missed opportunities for prevention or early intervention, ineffective referrals, incomplete treatment, high rates of hospital and emergency department readmissions, and individual tragedies that could have been prevented. For example, a recent study found that doctors continue to prescribe opioids for 91 percent of patients who suffered a non-fatal overdose, with 63 percent of those patients continuing to receive high doses; 17 percent of these patients overdosed again within 2 years.[6] Effective coordination between emergency departments and primary care providers can help to prevent these tragedies.

Other tragedies occur when patients complete treatment and the health care system fails to provide adequate follow-up and coordination of the wrap-around services or recovery supports necessary to help them maintain their recovery, leading to relapse. The risk for overdose is particularly high after a period of abstinence, due to reduced tolerance—patients no longer know what a safe dose is for them—and this all too often results in overdose deaths. This is a common story when patients are released from prison without a coordinated plan for continuing treatment in the community. One study from the Washington State Department of Corrections found that during the first 2 weeks after release, the risk of death among former inmates was 12.7 times higher than among state residents of the same age, sex, and race. Health care systems play a key role in providing the coordination necessary to avert these tragic outcomes.[7]

> **KEY TERMS**
>
> **Wrap-Around Services.** Wrap-around services are non-clinical services that facilitate patient engagement and retention in treatment as well as their ongoing recovery. This can include services to address patient needs related to transportation, employment, childcare, housing, and legal and financial problems, among others.

Substance Use Disorder Services Have Traditionally Been Separate From Mental Health and General Health Care

The separation of the treatment systems for substance use disorders, mental illness, and general health care has historical roots.[8-10] For example, Alcoholics Anonymous (AA) was founded in 1935 in part because mainstream psychiatric and general medical providers did not attend to substance use disorders. If treated at all, alcoholism was most often treated in asylums, separate from the rest of health care. The separation of substance use disorder treatment and general health care was further influenced by social and political trends of the 1970s. At that time, substance misuse and addiction were generally viewed as social problems best dealt with through civil and criminal justice interventions such as involuntary commitment to psychiatric hospitals, prison-run "narcotic farms," or other forms of confinement.[11] However, when many college students and returning Vietnam veterans were misusing alcohol, using drugs, and/or becoming addicted to illicit substances, high numbers of arrests and other forms of punishment became politically and economically infeasible. At this time, there was a major push to significantly expand substance misuse prevention and treatment services.

Despite the compelling national need for treatment, the existing health care system was neither trained to care for, nor especially eager to accept, patients with substance use disorders. For these reasons, new substance use disorder treatment programs were created, ultimately expanding to programs in more than 14,000 locations across the United States. This meant that with the exception of withdrawal management in hospitals (detoxification), virtually all substance use disorder treatment was delivered by programs that were geographically, financially, culturally, and organizationally separate from mainstream health care.

> **FOR MORE ON THIS TOPIC**
>
> See Chapter 4 - *Early Intervention, Treatment, and Management of Substance Use Disorders.*

Even though these programs were separate from the rest of health care, these new delivery sites were a critical step toward better addressing the growing problems related to substance misuse and substance use disorders. One positive consequence was the initial development of effective and inexpensive behavioral change strategies rarely used in the treatment of other chronic illnesses. However, the separation of substance use disorder treatment from general health care also created unintended and enduring impediments to the quality and range of care options available to patients in both systems. For example, it tended to reinforce the notion that substance use disorders were different from other medical conditions. Despite numerous research studies documenting high prevalence rates of substance use disorders among patients in emergency departments, hospitals, and general medical care settings, mainstream health care generally failed to recognize or address substance use-related health problems.[8,12-15]

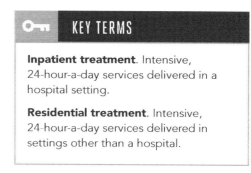

KEY TERMS

Inpatient treatment. Intensive, 24-hour-a-day services delivered in a hospital setting.

Residential treatment. Intensive, 24-hour-a-day services delivered in settings other than a hospital.

The continued separation of substance use and general health care services has been costly, often harmful, and for some individuals even fatal. A recent study of world health settings showed that the presence of a substance use disorder often doubles the odds that a person will develop another chronic and costly medical illness, such as arthritis, chronic pain, heart disease, stroke, hypertension, diabetes, or asthma.[16] Yet despite the impact of substance use on physical health, few medical, nursing, dental, or pharmacy schools teach their students how to identify, prevent, and treat substance use disorders;[17-19] and, until recently, few insurers offered comparable reimbursement for substance use disorder treatment services.[20-23]

Even now, there are health care professionals who continue to be hesitant to provide patients with medication-assisted treatment (MAT), especially maintenance medications (methadone and buprenorphine) for opioid use disorders, because of deeply ingrained but erroneous misconceptions about these treatments, such as the idea that they "substitute one addiction for another."[24] This has hindered the adoption of these effective medications even by substance use disorder treatment facilities; and when they are used by substance use disorder treatment providers, they are often prescribed at insufficient doses, for insufficient durations, contributing to treatment failure and reinforcing a belief that they are not effective.[25,26] In fact, ample research shows that, when used correctly, MAT can reduce or eliminate illicit drug use and associated criminality and infectious disease transmission and restore patients to healthy functioning.[25,27,28]

A Growing Impetus for Integration

An integrated system of prevention, early intervention, treatment, and recovery that can address the full spectrum of substance use-related health problems is a logical and necessary shift that our society must make to prevent substance misuse and its consequences and meet the needs of individuals with substance use disorders. Providing services to people with mild and moderate substance use disorders—by far the largest proportion of all those diagnosed—in general health care settings will likely lessen the need for intensive and costly substance

FOR MORE ON THIS TOPIC

See Chapter 4 - *Early Intervention, Treatment, and Management of Substance Use Disorders.*

use disorder treatment services later, even though specialty care is still essential for people with serious substance use disorders, just as it is for patients with other severe diseases and conditions.

Beginning in the 1990s, a number of events converged to lay the foundation for integrated care. First, a number of IOM reports and other major articles established that substance use disorders are inherently health conditions that require a collaboration between general health care settings and specialty care[29] to improve treatment[30] and reduce gaps in quality for health care broadly[31] and for mental disorders and substance use disorders in particular.[29,32] This was followed, in more recent years, by legislation that aims to transform the way services are provided and to facilitate access to prevention and treatment services through expanded insurance coverage. The Paul Wellstone and Pete Domenici Mental Health Parity and Addiction Equity Act of 2008 (MHPAEA) requires the financial requirements and treatment limitations imposed by most health plans and insurers for substance use disorders be no more restrictive than the financial requirements and treatment limitations they impose for medical and surgical conditions.

Further, the Affordable Care Act, passed in 2010, requires that non-grandfathered health care plans offered in the individual and small group markets both inside and outside insurance exchanges provide coverage for a comprehensive list of 10 categories of items and services, known as "essential health benefits." One of these essential health benefit categories is mental health and substance use disorder services, including behavioral health treatment. This requirement represents a significant change in the way many health insurers respond to these disorders. The Affordable Care Act also reaffirmed MHPAEA by requiring that mental health and substance use disorder benefits covered by plans offered through the exchanges be offered consistent with the parity requirements under MHPAEA.

Medicaid Expansion under the Affordable Care Act

To more broadly cover uninsured individuals, the Affordable Care Act includes a provision that allows states to expand Medicaid coverage. In those states ("Medicaid expansion states"), individuals in households with incomes below 138 percent of the federal poverty level are eligible for Medicaid. Benefits include mental health and substance use disorder treatment services with coverage equivalent to that of general health care services.

Medicaid expansion is a key lever for expanding access to substance use treatment because many of the most vulnerable individuals with substance use disorders have incomes below 138 percent of the federal poverty level. As of fall 2015, an estimated 3 million adults have incomes that make them eligible for Medicaid under the Affordable Care Act but live in a state that has declined to expand Medicaid eligibility as permitted under the new law.[36,37]

A major goal of the Affordable Care Act is to expand insurance coverage and reduce the number of uninsured individuals.[33] As of March 2016, more than 20 million previously uninsured individuals (including children on parents' plans) had new benefits under the Affordable Care Act.[34] These enrollment figures include those who were previously uninsured, as well as 1 million who previously had employer-based coverage and 3 million who previously had non-group and other insurance coverage.[33] Individuals with substance use disorders are overrepresented in the newly insured population (including children now on parents' plans), because they were previously disproportionately uninsured, young adults without dependent children. They now are eligible for coverage under the Affordable Care Act, which will enable them to receive substance use disorder prevention, treatment, and RSS.[35]

Most recently, Congress passed the Protecting Access to Medicare Act, which, in addition to its Medicare provisions, funds pilot programs to increase access to, and Medicaid payment for, community mental health and substance use disorder treatment services. This is an important opportunity for integration.

Other changes, described later in this chapter, are also helping to create momentum for integration. These include new or improved organizational structures, such as medical homes, health homes, and ACOs; improved health IT, such as EHRs; clinical approaches, such as new substance use disorder treatment medications that can be prescribed in primary care settings; and effective approaches to identifying and preventing substance misuse problems. In addition, organizations including the American College of Physicians and the American Society of Addiction Medicine (ASAM) now recommend integration of substance use-related and mental health services with primary care.[38] Of historical note, although the World Health Organization and the American Medical Association have long identified alcohol and drug use disorders as medical conditions, it was only in 2016 that addiction medicine was formally recognized as a new subspecialty by the American Board of Medical Specialties under the American Board of Preventive Medicine.

Figure 6.1 summarizes a few of the key changes that are occurring as substance use disorder treatment services are integrated into mainstream health care.

Figure 6.1: Substance Use Disorders Services: Past and Future

Past	Future
Substance use mainly ignored in primary care	Substance use screened and monitored in primary care
Focus on the most severe problems	Addresses full spectrum of problems
Paper charts: little contact between specialty substance use disorders and health care	EHR, clinical coordination, patient portals, health IT treatment options that focus on coordination of care
Limited use of health IT	Leveraging technologies including patient portals, HIEs, technology delivered treatments
Little focus on physical health issues	Addresses medical problems with focus on whole person wellness
Medications seldom available	Medications readily available
Separate oversight structures and reporting	Performance and outcomes measurement, ongoing quality improvement
12-step programs	12-step and other RSS, social network innovations

Health care professionals are being encouraged to offer prevention advice, screen patients for substance misuse and substance use disorders, and provide early interventions in the form of motivational approaches, when appropriate.[39,40]

Primary care has a central role in this process, because it is the site for most preventive and ongoing clinical care for patients—the patient's anchor in the health care system. For example, primary care settings can serve as a conduit to help patients engage in and maintain recovery. Also, approaches such as screening, brief intervention, and referral to treatment (SBIRT) provide primary care providers with tools for addressing patients' substance misuse. Based upon the strength of the evidence for their effectiveness, the U.S. Preventive Services Task Force (USPSTF) has recommended alcohol screening and brief behavioral counseling interventions for adults in primary care and given the supporting evidence for these services a "B" grade. This is significant because under the Affordable Care Act, preventive services given a grade of A or B by the USPSTF must be covered by most health plans without cost-sharing.[41-43] The USPSTF recommendation supports the expectation that primary care providers will soon routinely screen adults of all ages for unhealthy alcohol use as they now do for blood pressure and weight. Relatedly, the National Commission on Prevention Priorities of the Partnership for Prevention ranks primary care-based interventions to reduce alcohol misuse among the most valuable clinical preventive services.[44,45]

> **FOR MORE ON THIS TOPIC**
>
> See Chapter 4 - *Early Intervention, Treatment, and Management of Substance Use Disorders.*

The literature on the effectiveness of drug-focused brief intervention in primary care and emergency departments is less clear, with some studies finding no improvements among those receiving brief interventions.[46,47] However, at least one study found significant reductions in subsequent drug use.[48] Trials evaluating different types of screening and brief interventions for drug use in diverse settings with a range of patient groups are lacking. The USPSTF's current rating for illicit drug screening and brief intervention remains "I" for insufficient evidence to support its use as a preventive service. However, assessment for drug use is recommended under numerous circumstances, including treating any condition for which drug use might interfere with the treatment; considering potential interactions with prescribed medications; supporting integration of behavioral health care; and monitoring patient risk when prescribing opioid pain medications or sedatives/tranquilizers.

It is also important to emphasize that brief primary care-based interventions by themselves are likely not sufficient to address severe substance use disorders. However, primary care providers can use other interventions with this population, including providing MAT, providing more robust monitoring and patient education,[49,50] and importantly, referring individuals to specialty substance use disorder treatment. Effective referral arrangements that include motivating patients to accept the referral are critical elements to encourage individuals to engage in treatment for their substance use disorder.

Reasons Why Integrating Substance Use Disorder Services and Mainstream Health Care Is Necessary

A number of strong arguments underpin the growing momentum to integrate substance use disorder services and mainstream health care. The main argument is that substance use disorders are medical conditions like any other—the overarching theme of much of this *Report*. Recognition of that fact means it no longer makes sense to keep substance use disorders segregated from other health issues. A number of other realities support the need for integration:[63]

- Substance use, mental disorders, and other general medical conditions are often interconnected;
- Integration has the potential to reduce health disparities;
- Delivering substance use disorder services in mainstream health care can be cost-effective and may reduce intake/treatment wait times at substance use disorder treatment facilities; and
- Integration can lead to improved health outcomes through better care coordination.

Health Systems and Opioids

Physician prescribing patterns, patient drug diversion (selling, sharing, or using medications prescribed for another person), and doctor shopping behaviors have all contributed to the ongoing opioid overdose epidemic.[51] For example, evidence indicates that chronic pain patients with substance use disorders are prescribed opioids more often than other individuals with chronic pain, with the trend increasing over time.[52] Also, a study in two health systems found opioid prescription rates for older persons, particularly older women,[53] to be higher over time than for other individuals with long-term chronic pain.

In March 2015, the U.S. Department of Health and Human Services (HHS) made addressing the opioid misuse crisis a high priority, announcing a national opioid initiative focused on three priority areas: (1) providing training and educational resources, including updated prescriber guidelines, to assist health professionals in making informed prescribing decisions; (2) increasing use of the opioid overdose reversal drug naloxone; and (3) expanding the use of MAT. Since then, HHS has initiated many efforts to help reduce prescription opioid misuse and use disorders. Improving prescribing practices is one of these important efforts.[54] In March 2016, the CDC released the *Guideline for Prescribing Opioids for Chronic Pain*, which provides recommendations about the appropriate prescribing of opioid pain relievers and other treatment options to improve pain management and patient safety.[55] The guideline is not intended to regulate necessary and appropriate opioid prescribing. Rather, the guideline is meant to inform health care professionals about some of the consequences of treatment with opioids for chronic pain and to consider, when appropriate, tapering and changing prescribing practices, as well as considering alternative pain therapies. The same month, HHS also released the National Pain Strategy, which outlines the federal government's first coordinated plan for addressing chronic pain that affects so many Americans.[56] The goals of the National Pain Strategy will be achieved through a broad effort that includes improved pain care and safer prescribing practices, such as those recommended by the CDC Guideline.

The National Heroin Task Force, which consisted of law enforcement, doctors, public health officials, and education experts, was convened to develop strategies to confront the heroin problem and decrease the escalating overdose epidemic and death rate.[57] In 2015, the Task Force developed a report outlining the steps being taking to address the opioid problem. This included a multifaceted strategy of enforcement and prevention efforts, as well as increased access to substance use disorder treatment and recovery services. Although only about 4 percent of those who misuse prescription opioids transition to using heroin, concern is growing that tightening restrictions on opioid prescribing could potentially have unintended consequences resulting in new populations using heroin.[58] The Task Force states that "evidence shows that some people who misuse opioid medications migrate to heroin because heroin is more accessible and less costly than prescription opioids."[59] In fact, nearly 80 percent of recent heroin initiates reported that they began their opioid use through the nonmedical use of prescription opioid medications."[58]

The concern about opioid overdoses has also triggered efforts by health systems to increase access to naloxone, an opioid antagonist that prevents overdose fatalities by rapidly restoring normal respiration to a person whose breathing has slowed or stopped as a result of opioid use. Since 1996, community-based organizations in many states have implemented overdose education and naloxone distribution programs for people who use heroin or misuse pharmaceutical opioids and efforts are underway to expand access to naloxone to patients who are prescribed opioids for pain. Expanded access to naloxone through large health systems could prevent overdose fatalities in broad populations of patients, including patients who may experience accidental overdose from misusing their medications. The Substance Abuse and Mental Health Services Administration (SAMHSA) has developed an easy-to-use toolkit to be distributed with naloxone.[60] Prior research has suggested the potential to translate overdose education and naloxone distribution into routine primary care practice[61] and examination of the perspectives of primary care providers on this practice revealed knowledge gaps about naloxone but also a willingness to follow standardized naloxone prescribing practices when they emerge.[62]

> **FOR MORE ON THIS TOPIC**
>
> See Chapter 4 - *Early Intervention, Treatment, and Management of Substance Use Disorders.*

Substance Use Disorders, Mental Disorders, and Other Medical Conditions Are Interconnected

Many individuals who come to mainstream health care settings, such as primary care, obstetrics and gynecology, emergency departments, and hospitals, also have a substance use disorder. In a study within one health plan, one third of the most common and costly medical conditions were markedly more prevalent among patients with substance use disorders than they were among similar health system members who did not have a substance use disorder.[64] Similarly, many individuals who present at specialty substance use disorder treatment programs have other medical conditions,[65,66] including hypertension, HIV/AIDS, coronary artery disease, hepatitis, chronic liver disease, and psychiatric disorders.[67]

Because substance use complicates many other medical conditions, early identification and management of substance misuse or use disorders presents an important opportunity to improve health outcomes and reduce health care costs.[68] Research shows that primary care patients with mild or moderate substance use have higher rates of other medical problems, including injury, hypertension, and psychiatric disorders, as well as higher costs.[69] For example, cocaine use is associated with cardiovascular complications[67,70,71] and neurological and psychiatric disorders,[67,71] and long-term marijuana use has been associated with chronic bronchitis and cardiovascular problems.[72-74] Alcohol misuse is associated with liver and pancreatic diseases; hypertension; reproductive system disorders; trauma; stroke;[75] and cancers of the oral cavity, esophagus, larynx, pharynx, liver, colon, and rectum.[76,77] Even one drink per day may increase the risk of breast cancer.[67,76,78]

In addition to the health problems faced by individuals engaged in substance use mentioned above, substance use can adversely affect a developing fetus. In the United States, fetal alcohol spectrum disorders (FASD) remain highly prevalent and problematic, even though they are preventable.[79] A study of children in public and private schools in a Midwestern community calculated rates of FASD to be as high as 6 to 9 per 1,000.[80]

Opioid pain reliever use among pregnant women has also become a major concern due to neonatal abstinence syndrome (NAS), a treatable condition that newborns experience after exposure to drugs while in the mother's womb.[81] NAS may cause neurological excitability, gastrointestinal dysfunction, and autonomic dysfunction. Newborns with NAS are more likely than other babies to also have low birthweight and respiratory complications. The incidence of NAS has increased dramatically in the last decade along with increased opioid misuse.[82] In 2012, an estimated 21,732 infants were born with NAS, a five-fold increase since 2000. Moreover, in 2012, newborns with NAS stayed in the hospital an average of 16.9 days, more than eight times the number of days other newborns stay in the hospital (2.1 days).[83] These newborns with NAS cost hospitals an estimated $1.5 billion, and 81 percent of these costs were paid by state Medicaid programs.[83] These data suggest the need to develop and test measures to reduce newborn exposure to opioids. For women who are considering getting pregnant or are already pregnant, abstaining from all substances is recommended, since NAS is not exclusively caused by opioids.[84]

Adolescents with substance use disorders experience higher rates of other physical and mental illnesses, as well as diminished overall health and well-being.[85-88] Sexually transmitted infections and HIV/AIDS,[89] appetite changes and weight loss, dermatological problems, gastrointestinal problems, headaches,[86] insomnia and chronic fatigue,[90] and heart, lung, and abdominal abnormalities are only some of the problems that affect the health of young people who misuse alcohol and drugs.[87] A study of adolescents entering specialty substance use disorder treatment—as compared with age-matched adolescent patients without a substance use disorder—found higher rates of clinically diagnosed sinusitis, asthma, abdominal pain, sleep disorders, injuries and overdoses.[91]

In addition to the physical health problems described above, mental health problems are also over-represented among adolescents with substance use disorders,[92,93] particularly attention-deficit hyperactivity disorder,[94-98] conduct disorders,[99] anxiety disorders,[100] and mood disorders.[101-103] In addition, alcohol and drug use are associated with serious personal and social problems for users and for those around them including elevated rates of morbidity and mortality related to traffic crashes, intimate partner violence, risky sex, and unintentional injuries, including death from overdose.[104-110]

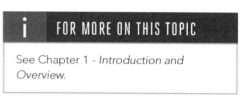

FOR MORE ON THIS TOPIC

See Chapter 1 - *Introduction and Overview.*

Integration Can Lead to Improved Health Outcomes through Better Care Coordination

Treatment of substance use disorders has historically been provided episodically, when a person experiences a crisis or a relapse occurs.[32] This is neither good quality nor efficient care, because severe substance use disorders are chronic health problems, similar to other health conditions and with similar outcomes.[12,111] Studies conducted over extended periods of time have found that annual primary care visits were associated with better outcomes and reduced health care costs following substance use disorder treatment,[112-115] but research on models of chronic care management is only beginning and thus far no consensus has emerged on the best approach.[116-119] These types of long-term studies will be more informative as the substance use disorder treatment, health care, and mental health systems become more integrated and as researchers build on disease management models that are effective for other medical conditions.

In addition to chronic care management for severely affected individuals, coordinating services for those with mild or moderate problems is also important. Studies of various methods for integrating substance use services and general medical care have typically shown beneficial outcomes.[66,120,121] The effectiveness of providing alcohol screening and brief counseling in primary care is supported by a robust evidence base,[122] and a growing literature is showing its benefits as a first tool in managing chronic health conditions that may arise from, or be exacerbated by, alcohol use.[123-125] Primary care-based alcohol use disorder case management involving pharmacotherapy and psychosocial support has been found to increase engagement in specialty substance use disorder treatment and to decrease heavy drinking.[126]

Care coordination is an essential part of quality in all health care. The Healthcare Effectiveness Data and Information Set (HEDIS), The Joint Commission, and organizations such as the National Committee for Quality Assurance emphasize coordination and accountability and the use of evidence-based care and performance indicators to establish and monitor quality and value. This approach to care delivery proceeds on the assumption that services for the range of substance use disorders should be fully integrated components of mainstream health care.

Quality and Performance Measurement and Accountability

Publicly available quality measurement information helps consumers, health care purchasers, and other groups make informed decisions when choosing services, providers, and care settings. Performance measurement has the dual purpose of accountability and quality improvement.

A 2015 IOM study on *Psychosocial Interventions for Mental and Substance Use Disorders* recommended that the substance use disorder field develop approaches to measure quality, similar to approaches used for other diseases. This includes the development of performance measures, use of health IT for standardized measurement, and utilization of these measures to support quality improvement.[127]

Measures have been proposed by a variety of organizations, including SAMHSA, as part of its 2013 National Behavioral Health Quality Framework; by the ASAM, as part of its development of standards of care for specialist addiction medicine physicians; by the Behavioral Health Steering Committee of the National Quality Forum; and by accrediting bodies such as The Joint Commission. Many measures are being tested by public and private health plans, though most have not been adopted widely for quality improvement and accountability. The single substance use measure included in HEDIS is "initiation and engagement of alcohol and other drug dependence treatment." Although the HEDIS measure is limited, it does provide health systems a beginning benchmark for tracking substance use disorders. A measure of care continuity after emergency department use for substance use disorders is in process.

Because substance use disorder treatment is currently not well integrated and services are often provided by multiple systems, it can be challenging to effectively measure treatment quality and related outcomes. The ability to track service delivery across these multiple environments will be critical for addressing this challenge. For example, community monitoring systems to assess risk and protection for adolescents are being developed.[128-130]

Pay-for-performance is an approach for improving quality and for incentivizing programs or health care professionals to produce particular outcomes (for example, treatment retention and treatment outcomes). It has been used more in general health care than in substance use disorder treatment. However, Delaware and Maine have experimented with it in their public substance use disorder treatment systems, and several studies have found improvement in retention and outcomes.[131,132] Potential concerns with pay-for-performance are that treatment programs may not accept the most severe patients and that methods of risk adjustment to compensate programs that accept those patients are not well-established. Although pay-for-performance is a promising approach, more research is needed to address these concerns.

A fundamental concept in care coordination between the health care, substance use disorder treatment, and mental health systems is that there should be "no wrong door."[133] This means that no matter where in the health care system the need for substance use disorder treatment is identified the patient will be effectively linked with appropriate services.

Several models of coordination have been described by researchers. In one such model, coordination ranges from referral agreements to co-located substance use disorder, mental health, and other health care services. Onsite programs had the highest rates of treatment engagement.[134] A recent meta-analysis concluded that integrated treatment of adolescent substance use disorders, along with mental disorders and medical care, produced better outcomes than when treatment was provided separately.[135] Other observational research has found that co-location of specialty substance use disorder treatment and mental health care is associated with better outcomes in adolescents.[93] SAMHSA and the Health Resources and Services Administration (HRSA) have also developed a model with six levels of coordination (Figure 6.2).

Figure 6.2: A Continuum of Collaboration between Health Care and Specialty Services

Coordinated Key Element: Communication		Co-located Key Element: Physical Proximity		Integrated Key Element: Practice Change	
LEVEL 1	LEVEL 2	LEVEL 3	LEVEL 4	LEVEL 5	LEVEL 6
Minimal Collaboration	Basic Collaboration at a Distance	Basic Collaboration Onsite	Close Collaboration Onsite with Some System Integration	Close Collaboration Approaching an Integrated Practice	Full Collaboration in a Transformed/ Merged Integrated Practice
Behavioral health, primary care, and other health care professionals work:					
In separate facilities, where they:	In separate facilities, where they:	In same facility not necessarily same offices, where they:	In same space within the same facility, where they:	In same space within the same facility (some shared space), where they:	In same space within the same facility, sharing all practice space, where they:
• Have separate systems • Communicate about cases only rarely and under compelling circumstances • Communicate, driven by provider need • May never meet in person • Have limited understanding of each other's roles	• Have separate systems • Communicate periodically about shared patients • Communicate, driven by specific patient issues • May meet as part of a larger community • Appreciate each other's roles as resources	• Have separate systems • Communicate regularly about shared patients, by phone or e-mail • Collaborate, driven by need for each other's services and more reliable referral • Meet occasionally to discuss cases due to close proximity • Feel part of a larger yet non-formal team	• Share some systems, like scheduling or medical records • Communicate in person as needed • Collaborate, driven by need for consultation and coordinated plans for difficult patients • Have regular face-to-face interactions about some patients • Have a basic understanding of roles and culture	• Actively seek system solutions together or develop work-a-rounds • Communicate frequently in person • Collaborate, driven by desire to be a member of the care team • Have regular team meetings to discuss overall patient care and specific patient issues • Have an in-depth understanding of roles and culture	• Have resolved most or all system issues, functioning as one integrated system • Communicate consistently at the system, team, and individual levels • Collaborate, driven by shared concept of team care • Have formal and informal meetings to support integrated model of care • Have roles and cultures that blur or blend

Source: Heath, et al., (2013).[136]

These models, as well as recovery-oriented systems of care, provide opportunities for substance use disorder services and mainstream health care to engage in various types of collaborative efforts to integrate their services at all stages: prevention, treatment, and recovery. Importantly, the models all emphasize the relationship between person-centered, high-quality care and fully integrated models. Innovative financing mechanisms now being explored also allow for formal arrangements to implement some of the models discussed above, including linking to off-site health professionals in specialty substance use disorder treatment settings (and vice versa) when locating multiple services at one site is not feasible.

Integration Can Help Address Health Disparities

Integrating substance use services with general health care (e.g., in community health centers) provides opportunities to address longstanding health disparities. Prevalence of substance misuse and substance use disorders differs by race and ethnicity, sex, age, sexual orientation, gender identity, and disability, and these factors are also associated with differing rates of access to both health care and substance use disorder treatment. These differences are often exacerbated by socioeconomic variables.[137,138] Some racial and ethnic groups experience disparities in entering and engaging in treatment. A study of a large health system found that Black or African American women but not Latina or Asian American women were less likely to attend substance use disorder treatment, after controlling for other factors; there were no ethnicity differences for men.[139]

In addition, an analysis of longitudinal data from the *National Epidemiologic Survey on Alcohol and Related Conditions* showed that individuals from most racial and ethnic groups were less likely to receive an alcohol intervention than were White individuals over a 3 year period.[140] Controlling for socioeconomic status and clinical conditions increased the disparity, and Hispanic or Latino individuals were the least likely to receive services. Differences within the various racial and ethnic groups by sex were not studied.

A fundamental way to address disparities is to increase the number of people who have health coverage. The Affordable Care Act provides several mechanisms that broaden access to coverage. As a result, more low-income individuals with substance use disorders have gained health coverage, changed their perceptions about being able to obtain treatment services if needed, and increased their access to treatment.[141] However, in states that have elected not to expand Medicaid, some low-income adults who need substance use disorder treatment, especially single childless adults, are unable to receive these services. Individuals whose incomes are too high to qualify for Medicaid but are not high enough to be eligible for qualified health plan premium tax credits also rarely have coverage for substance use disorder treatment.[142] As **Figure 6.3** shows, more Blacks or African Americans are in the coverage gap than other groups, and more Hispanics or Latinos are ineligible due to immigration status.[142] One study conducted by The Pew Charitable Trusts reported that 14 percent of the low-income adults who are newly eligible for Medicaid under the Affordable Care Act have drug and alcohol addictions, compared to 10 percent in the general population. Because the new Medicaid population includes large numbers of young, single men—a group at much higher risk for alcohol and drug misuse—Medicaid enrollees needing treatment could more than double, from 1.5 million prior to the 2014 Medicaid expansion to about 4 million in the next five years.[8,143,144]

HEALTH CARE SYSTEMS

Figure 6.3: Eligibility for Affordable Care Act Coverage Among the Nonelderly Uninsured by Race and Ethnicity, as of 2015

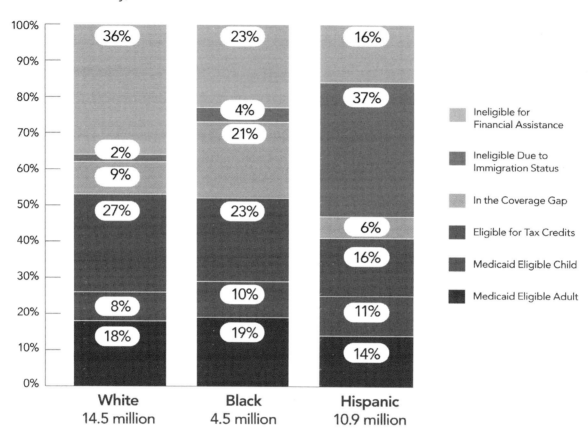

Notes: Totals may not sum to 100 percent due to rounding. Ineligible for Financial Assistance share includes those ineligible due to offer of employer sponsored insurance or income. Tax Credit Eligible share includes adults in MN and NY who are eligible for coverage through the Basic Health Plan.

Source: Kaiser Family Foundation analysis based on 2015 Medicaid eligibility levels and 2015 Current Population Survey.[142]

Another way to address disparities is to ensure that substance misuse prevention, interventions, treatments, and recovery services are tailored and relevant to the populations receiving them. Several interventions have been adapted explicitly to address differences in specific populations; they were either conducted within health care settings or are implementable in those settings. The list below provides examples of such programs that have been shown to be effective in diverse populations:

- An evidence-based prevention intervention focused on women who are at risk for an alcohol-exposed pregnancy because of risky drinking and not using contraception consistently and correctly.[145] The program has been adapted to serve American Indian women of the Oglala Sioux Tribe.[146] Implementation of this intervention in health care settings has high potential for improving outcomes.

> **i   FOR MORE ON THIS TOPIC**
>
> See Chapter 3 - Prevention Programs and Policies and Chapter 4 - Early Intervention, Treatment, and Management of Substance Use Disorders.

- A study of a computerized screening and brief intervention in both Spanish and English used in a public health center's obstetrics-gynecology department was shown to be feasible and accepted by patients.[147]
- A small trial of Latino heavy drinkers compared culturally adapted motivational interviewing to motivational interviewing that was not culturally adapted. The trial suggested stronger results for the culturally adapted program.[148]
- A study comparing rural and urban differences in screening for substance use disorders in mental health clinics did not find significant differences in screening outcomes. However, rural clinics did significantly less following up for substance use problems in their patients than their urban counterparts. Larger rural clinics did better than small ones.[149]

Importantly, if health care systems systematically screen to identify individuals with risky use or potential substance use disorders, and respond appropriately to the level of the identified problem (with brief interventions, medications, and/or referral to specialty substance use disorder treatment), disparities in the use of treatment among those populations should lessen dramatically. In other words, it is expected that the number of people who seek treatment across all racial and ethnic groups will increase.

Few studies have directly compared treatment populations by race and ethnicity. However, some studies have examined race and ethnicity as predictors of outcomes in analyses controlling for many other factors (such as age, substance use disorder severity, mental health severity, social supports), and they showed that after accounting for these socioeconomic factors, outcomes did not differ by race and ethnicity. Some examples from an integrated health system include adolescent studies comparing Blacks or African Americans, American Indians or Alaska Natives, Hispanics or Latinos, and Whites.[150-152] The same is true for short-term and long-term treatment outcomes of adults.[112,153-155]

This body of research has some key caveats. For example, studies have found that matching programs and providers by race or ethnicity may produce better results for Hispanics or Latinos than for other racial and ethnic groups.[156] However, this research also suggests that all racial and ethnic groups can benefit equally from substance use disorder treatment. At the same time, offering programs that are tailored to patient characteristics or that incorporate health care professionals who share similarities with their patients in sex, age, or race or ethnicity may improve willingness to enter and engage in treatment.[157-159]

> **FOR MORE ON THIS TOPIC**
>
> See the section on "Considerations for Specific Populations" in Chapter 4 - Early Intervention, Treatment, and Management of Substance Use Disorders.

It should also be noted that civil rights laws, such as Section 504 of the Rehabilitation Act, the Americans with Disabilities Act (ADA), and Section 1557 of the Affordable Care Act, protect many people with substance use disorders and impose requirements on substance use disorder treatment programs. These laws require individual assessment of a person with a disability, identifying and implementing needed reasonable modifications of policies and practices when necessary to provide an equal opportunity for a person with a disability to participate in and benefit from treatment programs. More generally, these laws prohibit programs from excluding individuals from treatment programs on the basis of a co-occurring disability, if the individual meets the qualifications for the program. Additionally, under Title

VI of the Civil Rights Act and Section 1557 of the Affordable Care Act, providers who receive federal financial assistance must address the needs of people with limited English proficiency. The ADA and Section 504 also apply to discriminatory zoning laws and decisions that operate as a barrier to providers seeking to open or expand substance use disorder treatment programs.[160]

As the section on **Electronic Health Records and Health Information Technology** shows, health IT holds tremendous promise to provide culturally appropriate services in multiple languages and that incorporate health care professionals with characteristics similar to the target patients' population. One example with cultural relevance is a pilot randomized trial of a computer-delivered brief intervention in a prenatal clinic, which matched health care professionals and patients on race/ethnicity; patients found the intervention to be easy to use and helpful.[161] Such services have the potential to be cost-effective and to reach individuals in rural or urban settings and those who have difficulty attending treatment, including those with disabilities.

Integration Can Reduce Costs of Delivering Substance Use Services

With scarce resources and many social programs competing for limited funding, cost-effectiveness is a critical aspect of substance use-related services. Over the past 20 years, several comprehensive literature reviews have examined the economics of substance use disorder treatment.[162-165]

Although the United States spends roughly $35 billion across public and private payors to treat substance use disorders,[166,167] the social and economic costs associated with these disorders are many times higher: Annual costs of substance misuse and substance use disorders in the United States are estimated at more than $400 billion.[168,169] Thus, treating substance use disorders has the potential for positive net economic benefits, not just in regard to treatment services but also general health care.[162,170-172] For example, on average individuals with chronic medical conditions incur health care costs two to three times higher when they have a comorbid substance use disorder compared with individuals without this comorbidity.[173] The net benefits of integrated treatment include improved health care outcomes and reduced health care costs, as well as reduced crime, improved child welfare, and greater employment productivity.[125,174-178] Major individual and societal savings also stem from fewer interpersonal conflicts, greater workplace productivity, reduced infectious disease transmission, and fewer drug-related accidents, including overdoses and deaths.[179]

> **KEY TERMS**
>
> **Net economic benefit.** The value of total benefits minus total costs.

Evaluations of Medicaid expenditures for substance use disorder treatment show that the costs of treating substance use disorders are more than offset by the accompanying savings to Medicaid in reduced health care costs, such as reductions in future substance use disorder-related hospitalizations and residential treatment costs.[188-190] For example, as discussed below, an analysis of Washington State Medicaid found that providing substance use disorder treatment resulted in aggregate net savings to the Medicaid program, in the millions of dollars.[190] These and other studies point out that investments in engaging people into effective treatment for substance use disorders will reduce costs in many areas.

Costs of Substance Use Disorders in Other Service Systems

Costs associated with substance use disorders are not limited to health care. The accumulated costs to the individual, the family, and the community are staggering and arise as a consequence of many direct and indirect effects, including compromised physical and mental health, loss of productivity, reduced quality of life, increased crime and violence, misuse and neglect of children, and health care costs.

Criminal Justice System

As described elsewhere in this *Report*, a substance use disorder is a substantial risk factor for committing a criminal offense. Reduced crime is thus a key component of the net benefits associated with prevention and treatment interventions. Overall, within the criminal justice system, more than two thirds of jail detainees and half of prison inmates experience substance use disorders.[180,181] Many require treatment interventions, although only approximately 10 percent of prison inmates receive substance use disorder treatment services.[181] Applying inflation-adjusted estimates of the costs of in-prison care, the public sector spends approximately $400 million on such prison-based services, with substantial additional costs for after-care.[182]

Child Welfare and Related Service Systems

Substance use-related costs are also prominent within child welfare and related services. The estimated prevalence of substance use disorders among parents involved in the child welfare system varies across service populations, time, and place. One widely cited estimate is that between one-third and two-thirds of parents involved with the child welfare system experience some form of substance use problem.[183]

The *National Survey of Child and Adolescent Well-Being* found that caseworkers perceived substance misuse problems in 23 percent of cases, which was correlated with significantly higher probabilities of severe harm to children (24 percent), compared with parents with no such indication (5 percent).[184] Consistent with these findings, caseworker-perceived substance misuse problems were associated with more than twice the risk of out-of-home, or foster care, placement (38 percent vs. 16 percent) within this sample. Children of parents with substance use problems were more likely than others to require child protective services at younger ages, to experience repeated neglect and abuse from parents, and to otherwise require more intensive and intrusive services.[183] An estimated 19 percent of adolescents served by the child welfare system have experienced some substance use disorder, highlighting another challenge facing these service systems.[185]

In fiscal year 2016, approximately $5.2 billion was proposed for Federal Title IV-B, IV-E, and child abuse prevention services. Substance use disorders appear to account for a large proportion of child welfare, foster care, and related expenditures in the United States.

Military Health System

The United States military health system includes Department of Defense (DoD), Army, Navy, Air Force, and Marine Corps programs as well as health care outside the direct care system (TRICARE) for military members and their dependents, both in the United States and abroad. It is one of the largest health care systems in the United States. The IOM conducted a comprehensive study of military prevention and treatment services for substance use disorders.[186] As found in other health systems discussed in this *Report*, the prevalence of alcohol problems is high. A study of the economic impact of alcohol misuse among beneficiaries of the DoD's TRICARE insurance program found that the DoD spent approximately $1.2 billion to address problems related to alcohol use in 2006: $425 million in medical costs and $745 million in reduced readiness and misconduct.[187] In addition, opioid use disorders, often initiated when opioids are prescribed following injuries during deployment, are increasing at a high rate and are of high concern. Further, service members and veterans suffer from high rates of co-occurring health problems that pose significant treatment challenges, including traumatic brain injury, post-traumatic stress disorder, depression, and anxiety. Along with other recommendations, the IOM report recommended conducting routine screening, integrating substance use treatment with other health care, and implementing evidence-based treatments.

Costs of Substance Use Disorders in Other Service Systems, continued

These illustrative examples underscore that the costs associated with substance use disorders are incurred across diverse service systems that serve vulnerable populations. These expenditures might be reduced through more aggressive measures to address substance misuse problems and accompanying disorders. Moreover, many substance use-related services provided through criminal justice, child welfare, or other systems seek to ameliorate serious harms that have already occurred, and that might have been prevented with greater impact or cost-effectiveness through the delivery of evidence-based prevention or early treatment interventions.

Economic Analyses can Assess the Value of Substance Use Interventions

Different kinds of economic analyses can be particularly useful in helping health care systems, community leaders, and policymakers identify programs or policies that will bring the greatest value for addressing their needs. Two commonly used types of analyses are cost-effectiveness analysis[199] and cost-benefit analysis. Both types of studies have been used to examine substance use disorder treatment and prevention programs. Studies have found a number of substance use disorder treatments, including outpatient methadone, alcohol use disorder medications, and buprenorphine, to be cost-effective compared with no treatment.[162,200-209] The same is true for outpatient services without MAT and residential levels of treatment.

Cost-effectiveness Analyses

Treatment Settings and Approaches. A 2003 study estimating the cost-effectiveness of four different treatment modalities—inpatient, residential, outpatient methadone, and outpatient without MAT—found that the treatment of substance use disorders is cost-effective compared to other health interventions, with outpatient programs without MAT being the most cost-effective. Estimated cost per abstinent case ranged from $11,411 for outpatient treatment without MAT to $28,256 in the inpatient setting, with an average cost across all modalities of $22,460 per abstinent study participant (adjusted to 2014 dollars).[205]

> **KEY TERMS**
>
> **Cost-effectiveness study.** A comparative analysis of two or more interventions against their health and economic outcomes. These outcomes could be lives saved, illnesses prevented, or years of life gained.
>
> **Cost-benefit study.** A study that determines the economic worth of an intervention by quantifying its costs in monetary terms and comparing them with the benefits, also expressed in monetary terms. Total benefits divided by total costs is called a cost-benefit ratio. If the ratio is greater than 1, the benefits outweigh the costs.

Methadone Maintenance versus Methadone Detoxification. A 2004 study evaluating the incremental cost-effectiveness of sustained methadone maintenance relative to a 180-day methadone detoxification enriched with intensive psychosocial services followed by drug-free substance use disorder treatment found that methadone maintenance yielded better outcomes, including reduced opioid use and lower subsequent behavioral health care costs, and had a cost-effectiveness ratio of approximately $20,000 per life year gained.[203]

Methadone Maintenance versus Maintenance with Other Medications. As the use of MAT options has grown, cost-effectiveness studies have compared alternative MAT interventions and MAT compared to medication-free behavioral therapies. For example, a 2015 study examining injectable, extended-release naltrexone compared with methadone maintenance treatment and buprenorphine maintenance treatment for opioid dependence found that extended release naltrexone was more effective among patients remaining in treatment but also more costly than the other options,[227] totaling an additional $72 per opioid-free day. However, extended-release naltrexone is not off-patent, and therefore these cost findings will likely change when it becomes generic.

Extended Buprenorphine-Naloxone Treatment versus Brief Detoxification. A 2010 study of extended buprenorphine-naloxone treatment for opioid-dependent youth estimated that the cost-effectiveness ratio for buprenorphine compared to detoxification was $29,415 (outpatient treatment program costs for up to 12 weeks) per Quality-Adjusted Life Year (QALY).[228] Results like this indicate that buprenorphine is highly cost-effective by the standard benchmarks often employed to evaluate clinical and population health interventions ($50,000 to $100,000 per QALY).

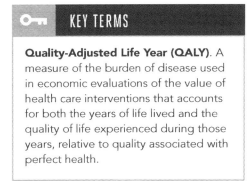

KEY TERMS

Quality-Adjusted Life Year (QALY). A measure of the burden of disease used in economic evaluations of the value of health care interventions that accounts for both the years of life lived and the quality of life experienced during those years, relative to quality associated with perfect health.

Buprenorphine-Naloxone versus No Treatment. A 2012 study examined individuals with opioid use disorders who had completed 6 months of buprenorphine-naloxone treatment within a primary care setting. It estimated that office-based buprenorphine-naloxone treatment for clinically stable patients has a cost-effectiveness ratio of $38,107 per QALY compared to no treatment after 24 months.[229] The cost-effectiveness ratio was measured by calculating the difference in treatment costs between those receiving buprenorphine-naloxone treatment and those that did not and dividing them by the difference in patients' health outcomes.

SBI. A 2014 review of cost-effectiveness studies for alcohol SBI in a primary care setting found considerable variability in the estimated cost-effectiveness ratios and cost savings across studies.[230] However, almost all the studies found SBI to be cost-effective or to produce cost savings. For example, a 2008 analysis of alcohol SBI in primary care settings found an incremental cost-effectiveness ratio for SBI of $2,413 per QALY gained compared to a do-nothing scenario (in 2014 dollars).[45] The authors compared the cost-effectiveness of alcohol SBI to 24 other preventive services that have been deemed effective by the USPSTF. Using that comparison, alcohol misuse screening achieved a combined score similar to screening for colorectal cancer, hypertension, or vision (for adults older than age 64), and to influenza or pneumococcal immunization. Because current levels of SBI delivery are much lower than desired, this service deserves special attention by health care professionals and care delivery systems.[45] Importantly, all of the interventions that have proved to be cost-effective are appropriate for implementation in primary care.

Cost-Benefit Analyses

Interventions that prevent substance use disorders can yield an even greater economic return than the services that treat them. For example, a recent study of prevention programs estimated that every dollar spent on effective, school-based prevention programs can save an estimated $18 in costs related to problems later in life.[231]

The Washington State Institute for Public Policy has used a standardized model to estimate the cost-benefit of diverse prevention, early intervention, and treatment programs. Benefit-per-dollar invested ratios for evidence-based interventions (EBIs) include $27.48 for every dollar invested in brief intervention in primary care; $36.71 for brief intervention in a medical hospital; $9.07 for brief intervention in an emergency department; $136.41 for cognitive behavior coping skills therapy; $33.71 for contingency management for substance use; $41.10 for motivational interviewing to enhance treatment engagement; $14.79 for brief marijuana dependence counseling; and $34.90 for brief cognitive behavioral intervention for amphetamine users.[232] Although some of the 30 interventions studied had smaller benefit-to-cost ratios than others (e.g., $2.18 for methadone maintenance treatment and $1.30 for buprenorphine/buprenorphine-naloxone treatment), all had benefits greater than their costs.

> **FOR MORE ON THIS TOPIC**
>
> See Chapter 3 - *Prevention Programs and Policies*.

How Much Does Alcohol or Drug Screening and Treatment Cost?

In a 2005 literature review of the economics of substance use disorder treatment, one study highlighted the variability in cost estimates for substance use disorder treatment delivered in specialty settings. For example, they reported per-patient weekly costs ranging from $90 to $208 for standard outpatient treatment; $682 to $936 for residential treatment; and $100 to $125 for methadone maintenance treatment.[162] Another study, estimated service costs in 170 methadone maintenance treatment programs and found that methadone dosing was $33 per patient per week, individual counseling was $49 per patient per session (approximately 43 minutes per session), and group counseling was $12 per patient per session (approximately 77 minutes per session).[191] A 2009 study estimated service costs for 70 standard outpatient programs and found that individual counseling was $75 per patient per hour and group counseling was $9 per patient per hour.[192]

A 2012 review of 17 studies on the cost of alcohol screening and brief intervention (SBI), found considerable variability, with costs ranging from $0.56 to $663.74 per screen and $3.76 to $268.16 per brief intervention.[193] Median costs were approximately $4 per screen and $53 per brief intervention. Costs were typically lower when activity-based costing (assigning the cost and amount of each activity that is part of the intervention) was employed and when the SBI occurred in a primary care setting or was performed by a provider who was not a physician. Additionally, variation was attributed to the wage of the person conducting the screening and the amount of time the screening took. A 2015 study examined costs of SBI for illicit drug use in primary care settings; they estimated that per-person costs were $16.43 for screening, $40.98 for a brief negotiated interview, and $265.49 for an adaptation of motivational interviewing.[194]

In recent years, use of MAT has increased. Recent studies have examined extended-release naltrexone, buprenorphine, and methadone for opioid use disorder treatment.[195-197] These studies found that health care costs were generally as low or lower for individuals receiving extended-release naltrexone compared to individuals receiving other treatments for opioid use disorder. Individuals with opioid use disorders who received extended-release naltrexone had $8,170 lower costs compared to those receiving methadone maintenance. Individuals receiving buprenorphine with counseling had significantly lower total health care costs than individuals receiving little or no treatment for their opioid use disorder ($13,578 compared to $31,055). However, those receiving buprenorphine plus counseling did not differ significantly in total health care costs when compared to those receiving only counseling (mean health care costs for those receiving counseling only were $17,017).[196] It is important to note, however, that while some treatments may be less costly, they may also be less effective.

Another study, the Combined Pharmacotherapies and Behavioral Interventions (COMBINE) trial, examined nine treatment alternatives for alcohol treatment, including MAT. They reported mean per-patient cost estimates of $631 for a combined behavioral intervention (CBI) without MAT, $766 for naltrexone with medical management, and $865 for acamprosate with medical management. Combining CBI with a MAT option increased cost estimates to $1,183 for naltrexone plus CBI and $1,285 for acamprosate plus CBI.[198] However, in the COMBINE study, naltrexone combined with medical management was found to be the most cost-effective treatment. While other treatments may be less costly, they are also somewhat less effective.

*All costs in this sidebar are calculated in 2014 dollars.

Financing Systems for Substance Use Disorder Services

In 2013, about three-quarters of all general health care purchased in the United States was paid for by private insurance, Medicare, or Medicaid. The rest was covered by consumers paying out-of-pocket, by other federal health grants, and by programs and other insurance provided by the DoD, Department of Veterans Affairs, and other state and local programs.[211] In the case of treatment for substance use disorders, only about 45 percent of spending was through private insurance, Medicare, or Medicaid. In 2014, the largest share of substance use disorder treatment financing was from state (non-Medicaid) and local governments (29 percent).[211]

Private Insurance

In 2014, 66.0 percent of individuals in the United States had private health insurance, either obtained through employers or individually.[212] Approximately 9 percent of insured individuals met criteria for a diagnosis of substance use disorder, as defined by the Fourth Edition of the *Diagnostic and Statistical Manual of Mental Disorders* (DSM-IV).[214] However, in 2013, only 7 percent of privately insured individuals aged 12 and older with a substance use disorder received treatment from specialty treatment providers,[214] and total spending on treatment for substance use disorders makes up only 0.6 percent of overall private insurance spending.

Coverage of substance use disorder services under private insurance has waxed and waned over the past 30 years. During the 1980s, insurance benefits and specialty addiction providers expanded,[215,216] and from 1986 to 1992, substance use disorder spending grew by 6.7 percent annually, a substantial increase but still significantly below the 10.3 percent annual growth rate of all health care spending over the same period. This expansion was followed by managed care restrictions on reimbursement for substance use disorder treatment in inpatient settings, such as limitations on length of residential rehabilitation stays (a common treatment regimen).[217,218] As a result, inpatient substance use disorder treatment services declined from accounting for 50 percent of total spending for substance use disorder treatment in 1986 to only 19 percent in 2014 (Figure 6.4). Further, the share of substance use disorder financing from private insurance dropped dramatically between 1986 and 2014, from 32 percent in 1986 to 13 percent in 2005; this was followed by an increase to 18 percent in 2014, likely due to MHPAEA and qualified health plan coverage now being available through the Affordable Care Act.[211]

Medicaid

Approximately 20 percent of people in the United States have health coverage through Medicaid, a joint federal and state health coverage program that provides medical assistance for children, families, and individuals with low income and limited resources; an estimated 12 percent of adult Medicaid beneficiaries have a substance use disorder.[212] The federal government finances approximately 60 percent (national average) of Medicaid and the states finance the balance.[220] The federal medical assistance percentages (or "match") vary significantly among states, based on the state's per capita income and other factors.

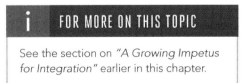

FOR MORE ON THIS TOPIC

See the section on *"A Growing Impetus for Integration"* earlier in this chapter.

HEALTH CARE SYSTEMS

Figure 6.4: Percentage Distribution of Spending on Substance Misuse Treatment by Setting, 1986–2014

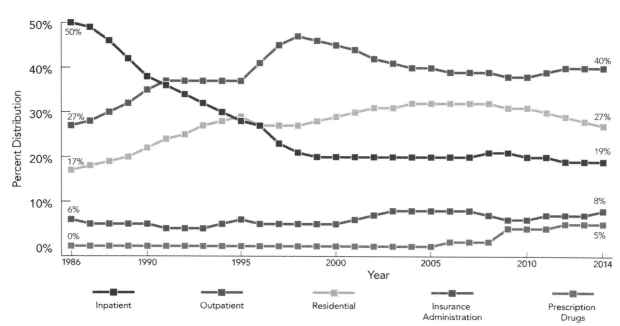

Source: Substance Abuse and Mental Health Services Administration, (2016).[167]

The federal government establishes basic requirements that states must follow in designing their Medicaid programs, including some mandated services that must be covered and guidance regarding payment rate-setting and contractual arrangements, eligibility and quality standards, and provision of optional services.[221] However, state implementation decisions can have a significant impact on what services are covered and for whom. States can choose to cover or not cover specific treatments or to place restrictions on covered services. In the past, some states have not included certain critical substance use disorder treatment options in their benefit packages (e.g., methadone), or they have restricted the doses or length of treatment, or added requirements such as prior authorization processes to obtain some treatments (e.g., buprenorphine). In many states, Medicaid also does not cover residential treatment, especially for adults.

For those who are eligible and have substance use disorders, Medicaid is an extremely important program, as it can cover many services that such individuals may need, such as crisis services and many preventive services. In addition, while Medicaid does not provide payments for housing (e.g., rental subsidies) or other room and board costs in the community, states can supplement Medicaid coverage with supportive services to help people maintain housing in collaboration with housing authorities.[222]

In states that did not expand Medicaid, racial and ethnic minorities are disproportionately affected. In addition, in these states, young adult single males—a group with high rates of substance use disorders—are ineligible for Medicaid benefits.[223]

An estimated 14 to 15 percent of uninsured individuals nationwide who could be newly eligible for Medicaid coverage under the Affordable Care Act have a substance use disorder.[35] If they obtain substance use disorder treatment, this will lead to an additional 450,000 previously uninsured individuals having access to affordable substance use disorder treatment.

Medicare

Medicare covers almost all individuals aged 65 or over as well as those eligible because of disabilities. Approximately 56.2 million, or 17 percent of individuals in the United States, have Medicare.[224] Approximately 3 percent of Medicare beneficiaries and 6 percent of those who are eligible for both Medicare and Medicaid have a substance use disorder in any given year.[226] Of these, 19.3 percent received specialty substance use disorder treatment, including individual, group, and/or family therapy.[225] In general, Medicare Parts A and B (or private Medicare Advantage plans under Part C) cover inpatient (but not residential) and outpatient services for substance use disorders, as well as substance use disorder screening and brief intervention. Prescription drug treatment is generally covered for beneficiaries enrolled in Medicare Part D (or a Medicare Advantage plan that includes drug coverage). Medicare does not cover outpatient use of oral methadone for substance use disorders, but Part D can include coverage for medications, such as disulfiram, naltrexone, acamprosate, and buprenorphine.

Other Federal, State, and Local Funding

Although insurance coverage is critical to improving access to and integration of services for individuals with substance use disorders, it is unlikely to cover all the services that such individuals may need, such as crisis services (e.g., emergency treatment intervention), housing, supported employment, and many community prevention programs and services (e.g., school-based prevention programs). These services are often supported by federal, state, and local governments and non-profit organizations, financed through general revenues and the SAMHSA Substance Abuse Prevention and Treatment Block Grant (SABG).

Uninsured Individuals

Research has shown that uninsured individuals have higher unmet medical needs than do insured individuals, and those without insurance also have higher rates of substance use disorders than do individuals with insurance.[226] Among uninsured individuals, 12 percent met DSM-IV criteria for a substance use disorder.[214]

Financing Community Prevention

Federal Funding Streams

Funds from federal block grants to states for substance use disorder treatment services (such as the SABG, which is often used for prevention activities) and for maternal, child, and adolescent health services (Title V of the Maternal and Child Health Services Block Grant) may be used to fill the gaps in treatment services not covered by insurance. These funds also finance treatment for people without insurance and support community prevention activities.[233]

In addition, federal funding for certain community prevention programs encourages public-private partnerships and community collaboration to improve health outcomes. Grants are used to increase screening, counseling, workplace wellness programs, and community prevention. In addition, federal funding for community prevention programs is available through the Drug Free Communities Support Program, which is funded by the White House Office of National Drug Control Policy and administered by SAMHSA.[234]

> **FOR MORE ON THIS TOPIC**
>
> See Chapter 3 - *Prevention Programs and Policies.*

Although investments in prevention have repeatedly demonstrated favorable economic returns,[235] primary prevention for all health conditions still accounts for less than 5 percent of overall health spending in the United States. Prevention should be seen as an appropriate health cost to be covered by insurance. Current funding options for community prevention, described below, include grants from hospital and health system foundations, hospital-based community benefit programs, tax earmarks, and targeted state programs.

Hospital and Health System Foundation Grants

Foundations formed from the conversion of tax-exempt non-profit hospitals and health systems into for-profit entities are required by federal law to invest in health-related activities within the community area served by that hospital.[236] These "health conversion foundations" or "new health foundations" now exist in more than 200 communities in the United States, and they are a potential source of funding for programs relating to the prevention and treatment of substance misuse.[237]

Non-profit Hospital Community Benefits

Beginning in 1994, tax-exempt hospitals have been required to provide benefits to the community in return for not paying taxes.[238] The Affordable Care Act clarified community benefit expectations for all non-profit hospitals. Tax-exempt hospitals must: (1) conduct a community health needs assessment at least once every 3 years; (2) involve public health experts and representatives of the community served by the facility in the needs assessment; (3) make the results of the assessment available to the public; (4) develop an implementation strategy to address each of the community health needs identified through the assessment; and (5) report yearly to the Internal Revenue Service.[239] The Secretary of the Treasury, in collaboration with the Secretary of Health and Human Services, must report annually to Congress on, among other things, hospitals' levels of charity care, related costs, and community benefit activities.

Although hospitals have flexibility in their definition of "community served by the facility," they are expected to define community by the geographic location, not by the demographic or geographic profiles, of patient discharges. Many states also have community benefit programs that must be synchronized with the requirements of the Affordable Care Act.[240] The 1997 IOM report *Improving Health in the Community* outlined how multiple stakeholders can conduct a community health assessment and share accountability for health outcomes of specific populations.[241]

Local or State Substance Use Tax Earmarks

In certain jurisdictions, direct funds from a local or state tax can be earmarked for substance misuse prevention in the same way as tobacco taxes are currently used for public health and health programming in many states.[242] Jackson County, Missouri, is an example of a local jurisdiction with a dedicated funding stream for substance use problem prevention.[243]

> ### Financing Community Prevention, continued
>
> Jackson County, Missouri, first introduced a dedicated sales tax in 1989 to tackle drug use and drug-related crime. This later became known as COMBAT—Community-Backed Anti-Drug Tax—and enabled Jackson County to approach the impact of drugs on individuals and communities as both a legal issue and a public health crisis. It was renewed for seven years in 2009, and the one-quarter of one-cent sales tax generates over $20 million per year. The funds are used for a variety of prevention, treatment, and anti-drug and drug-related crime prevention programs. In addition, Florida and Indiana, among other states, earmark alcohol taxes for child and adolescent substance use-related services.[244]
>
> ### State Prevention Trust Funds
>
> The Massachusetts Legislature passed the first state-based prevention fund, called the Prevention and Wellness Trust Fund, in 2012 as part of a health cost control bill. Funded through a one-time $57 million assessment, the Trust Fund is used to reduce the prevalence of preventable health conditions and lower health care costs. Grantees have a strong focus on extending care beyond clinical sites into the community.[245]

Challenges Facing the Integration of Substance Use Services and Health Care

It is clear that integrating substance use disorder services with mainstream health care is beneficial for individuals and communities and that health reform is encouraging this trend. However, several key challenges must be addressed if integration is to be fully successful. Specifically:

- The substance use disorder treatment system is underprepared to support care coordination;
- The primary care system has been slow to implement MAT as well as prevention, early identification, and other evidence-based recommendations;
- The existing health care workforce is already understaffed and often lacks the necessary training and education to address substance use disorders; and
- The need to protect patient confidentiality creates hurdles for sharing of information.

The Infrastructure of the Substance Use Disorder Treatment System Is Underdeveloped

The Congressional Budget Office currently estimates that by 2026, 24 million Americans who would otherwise be uninsured will obtain health insurance coverage as a result of the Affordable Care Act.[246] For those insured by insurance plans sold to small employers and in the individual market, substance use disorder services are considered an essential health benefit. As a result, the Affordable Care Act, coupled with MHPAEA is projected to expand access to mental and behavioral health services to more than 60 million Americans.[247]

However, the specialty care substance use disorder treatment system faces challenges along with these new opportunities.[248] That system is changing as health systems respond to new requirements, begin to provide services internally, and develop new contracting mechanisms.[249] Public substance use disorder systems are also changing as they are presented with new funding options under Medicaid and other funding sources.[248]

Nationally representative data from the 2014 *National Drug Abuse Treatment System Survey* underscore the importance (but also the difficulty) of integrated care efforts.[250] Directors at only 15 percent of responding units reported signed contracts to work with a medical home, meaning that less than 50 percent of patients were receiving treatment in a program that was prepared to integrate general health care.[250] These data showed particularly dramatic differences between Medicaid expansion and non-expansion states,[250] with Medicaid expansion acting as a key driver of integrated care. Fifty-five percent of addiction treatment patients in expansion states are receiving care in organizations that at least have contractual linkages to some medical or health home arrangement.[251]

Substance use disorder treatment organizations currently face significant challenges in engaging in care coordination with other types of providers. Because these organizations have traditionally been organized and financed separately from general health care systems, the two systems have not routinely exchanged clinical information. Efforts to increase HIE are constrained by the relatively low use of EHRs. In a 2012 survey of treatment programs to assess their readiness for health reform, 63 percent described their organizations' adoption of EHRs as having not yet begun, or only in the early stages.[252] A 2015 study reported that substance use disorder treatment organizations across the nation are poorly positioned to work effectively with health homes or other health professionals.[253] Not surprisingly, organizations with annual budgets less than $5 million were less likely than larger ones to report high readiness.[254] Some evidence also suggests that publicly funded substance use disorder treatment centers are less technically proficient and less responsive to making changes than for-profit treatment facilities. For example, private, for-profit treatment facilities were significantly more likely to be early adopters of buprenorphine therapies than were their public or private non-profit peers.[255] Substantial technical assistance and investments in staff and information technology are needed, yet substance use disorder treatment providers receive relatively little assistance or resources from federal or state agencies to make these changes.[253] However, a February 29, 2016 State Medicaid Director Letter outlined that states, subject to prior approval by the Centers for Medicare & Medicaid Services (CMS), may use federal matching funds to connect Meaningful Use Eligible Medicaid Providers to other providers including substance use disorder treatment providers to support HIE and care coordination. This offers promise for increasing adoption and use of health IT by behavioral health providers.[256]

Another challenge for effectively coordinating care relates to the need for specialty substance use disorder treatment programs to comply with substance abuse confidentiality regulations (42 CFR Part 2) and state privacy laws when implementing health IT systems. In addition, substance use disorder treatment organizations face the challenge of communicating with non-health care personnel including those in social service, criminal justice, and educational facilities and even when EHRs are in place these systems lack interoperability (the ability to effectively exchange digital health information from an EHR in a common format) with the information systems used by social service organizations, hindering communication.

Medical homes are most likely to pursue contractual arrangements with large and technologically sophisticated organizations that are best equipped to meet their needs for timely clinical and administrative information. The move toward integrated care is therefore likely to accelerate consolidation of substance use disorder treatment programs, which may hasten the adoption of new technologies and processes among sophisticated providers. Particularly in combination with expanded insurance coverage, this trend may attract new partnerships, for example between ACOs, which are integrated delivery systems, and more sophisticated specialty addiction providers. Yet, the same patterns may harm smaller providers, some of whom offer the only culturally competent services for particular patient groups, such as services tailored for specific racial and ethnic populations, sexual and gender minorities, or women in need of trauma-related residential services.[257-259]

Slow Implementation of Pharmacotherapies for Use in Treatment

One key challenge for integrating substance use treatment and health care is that implementation of pharmacotherapies (i.e., MAT) in primary care has been slow.[260] In part, this is due to the fact that health insurers individually determine whether they cover substance use medications[261] and treatment providers may not offer medications to patients with substance use disorders. A study of 2009–2010 national treatment center data found that only 25 percent of substance use disorder treatment centers offered medications for alcohol and/or drugs: 24.5 percent offered buprenorphine, 18.7 percent offered acamprosate, 17.3 percent offered tablet naltrexone, 15.9 percent offered disulfiram, 9.1 percent offered injectable naltrexone, and 9.0 percent offered methadone.[262] Studies have found that only 25 percent of private, for-profit treatment centers used buprenorphine, 15.6 percent used acamprosate, and 15.7 percent used disulfram. Research suggests that whether treatment programs offer MAT is influenced by a number of organizational and state-level factors, including differences in organizational size, whether the treatment program is in a hospital setting, whether psychiatric medications are prescribed, whether the program has access to prescribing staff, and whether state Medicaid policies support the use of generic drugs.[263-266]

Another medication, extended-release injectable naltrexone, approved by the FDA for use in treating individuals with opioid use disorders, is underutilized by programs. For example, one study found that only three percent of United States treatment programs used it for opioid use disorders.[267] In contrast, buprenorphine for opioid use disorder is becoming more established, although it too is underused. One study found that between 2005 and 2011, its use for detoxification in specialty opioid treatment programs (OTPs) increased from 36 percent of programs in the sample to 46 percent; its use for maintenance increased from 37 percent of programs in the sample to 53 percent.[268] One deterrent to rapid expansion of access to buprenorphine has been the limit on the number of patients a certified physician can treat with buprenorphine. A recent study found that raising this limit further, rather than increasing the number of specialty addiction programs or waivered physicians, may be the most effective way to increase buprenorphine use.[269] Up until July 2016, qualified practitioners were allowed to treat a maximum of 30 patients at a time the first year and up to 100 patients at a time thereafter. On July 6, 2016, HHS issued a final rule for "Medication Assisted Treatment for Opioid Use Disorders," which increased access to buprenorphine medications in the office-based setting as authorized under the Controlled Substances Act 21 U.S.C. 823(g)(2).[270] The rule allows eligible practitioners to request approval to treat up to 275 patients under section 303(g)(2) of the Controlled Substances Act.

Limited Implementation of Prevention, Early Identification, and Other Evidence-based Recommendations

Another key challenge is that primary care settings have not yet routinely implemented recommended preventive health and intervention services related to substance misuse. Currently, the Affordable Care Act requires that all non-grandfathered health plans must cover, without cost-sharing, certain preventive health services recommended by the USPSTF,[271] and women's preventive services and preventive services for infants, children, and adolescents in guidelines supported by HRSA. As discussed earlier, the USPSTF recommends alcohol screening and counseling for adults. However, none of the 22 women's health guidelines, which are being updated at the time of this *Report*, or 26 children/adolescent guidelines supported by HRSA include a screening requirement related to alcohol use.[42,43]

Studies of SBIRT for alcohol use problems have identified many implementation challenges.[272-277] Some of the most commonly noted challenges include the intense time constraints experienced in modern clinical settings,[276] the multiple competing preventive and clinical priorities faced by providers,[278] inadequate health care professional training on alcohol SBI techniques,[277] and providers' feelings that they are unable to address sensitive health issues adequately.[279] Currently, only about one in six adults in the United States reports being asked about their drinking,[280] and less than 10 percent of health plans verify that screening is performed.[281] In pediatric health care settings, other issues, especially restrictions on disclosure of confidential information to parents (which varies by state), also pose challenges.[282]

The USPSTF currently considers the evidence to be insufficient to support screening or behavioral interventions for substance misuse problems in pediatrics.[43,283] However, a number of studies, funded by the National Institutes of Health (NIH) and foundations such as The Conrad N. Hilton Foundation, are currently underway that could add to the evidence base. Major pediatric medical organizations, including the American Academy of Pediatrics, strongly recommend addressing these issues regularly at each well-adolescent visit and appropriate urgent care visits.[284] *Bright Futures*, a HRSA-funded program, sets Recommendations for Preventive Pediatric Health Care and includes alcohol and drug use screening within its recommended schedule for an annual clinical preventive visit for adolescents and young adults between the ages of 11 and 21. The Affordable Care Act requires health plans to cover, at no out-of-pocket cost to families, the preventive care services outlined in this schedule. *Bright Futures* discusses how to incorporate screening into the preventive services visit for these age groups. In addition, SAMHSA recommends universal screening and brief intervention and referral to treatment at each well-visit,[285] and the National Institute on Alcohol Abuse and Alcoholism (NIAAA) recommends universal screening for alcohol misuse.

Screening and brief intervention for substance misuse is also consistent with the prevention activities recommended in the 2009 IOM report *Preventing Mental, Emotional, and Behavioral Disorders Among Youth: Progress and Possibilities*.[286] Yet screening is seldom addressed according to guidelines or with appropriate evidence-based practices,[287,288] and even when screenings are conducted, appropriate follow-up is often not provided.[289,290] However, SBIRT can be effectively implemented, both for adults and adolescents,[291,292] and it is likely that many more systems will do so to comply with new requirements by

The Joint Commission and in the Affordable Care Act. The Joint Commission Requirements mandate that hospitals offer inpatients brief counseling for alcohol misuse and follow-up, and measure the provision of counseling as one of the core measures for hospital accreditation. Primary care teams that include non-physician providers (e.g., nurses, health educators) are increasingly used for substance use disorder, mental health, and other disease management, and they have proved to be a viable approach for implementing alcohol SBIRT.[291,293-298]

Meeting Challenges in Primary Care

Several large health systems, such as the Veterans Health Administration and Kaiser Permanente, have successfully implemented primary care-based alcohol SBI in a sustainable manner.[299-302] They have used a variety of approaches to accomplish this goal, including:

- Integrating screening, assessment, and clinical decision support tools in the EHR;
- Establishing interdisciplinary (primary care, substance use disorder treatment, and mental health) teams to guide integration and collaboration;
- Ensuring health system leadership support; and
- Using training curricula, targeted communications materials, robust performance feedback reporting for physicians and other staff, and existing financial incentives.[278,291,303-305]

These approaches can also be implemented in emergency departments and in obstetrics and gynecology departments.

The Health Care Workforce Is Limited in Key Ways

Workforce Shortages

Data on the substance use workforce are incomplete.[306] Although HRSA collects data on mental health workforce shortage areas, the agency does not collect similar data on the substance use disorder treatment workforce. Nevertheless, it is clear that the workforce is inadequate, as evidenced by its uneven geographic distribution (with rural areas underserved), access barriers for adolescents and children, and recruitment challenges across the treatment field. Moreover, the workforce is aging. For example, 46 percent of psychiatrists are older than age 65.[307,308] As of June 2016, more than three-quarters of United States counties had severe shortages of psychiatrists and other types of health care professionals needed to treat mental health and substance use disorders.[309] The scarcity of providers who can provide culturally competent services for minority populations and the high turnover rate, both noted in SAMHSA's 2013 Report to Congress[307] and other studies, exacerbate the workforce shortage.[310,311]

Recent reforms may strain the current workforce in an already overstretched health care system working to address treatment and prevention strategies. A recent study documented staffing models in primary care practices and determined that, even among those designated as patient-centered medical homes, fewer than 23 percent employed health educators, pharmacists, social workers, nutritionists, or community service coordinators, and fewer than half employed care coordinators.[312] The opioid epidemic has made the shortage of these types of health care professionals an even larger problem.[310]

Thus, it is crucial that health care professionals are given comprehensive training on the prevention and treatment of substance use disorders when patients present with comorbid conditions.[32]

The IOM's 2006 report *Improving the Quality of Health Care for Mental and Substance Use Conditions*,[32] which adapted *Crossing the Quality Chasm* to address mental and substance use conditions, noted that a critical concern in attracting a skilled workforce is the low salary structure of the substance use disorder treatment workforce. Much of the public treatment system is funded by Medicaid and SAMHSA's SABG. In practice, the Block Grant is used broadly, and Medicaid less and only with a subset of providers. It is not yet clear whether the integration of substance use disorder treatments in general health care will help to address salary structure.

Composition and Education

An integrated health and substance use disorder treatment system requires a diverse workforce that includes substance use disorder specialists, physicians, nurses, mental health treatment providers, care managers, and recovery specialists. This workforce also includes peer recovery coaches (a reimbursable service under some state Medicaid programs), health educators, social workers, and other staff who are trained to deliver timely mental health and substance use-related health interventions, such as SBI.[32] However, Medicare, and in some states Medicaid, restricts "billable" health care professionals to physicians (including psychiatrists), nurse practitioners and clinical nurse specialists, physician's assistants, clinical psychologists, clinical social workers, and certain other specified practitioners, and does not include as billable the multiple other licensed and certified professionals who are trained to provide services for substance use disorders.

As substance use disorder treatment and general health care become more integrated, clinical staff in both systems will need to expand their scope of work, operate in an integrated manner with a variety of populations, and shift their treatment focus as needed.[313-315] Being able to assess substance use disorder severity and co-occurring mental health and physical health problems will be important in each setting. Health care professionals moving from the specialty workforce into integrated settings will require specific training on treatment planning and care coordination and an ability and willingness to work under the leadership of medical staff. This transition to a highly collaborative team approach, offering individually tailored treatment plans, presents challenges to the traditional substance use disorder treatment workforce that is used to administering standard "programs" of services to all patients. Working in teams with the broad mandate of improved health is not currently commonplace and will require collaboration among professional and certification bodies. Incorporating peer workers, who bring specific knowledge of patients' experiences and needs and can encourage informed patient decision making, into teams will also require further adjustment.

Improving the Quality of Health Care for Mental and Substance Use Conditions also discussed the shortage of skills both in specialty substance use disorder programs and in the general health care system.[32] Of special concern was the inadequacy of substance use education as part of medical school training: Only 8 percent of medical schools had a separate required course on addiction medicine and 36 percent had an elective course;[32,316] on average, the residency curriculum for psychiatrists included only 8 hours on substance use disorders.[32,317] Schools of social work and psychology also provided little, and sometimes no, mandatory education on substance use-related problems.[32] The situation does not appear to have substantially changed since that report was released, although the recent recognition of addiction medicine as a subspecialty by the American Board of Medical Specialties should provide increased focus and perhaps attract more physicians to this field.

Workforce Development and Improvement

The Annapolis Coalition on the Behavioral Health Workforce provided a framework for workforce development in response to the challenges described above,[318] focusing on broadening the definition of "workforce" to address needed changes to the health care system. Currently, 66 organizations license and credential addiction counselors,[319,320] and although a consensus on national core competencies for these counselors exists,[321] they have not been universally adopted. Credentialing for prevention specialists exists through the International Certification & Reciprocity Consortium,[322,323] but core competencies for prevention professionals have not been developed. Without a comprehensive, coordinated, and focused effort, workforce expansion and training will continue to fall short of the challenge of meeting the needs of individuals across the continuum of service settings.

HRSA has taken a number of steps to address these workforce challenges as part of its mission to prepare a diverse workforce and improve the workforce distribution to increase access for underserved communities. Among its many programs, HRSA awards health professional and graduate medical education training grants and operates scholarship and loan repayment programs. Of particular note is the National Health Service Corps, where, as of September 2015, roughly 30 percent of its field strength of 9,683 was composed of behavioral health providers, meeting service obligations by providing care in areas of high need.[324] HRSA is also putting increased emphasis on expanding the delivery of medication-assisted treatment, increasing SBI, and coordinating RSS. The development of the workforce qualified to deliver these services and services to address co-occurring medical and mental disorders will have significant implications for the national workforce's ability to reach the full potential of integration.

Protecting Confidentiality When Exchanging Sensitive Information

Effectively integrating substance use disorder treatment and general health care requires the timely exchange of patient health care information. In the early 1970s, the federal government enacted Confidentiality of Alcohol and Drug Abuse Patient Records (42 U.S.C. § 290dd-2), and released regulations (42 CFR Part 2) to protect the confidentiality of substance use disorder treatment data. These privacy protections were motivated by the understanding that discrimination attached to a substance use disorder might dissuade people from seeking treatment, and were enacted in the context of patient methadone records being used in criminal cases. Due to its targeted population, 42 CFR Part 2 provides more stringent federal protections than most other health privacy laws, including the Health Insurance Portability and Accountability Act (HIPAA – 45 CFR Part 160 and 164). HIPAA does not require patient authorization to share health information for purposes of treatment, payment, or health care operations. With 42 CFR Part 2, patient consent is required to share and use patient identifying information and any information that could be used to identify someone as having, or having had, a substance use disorder, such as payment data.

Given the long and continuing history of discrimination against people with substance use disorders, safeguards against inappropriate or inadvertent disclosures are important. Disclosures to legal authorities can lead to arrest, loss of child custody, or relinquished parental rights. Disclosures to insurers or to employers can render patients unable to obtain disability or life insurance and can cost patients their jobs. Currently, persons with substance use disorders involving illicit drugs are not protected under anti-discrimination laws, such as the ADA.

However, exchanging treatment records among health care providers has the potential to improve treatment and patient safety. For example, in the case of opioid prescribing, a study in health systems of long-term opioid users found those with a prior substance use disorder diagnosis received higher dosages and were co-prescribed sedative-hypnotic medications—which can increase the risk for overdose—more often. Because of privacy regulations, it is likely that physicians were not aware of their patients' substance use disorders.[52] In most states, these challenges are now partially addressed through prescription drug monitoring programs (PDMPs), which are also helping to support care coordination.

PDMPs are state-run databases that collect prescribed and dispensed controlled prescription drug information and give prescribers and pharmacists access to a person's controlled substance prescription history. Authorized providers can check the database before prescribing or dispensing. However, PDMPs have many limitations. They do not include information about methadone used for opioid use disorders, which is exclusively dispensed at OTPs, or from programs covered by 42 CFR Part 2. While disclosure of patient-identifying information that is subject to 42 CFR Part 2 is allowable, it would require written patient consent, and re-disclosures of this information would not be permitted unless the patient consents. However, any information in the PDMP database could be potentially seen by anyone who has access to the state PDMP data and therefore may be in violation of Part 2. In addition, PDMPs only collect prescription information as allowed by their state laws, in most cases controlled substances Scheduled II through IV or V, and thus health care professionals may not be aware of other prescriptions their patients are receiving.[326] Further, the extent to which the PDMP systems are effectively designed and used is not fully known.[327]

As EHR interoperability and the exchange of health information increases, best practices must be developed for handling substance use disorder treatment data, consistent with state and federal privacy laws. It will be important that EHR technologies develop the functionality to share health information electronically while complying with HIPAA, 42 CFR Part 2, and state privacy statutes. One approach to sharing protected data electronically is called Data Segmentation for Privacy (DS4P), an optional criterion under the Office of the National Coordinator for Health Information Technology's (ONC's) 2015 Edition Health IT Certification Criteria.[325] SAMHSA recently developed an open source tool called Consent2Share (C2S), which is based on DS4P and allows patients to electronically create and manage consent directives specifying which providers can access their data.

Promising Innovations That Improve Access to Substance Use Disorder Treatment

Clearly, integrating health care and substance use disorder treatment within health care systems, as well as integrating the substance use disorder treatment system with the overall health care system, are complex undertakings. The good news, however, is that a range of promising health care structures, technologies, and innovations are emerging, or are being refined and strengthened, under health reform. These developments are helping to address challenges and facilitate integration. In so doing, they are broadening the focus of interventions beyond just the treatment of severe substance use disorders to encompass the entire spectrum of prevention, treatment, and recovery. These promising developments include:

- Medicaid innovations;
- EHRs and health IT;
- Disease registries; and
- Substance misuse and substance use disorder prevention through a public health approach.

Medicaid Innovations

Medicaid is not only an increasing source of financing for substance use disorder treatment services, it has become an important incubator for innovative substance use disorder financing and delivery models that can help integrate substance use disorder treatment and mainstream health care systems. Within the substance use disorder treatment benefit, and in addition to providing the federally required set of services, states also may offer a wide range of recovery-oriented services under Medicaid's rehabilitative services option. These services include therapy, counseling, training in communication and independent living skills, recovery support and relapse prevention training, skills training to return to employment, and relationship skills. Nearly all states offer some rehabilitative mental health services, and most states offer the rehabilitation option for substance use disorder services.[328]

CMS provides various authorities by which states can structure their Medicaid programs, thus providing mechanisms for states to expand and improve their substance use disorder treatment delivery system: This includes authorities to:[328-330]

- Offer coordinating, locating, and monitoring activities broadly and create incentive payments for providers who demonstrate improved performance on quality and cost measures (section 1905(t));
- Establish Alternative Benefit Plans (ABPs), which require that substance use disorder services are included and comply with mental health parity standards (section 1937);
- Establish voluntary or mandatory managed care plans, which require parity protections for enrolled individuals (sections 1915(a) and 1915(b) authorities, and section 1932 State Option to Use Managed Care);
- Provide home and community-based services and supports (sections 1915(c), 1915(i), 1915(j), and 1915(k));
- Develop health homes (section 1945 Health Home State Plan Option); and
- Conduct demonstrations to test policy innovations (section 1115).

Recently, CMS gave states new opportunities to design service delivery systems for substance use disorders through demonstration projects under section 1115. This initiative is designed to support states to provide coverage for the full continuum of care; ensure that care is delivered consistent with the ASAM Treatment Criteria; design strategies to coordinate and integrate care; and support quality improvement programs. In 2014, CMS launched the Medicaid Innovation Accelerator Program, which aims to improve "health and health care for Medicaid beneficiaries by supporting states' efforts to accelerate new payment and service delivery reforms."[331] CMS identified substance use disorders as the program's first area of focus. The agency is providing technical and program support to states to introduce policy, program, and payment reforms to identify individuals with substance use disorders, expand coverage for effective treatment, expand access to services, and develop data collection, measurement, and payment mechanisms that promote better outcomes. Medicaid is also encouraging the trend to integration in other ways, including supporting new models for delivering primary care, expanding the role of existing community-based care delivery systems, enacting mental health and substance use disorder parity for Medicaid and Children's Health Insurance Program (CHIP) as included in the final rule that CMS finalized in March 2016. This rule requires that Medicaid enrollees in managed care organizations (MCOs) and in ABPs have access to coverage for mental health and substance use services that is in parity to coverage of medical benefits and will benefit the over 23 million people enrolled in MCOs, Medicaid ABPs, and CHIP.

Health Homes

Health homes are grounded in the principles of the primary care medical home, which focuses on primary care-based coordination of diverse health care services, and patient and provider engagement. The Affordable Care Act created an optional Medicaid State Plan benefit allowing states to establish health homes to coordinate care for participants who have chronic health conditions. Health homes operate under a "whole-person" philosophy that involves integrating and coordinating all primary, acute, behavioral health, and long-term care services to address all the individual's health needs.

Beneficiaries with chronic conditions are eligible to enroll in health homes if they experience (or are at risk for) a second chronic condition, including substance use disorders, or are experiencing serious and persistent mental health conditions.[332] Such care arrangements are particularly pertinent to individuals with substance use disorders who experience severe co-occurring physical and/or mental disorders. These arrangements emphasize integration of care, targeting of health home services to high-risk populations with substance use and mental health concerns, and integration of social and community supports with general health services.

As of January 2016, 19 states and the District of Columbia had established Medicaid health home programs – covering nearly one million individuals – and nearly a dozen additional states had plans for establishing them. States such as Vermont, Maryland, and Rhode Island have implemented health home State Plan Amendments (SPAs) with substance use-related provisions.[333] Seven other states specifically identify individuals with substance use disorders as a target population.[334] Many other SPAs include behavioral health care arrangements that encompass substance use disorders.[334,335]

States that implement Medicaid health homes receive substantial federal subsidies, including 90 percent federal matching rates for health home services during the first eight quarters after the effective date of health home coverage under the Medicaid state plan, covering comprehensive case management, coordinating services and health promotion, comprehensive transitional care from inpatient to other settings, individual and family support services, linkage and referrals to community-based services, and health IT.[336,337]

In some settings, these integrated care models are associated with reduced cost and improved cost-effectiveness,[338] and research is underway to test new models. Recognizing the important role that these kinds of integrated care arrangements can play, the American Academy of Family Physicians and SAMHSA have issued reports promoting the inclusion of substance use and mental health services in patient-centered medical homes and related efforts.[248,339,340] Much remains to be implemented in both public and private systems, but health systems are responding in a variety of ways to address substance use issues and their efforts will be key in improving treatment quality and outcomes.[249,341]

Accountable Care Organizations

Another Affordable Care Act provision created opportunities to encourage the integration of primary and specialty care, as well as community and public health systems, by establishing integrated delivery systems known as ACOs.[238] ACOs include health care professionals and hospitals that are responsible, together, for the total health of their patient populations. The motivation behind ACOs is that by being responsible for the overall health of patients and coordinating the care they provide, the collaborating health systems can achieve the "three part aim" of better quality care for individuals, reduced per capita costs, and improved population health.[342] Because ACOs can include a range of different types of providers across a defined region, they interpret "population health" in two broad ways: as a "panel population," referring to all the patients participating in the health delivery system, and as a "geographic population," referring to all who live in the ACO's defined geographic catchment area.[343]

An ACO that focuses on the larger community is called an accountable care community (ACC). ACCs are an important variation on the ACO model because, by focusing on the larger community, they can address the social determinants of health and health disparities that have such a profound impact on community members' health and well-being, including their risks for substance misuse, substance use disorders, and related health consequences.[344]

Initially developed as a model under Medicare, ACOs have now also been encouraged under Medicaid for its covered populations.[345-348] The CMS State Innovation Models (SIM) Initiative supports the development and testing of state-based models for multi-payor payment and health care delivery system transformation for improving the performance of health systems. An underlying assumption of the new service delivery and payment models funded in the SIM states is that they will be more effective and produce better outcomes when implemented as part of a broad-based, statewide initiative that brings together multiple payors and stakeholders, and when they use the levers of state government to effect change.

The SIM states are leading the implementation of accountable care systems for Medicaid populations that embrace population health (for SIM states, this is defined as health of the community in a geographic area as opposed to the population of patients in the health delivery system). Several states have adopted ACC models that support integration of medical health care services with public health and community-based programs.[238] For example, Akron in Summit County, Ohio, set up one of the first ACCs to implement community-wide public-private partnerships to improve the health of the overall population.[349] Maine's accountable communities, Oregon's CCOs, and Minnesota's accountable communities are partnering with local public health authorities and other community entities to achieve this goal.[350]

Oregon's CCOs are a network of all types of health care professionals (physical health care, addiction and mental health care, and dental care providers) who have agreed to work together to serve people who receive health care coverage under Oregon's Medicaid plan, which is called Oregon Health Plan. The Oregon Health Authority publishes regular reports on quality, access, and progress toward benchmarks in both prevention and treatment.[351] Oregon Medicaid CCOs are currently reporting, and showing progress on, three quality measures specific to substance use: use of SBIRT, initiation of substance use treatment, and engagement in treatment.

Federally Qualified Health Centers

Increased insurance coverage and other provisions of the Affordable Care Act have sparked important changes that are facilitating comprehensive, high-quality care for people with substance use disorders. For example, the Affordable Care Act provided mandatory funding for Federally Qualified Health Centers (FQHCs) receiving grants under section 330 of the public health service act, including community health centers, migrant health centers, health care for the homeless health centers, and public housing primary care centers that is supporting the expansion of their activities and numbers of patients served.

These community health centers emphasize coordinated primary and preventive services that promote reductions in health disparities for low-income individuals, racial and ethnic minorities, rural communities, and other underserved populations. Two-thirds of health centers have been designated as PCMHs.[352] PCMHs emphasize care, coordination, and communication to improve health care quality, lower health care costs, and enhance both the patient and provider experience.

Community health centers provide primary and preventive health services to medically underserved areas and populations and may offer behavioral and mental health and substance use services as appropriate to meet the health needs of the population served by the health center. As such, they are well-equipped to address co-occurring physical, mental, and substance use disorders, and provide substance misuse prevention, treatment, and RSS to patients. Because they provide services regardless of ability to pay and are required to offer services on a sliding scale fee, they are well-positioned to serve low-income and economically vulnerable patients.

An example of the important role FQHCs can play in improving access to treatment for substance use disorders is their efforts in providing buprenorphine maintenance treatment for opioid-dependent patients within primary care. In 2016, $94 million was awarded by HRSA to 271 health centers in 45 states, the District of Columbia, and Puerto Rico with a focus on augmenting capacity to treat opioid use disorders in vulnerable populations. FQHCs have access to 340B drug pricing, making the purchase of substance use disorder medications less costly and thus more accessible than for providers who cannot take advantage of this pricing.[353] Recent services research indicates that such arrangements can achieve comparable outcomes to those achieved within the specialty addiction treatment sector.[354]

Electronic Health Records and Health Information Technology

EHRs and health IT have the potential to support better coordination of services across primary care and specialty substance use disorder treatment, greater safety by reducing harmful drug-drug interactions, and improved monitoring of treatment outcomes and relapse risk in general health care.

Strong health IT systems improve the organization and usability of clinical data, thereby helping patients, health care professionals, and health system leaders coordinate care, promote shared decision-making, and engage in quality improvement efforts. These systems have the capacity to easily provide information in multiple languages and to put patients in touch with culturally appropriate providers through telehealth.

"Meaningful use" rules from CMS now provide incentives for the use of certified health IT to facilitate care coordination. Medicare and Medicaid EHR Incentive Programs have thus far paid more than $34.5 billion in incentive payments for providers who adopt, implement, upgrade, and use certified EHR technology.[355] These incentives have worked: The *National Electronic Health Record Survey* found that as of 2014, more than 80 percent of primary care physicians had adopted an EHR, and more than half were using all basic functions.[356] These were the highest rates of any physician type using certified EHRs.

> **KEY TERMS**
>
> **Meaningful Use.** Using certified EHR technology to improve quality, safety, efficiency, and reduce health disparities; engage patients and family; improve care coordination and population and public health; and maintain privacy and security of patient health information.[2]

Health IT has shown benefits in improving care for patients with chronic conditions,[357] and use is expected to greatly increase because of the Affordable Care Act and related incentives, such as grants supporting health center networks with the implementation and adoption of health IT.[358-361] To further heighten uptake and implementation, CMS issued new rules to "ease the reporting burden for providers, support interoperability, and improve patient outcomes," including giving states and providers more time to comply with regulations and focusing on health information interoperability between providers and patients.[335,362] Additionally, CMS recently published its proposed rule on the Medicare Access and CHIP Reauthorization Act (MACRA) of 2015, providing incentives for using health IT to report quality measure results.

Health IT also holds great potential for improving services for individuals with substance misuse problems because they can provide up-to-date medical histories of patients to providers, and they can support care coordination by facilitating communications between primary and specialty care providers across health systems.[363] Clinical decision support tools can also help support improvements in care and include clinical guidelines, diagnostic support, condition-specific order sets, computerized alerts and reminders to care providers as well as patients, focused patient data reports and summaries, documentation templates, and contextually relevant reference information, among others. For example, educational and training materials including clinical guidelines for physicians (e.g., *Helping Patients Who Drink Too Much: A Clinician's Guide*[364]), can be made available through EHRs. Many health systems have additional information on wikis for patients and providers. Most have or will have patient portal websites, which can provide patients access to health, mental health, and substance use self-assessments; computerized interventions for reducing alcohol or drug use, anger management, dealing with depression, and other

> **KEY TERMS**
>
> **Clinical Decision Support.** A system that provides health care professionals, staff, patients, or other individuals with knowledge and person-specific information, intelligently filtered or presented at appropriate times, to enhance health and health care.

problems; referral sources for smoking quit-lines and self-help groups; information on medications for substance use disorders; and general health information.

Although research suggests that patients with substance use disorders are not using patient portals as much as individuals with other conditions,[365] they have great potential for reaching patients.[366-368] In particular, because they can be culturally relevant, these innovations may be helpful in providing substance use disorder services to individuals who do not have access to, or are hesitant to participate in, traditional services, or to augment those services, thereby helping to reduce health disparities.

To foster systems change, efforts are needed to increase adoption of EHR technology in substance use disorder and mental health treatment organizations. These programs currently lag and are likely to continue to lag behind the rest of medicine. It will be critical to facilitate the uptake of EHRs within the specialty substance use disorder treatment system, to implement common data standards to support interoperability across specialty substance use disorder treatment and mainstream health care, and to coordinate care across systems. The federal interagency Behavioral Health Coordinating Council recently created a quality metrics subcommittee tasked with ensuring that substance use and mental health performance and quality measures are consistently and appropriately included across payment systems of HHS, including diverse programs within CMS. The National Institute on Drug Abuse (NIDA) and NIAAA have developed common data elements for inclusion in EHRs, and SAMHSA supports the development of data standards for collecting behavioral health data in EHRs through the international standards development organization, Health Level 7, though none of these standards has been widely implemented to date.[364,369,370]

PDMPs are becoming an increasingly important health IT tool for preventing substance misuse and identifying patients with substance use disorders. As discussed above, PDMPs are state-run databases that collect prescribed and dispensed controlled prescriptions drug information and give providers and pharmacists access to information about a person's controlled substance prescription history. They are designed to help identify patients (as well as providers) who are misusing or diverting (i.e., channeling drugs into illegal use) these medications who would benefit from early interventions. This technology represents a promising state-level intervention for improving opioid prescribing, informing clinical practice, and protecting patients at risk in the midst of the ongoing opioid overdose epidemic. A number of states have passed legislation requiring prescribers to check their PDMP before prescribing controlled substances. Additional research is needed to identify best practices and policies to maximize the efficacy of these programs.

Disease Registries

Databases related to specific diseases or combinations of diseases have long been used by health care professionals to manage chronic conditions such as diabetes or HIV/AIDS. Now these disease registries are being developed for substance use disorders, such as opioid use disorder.[371] Although privacy concerns exist, disease registries can alert providers to the health care needs of those at risk because of substance misuse, including patients receiving opioids for chronic pain. Even low levels of alcohol and drug use are important factors in this population.[372]

Prevention of Substance Misuse and Substance Use Disorders Through Public Health Approaches

Because substance use disorders often first come to light in the context of school, law enforcement, and employment, communities have many opportunities to expand the delivery of prevention and treatment services to include schools and school-based health care clinics, jails and prisons, and places of employment. Services provided in these settings can range from prevention education to SBIRT to treatment for substance use disorders. For example, law enforcement and emergency medical services in many communities are already collaborating in the distribution and administration of naloxone to prevent opioid overdose deaths.

These efforts require a public health approach and the development of a comprehensive community infrastructure, which in turn requires coordination across federal, state, local, and tribal agencies. A number of states are developing promising approaches to address substance use in their communities. One recent example is Minnesota's 2012 State Substance Abuse Strategy, which includes a comprehensive strategy focused on strengthening prevention; creating more opportunities for intervening before problems become severe; integrating the identification and treatment of substance use disorders into health care reform efforts; expanding support for recovery; interrupting the cycle of substance use, crime, and incarceration; reducing trafficking, production, and sale of illegal drugs; and measuring the impact of various interventions.[373]

Comprehensive Addiction and Recovery Act (CARA)

On July 22, 2016, President Obama signed the Comprehensive Addiction and Recovery Act (CARA), into law. CARA aims to address the national epidemic of opioid addiction by creating and expanding federal grant programs to:

- Temporarily expand eligibility to prescribe buprenorphine-based drugs for MAT for substance use disorders to qualifying nurse practitioners and physician assistants, through October 1, 2021;
- Expand access to opioid overdose reversal drugs, by supporting the purchase and distribution of such medications and training for first responders;
- Increase awareness and educate the public regarding the misuse of prescription opioids;
- Reauthorize the National All Schedules Prescription Electronic Reporting (NASPER) Act, which provides grants to states to support and improve interoperability of PDMPs;
- Authorize Medicare prescription drug plans to develop a safe prescribing and dispensing program for beneficiaries that are at risk of misuse or diversion of drugs that are frequently abused or diverted;
- Create a comprehensive program at U.S. Department of Justice to improve efforts by law enforcement and the criminal justice system to address substance use disorders; and
- Establish an HHS-led task force to consolidate federal best practices for pain management.

These measures are important steps for reducing the impact of prescription drug misuse on America's communities by preventing and responding to opioid addiction. However, given the large number of Americans with untreated or inadequately treated opioid use disorders and the current scarcity of treatment resources, there is concern that the lack of funding for the bill will prevent this new law from having a substantial impact on the nation's ongoing opioid epidemic.

HEALTH CARE SYSTEMS

The opioid guideline published by the Washington State Agency Medical Directors' Group is another useful example. This group is composed of medical directors from seven state agencies, including the Department of Labor and Industries, the Health Care Authority, the Board of Health, the Health Officer, the Department of Veterans Affairs, the Office of the Insurance Commissioner, and the Department of Corrections. In 2007, the group developed its first opioid prescribing guideline in collaboration with practicing physicians, with the latest update released in 2015.[374] The guideline offers an approach to pain management that includes recommendations for appropriate opioid prescribing and management.

States' and localities' efforts to expand naloxone distribution provide another example of building a comprehensive, multipronged, community infrastructure. Many communities have recognized the need to make this potentially lifesaving medication more widely available. For example, community leaders in Wilkes County, North Carolina, implemented *Project Lazarus*, a model that expands access to naloxone for law enforcement, emergency services, education, and health services, and reduced the county overdose rate by half within a year. North Carolina also passed a law in 2013 that implemented standing orders, allowing naloxone to be dispensed from a pharmacy without a prescription.[375]

States have also expanded training on naloxone use for opioid users and their families and friends, as well as for a wide range of social service agency personnel. Federal partners have been instrumental in expanding access to naloxone training. HRSA established the Rural Opioid Overdose Reversal program in fiscal year 2015, awarding grants of $100,000 to 18 recipients representing 13 states to increase access to naloxone and train health care professionals and other social service personnel to administer the drug. In 2016, SAMHSA also provided $11,000,000 in funding to prevent prescription drug/opioid overdose-related deaths among individuals aged 18 or older by training first responders and other community stakeholders on prevention strategies.

A few states have passed legislation to make naloxone more readily available without a prescription if certain procedures are followed.[376,377] As of July 2015, 30 states have passed laws to provide legal protection to physician prescribers and to bystanders ("Good Samaritans") who administer naloxone when encountering an overdose situation.[378] Additionally, 48 states allow pharmacists to enter into Collaborative Pharmacy Practice Agreements with prescribers, which allow naloxone to be dispensed to those who may be able to use it to save lives.[379] For example, the Rhode Island Board of Pharmacy approved this type of agreement, which began in 2011 as a pilot program in five pharmacies. This program was expanded to all interested pharmacies in 2013 and formalized in regulation in 2014.[380,381]

States have also expanded naloxone coverage under Medicaid. The CDC reported more than 26,000 overdose reversals by lay people between 1996 and 2014, all using naloxone.[382] Health systems are developing protocols to dispense naloxone through primary care providers, pharmacies, and emergency departments. The need to engage individuals in services to address their opioid use is a critical next step following an overdose reversal. This becomes increasingly challenging as naloxone kits are distributed widely, rather than when distribution is limited to health care and substance use disorder treatment providers. In 2013, the State of Vermont implemented an innovative treatment system with the goal of increasing access to opioid treatment throughout the state. This model, called the "Hub and Spoke" approach, met this need by providing physicians throughout the state with training and supports for providing evidence-based buprenorphine treatment.

The result has been:[383,384]

- An increase in the number of physicians providing buprenorphine treatment by over 40 percent;
- The transition of several hundred individuals served in traditional OTP programs to certified physicians in primary care settings;
- Better access throughout the state to opioid treatment due to the expansion of entry points, and physician/OTP coordination; and
- An increased integration of primary care and addiction treatment.

Recommendations for Research

A key finding from this chapter is that the traditional separation of specialty addiction treatment from mainstream health care has created obstacles to successful care coordination. Research is needed in three main areas:

- Models of integration of substance use services within mainstream health care;
- Models of providing ongoing, chronic care within health care systems; and
- Models of care coordination between specialty treatment systems and mainstream health care.

In each of these areas, research is needed on the development of interventions and strategies for successfully implementing them. Outcomes for each model should include feasibility, substance use and other health outcomes, and cost.

Although a great deal of research has shown that integrating health care services has potential value both in terms of outcomes and cost, only a few models of integration have been empirically tested. Mechanisms through the Affordable Care Act make it possible to provide and test innovative structural and financing models for integration within mainstream health care. This research should cover the continuum of care, from prevention and early intervention to treatment and recovery, and will help health systems move forward with integration. This research should explore innovative delivery models including telemedicine and other health IT, as well as health or wellness coaching. Studies should focus on patient-centered approaches and should address appropriate interventions for individuals across race and ethnicity, culture, language, sex, sexual orientation, gender identity, disability, health literacy, and for those living in rural areas. So as not to limit health care systems to services for those with mild or moderate substance misuse problems and to offer support for individuals with severe problems who are not motivated to go to specialty substance use disorder treatment, it is also important to study how to implement medication and other evidence-based treatments across diverse health care systems.

This chapter pointed out that when substance use problems become severe, providing ongoing, chronic care is required, as is the case for many other diseases. Little research has studied chronic care models for the treatment of substance use disorders. Research is needed to develop and test innovative models of care coordination and their implementation. This research should use a more broadly defined workforce in both health care and substance use disorder treatment, develop models to share information electronically, and support coordination of care between health systems using health IT.

Finally, the chapter pointed out the gap in our understanding of how to implement models of care coordination between specialty addiction treatment organizations and social service systems, which provide important wrap-around services to substance use disorder patients. Many models are in existence, but have not been empirically tested. This area of research should involve institutions that provide services to individuals with serious co-occurring problems (specialty mental health agencies), individuals with legal problems (criminal justice agencies and drug courts), individuals with employment or other social issues, as well as the larger community, determining how to most effectively link each of these subpopulations with a recovery-oriented systems of care.

References

1. World Health Organization. (2015). Health systems strengthening glossary, G-H. *Health Systems.* Retrieved from http://www.who.int/healthsystems/hss_glossary/en/index5.html. Accessed on August 16, 2016.

2. HealthIT.gov. (2015). Meaningful use definition & objectives. Retrieved from https://www.healthit.gov/providers-professionals/meaningful-use-definition-objectives. Accessed on July 29, 2016.

3. SAMHSA-HRSA Center for Integrated Health Solutions. (2016). What is integrated care? Retrieved from http://www.integration.samhsa.gov/resource/what-is-integrated-care. Accessed on April 28, 2016.

4. Institute of Medicine (IOM). (2013). *Best care at lower cost: The path to continuously learning health care in America.* (0309260736). Washington, DC: The National Academies Press.

5. Puddy, R. W., & Wilkins, N. (2011). *Understanding evidence Part 1: Best available research evidence. A guide to the continuum of evidence of effectiveness.* Atlanta, GA: Centers for Disease Control and Prevention.

6. Larochelle, M. R., Liebschutz, J. M., Zhang, F., Ross-Degnan, D., & Wharam, J. F. (2016). Opioid prescribing after nonfatal overdose and association with repeated overdose: A cohort study. *Annals of Internal Medicine, 164*(1), 1-9.

7. Binswanger, I. A., Stern, M. F., Deyo, R. A., Heagerty, P. J., Cheadle, A., Elmore, J. G., & Koepsell, T. D. (2007). Release from prison—A high risk of death for former inmates. *New England Journal of Medicine, 356*(2), 157-165.

8. Baumohl, J., & Room, R. (1987). Inebriety, doctors and the state: Alcoholism treatment institutions before 1940. In M. Galanter (Ed.), *Recent Developments in Alcoholism* (Vol. 5, pp. 135-174). New York, NY: Plenum.

9. Baumohl, J., & Jaffe, J. H. (2001). Treatment, history of, in the United States. In R. Carson-DeSwitt (Ed.), *Encyclopedia of Drugs, Alcohol, and Addictive Behavior.* (2nd ed.). New York, NY: The Gale Group.

10. Weisner, C., & Morgan, P. (1992). Rapid growth and bifurcation: Public and private alcohol treatment in the United States. *Cure, care or Control: Alcoholism treatment in sixteen countries,* 223-251.

11. White, W. L. (1998). *Slaying the dragon: The history of addiction treatment and recovery in America.* Bloomington, IL: Chestnut Health Systems/Lighthouse Institute.

12. McLellan, A. T., Lewis, D. C., O'Brien, C. P., & Kleber, H. D. (2000). Drug dependence, a chronic medical illness: Implications for treatment, insurance, and outcomes evaluation. *JAMA, 284*(13), 1689-1695.

13. Soderstrom, C. A., Smith, G. S., Dischinger, P. C., McDuff, D. R., Hebel, J. R., Gorelick, D. A., . . . Read, K. M. (1997). Psychoactive substance use disorders among seriously injured trauma center patients. *JAMA, 277*(22), 1769-1774.

14. Wu, L.-T., Swartz, M. S., Wu, Z., Mannelli, P., Yang, C., & Blazer, D. G. (2012). Alcohol and drug use disorders among adults in emergency department settings in the United States. *Annals of Emergency Medicine, 60*(2), 172-180. e175.

15. Brown, R. L., Leonard, T., Saunders, L. A., & Papasouliotis, O. (1998). The prevalence and detection of substance use disorders among inpatients ages 18 to 49: An opportunity for prevention. *Preventive Medicine, 27*(1), 101-110.

16. Scott, K. M., Lim, C., Al-Hamzawi, A., Alonso, J., Bruffaerts, R., Caldas-de-Almeida, J. M., . . . de Jonge, P. (2016). Association of mental disorders with subsequent chronic physical conditions: World mental health surveys from 17 countries. *JAMA Psychiatry, 73*(2), 150-158.

17. Parish, C. L., Pereyra, M. R., Pollack, H. A., Cardenas, G., Castellon, P. C., Abel, S. N., . . . Metsch, L. R. (2015). Screening for substance misuse in the dental care setting: Findings from a nationally representative survey of dentists. *Addiction, 110*(9), 1516-1523.

18. Denisco, R. C., Kenna, G. A., O'Neil, M. G., Kulich, R. J., Moore, P. A., Kane, W. T., . . . Katz, N. P. (2011). Prevention of prescription opioid abuse: The role of the dentist. *The Journal of the American Dental Association, 142*(7), 800-810.

19. Krause, M., Vainio, L., Zwetchkenbaum, S., & Inglehart, M. R. (2010). Dental education about patients with special needs: A survey of US and Canadian dental schools. *Journal of Dental Education, 74*(11), 1179-1189.

20. O'Connor, P. G., Nyquist, J. G., & McLellan, A. T. (2011). Integrating addiction medicine into graduate medical education in primary care: The time has come. *Annals of Internal Medicine, 154*(1), 56-59.

21. McLellan, A. T., & Meyers, K. (2004). Contemporary addiction treatment: A review of systems problems for adults and adolescents. *Biological Psychiatry, 56*(10), 764-770.

22. Miller, N. S., Sheppard, L. M., Colenda, C. C., & Magen, J. (2001). Why physicians are unprepared to treat patients who have alcohol-and drug-related disorders. *Academic Medicine, 76*(5), 410-418.

23. D'Amico, E. J., Paddock, S. M., Burnam, A., & Kung, F.-Y. (2005). Identification of and guidance for problem drinking by general medical providers: Results from a national survey. *Medical Care, 43*(3), 229-236.

24. Knudsen, H. K., Abraham, A. J., & Oser, C. B. (2011). Barriers to the implementation of medication-assisted treatment for substance use disorders: the importance of funding policies and medical infrastructure. *Eval Program Plann, 34*(4), 375-381.

25. Mattick, R. P., Breen, C., Kimber, J., & Davoli, M. (2014). Buprenorphine maintenance versus placebo or methadone maintenance for opioid dependence. *Cochrane Database of Systematic Reviews, 2*.

26. MacDonald, K., Lamb, K., Thomas, M. L., & Khentigan, W. (2016). Buprenorphine maintenance treatment of opiate dependence: Correlations between prescriber beliefs and practices. *Substance Use & Misuse, 51*(1), 85-90.

27. Mattick, R. P., Breen, C., Kimber, J., & Davoli, M. (2009). Methadone maintenance therapy versus no opioid replacement therapy for opioid dependence. *Cochrane Database Syst Rev*(3), Cd002209.

28. Nunes, E. V., Krupitsky, E., Ling, W., Zummo, J., Memisoglu, A., Silverman, B. L., & Gastfriend, D. R. (2015). Treating opioid dependence with injectable extended-release naltrexone (XR-NTX): Who will respond? *Journal of Addiction Medicine, 9*(3), 238-243.

29. Institute of Medicine Division of Mental Health and Behavioral Medicine. (1990). *Broadening the base of treatment for alcohol problems.* Washington, DC: National Academy of Sciences.

30. Gerstein, D. R., & Lewin, L. S. (1990). Treating drug problems. *New England Journal of Medicine, 323*(12), 844-848.

31. Institute of Medicine Committee on Quality of Health Care in America. (2001). *Crossing the quality chasm: A new health system for the 21st century.* (0309073227). Washington, DC: National Academies Press.

32. Institute of Medicine, & Committee on Crossing the Quality Chasm. (2006). *Improving the quality of health care for mental and substance-use conditions.* Washington, DC: National Academies Press.

33. Congressional Budget Office. (n.d.). *Insurance coverage provisions of the Affordable Care Act: CBOS March 2015 baseline.*

34. U.S. Department of Health and Human Services. (2016). *Health insurance coverage and the affordable care act, 2010–2016.* Washington, DC: Assistant Secretary for Planning and Evaluation.

35. Mark, T. L., Wier, L. M., Malone, K., Penne, M., & Cowell, A. J. (2015). National estimates of behavioral health conditions and their treatment among adults newly insured under the ACA. *Psychiatric Services, 66*(4), 426-429.

36. Artiga, S., Stephens, J., & Damico, A. (2015). The impact of the coverage gap in states not expanding Medicaid by race and ethnicity. *The Henry J. Kaiser Family Foundation.* Retrieved from http://kff.org/disparities-policy/issue-brief/the-impact-of-the-coverage-gap-in-states-not-expanding-medicaid-by-race-and-ethnicity/. Accessed on October 8, 2015.

37. Garfield, R., Damico, A., & Cox, C. (2015). *New estimates of eligibility for ACA coverage among the uninsured.* Washington, DC: Kaiser Family Foundation.

38. Crowley, R. A., & Kirschner, N. (2015). The integration of care for mental health, substance abuse, and other behavioral health conditions into primary care: Executive summary of an American College of Physicians position paper. *Annals of Internal Medicine, 163*(4), 298-299.

39. Centers for Medicare & Medicaid Services. (2015). *Screening, brief intervention, and referral to treatment (SBIRT) services.* (ICN 904084). Washington, DC: U.S. Department of Health and Human Services.

40. Centers for Medicare & Medicaid Services. (2011). Decision memo for screening and behavioral counseling interventions in primary care to reduce alcohol misuse (CAG-00427N). Retrieved from https://www.cms.gov/medicare-coverage-database/details/nca-decision-memo.aspx?NCAId=249&ver=5&NcaName=Screening+and+Behavioral+Counseling+Interventions+in+Primary+Care+to+Reduce+Alcohol+Misuse&DocID=CAG-00427N&bc=gAAAAgAIAAA&. Accessed on April 6, 2016.

41. U.S. Department of Labor. (2013). FAQs about Affordable Care Act implementation part XII. Retrieved from http://www.dol.gov/ebsa/faqs/faq-aca12.html. Accessed on April 6, 2016.

42. Jonas, D. E., Garbutt, J. C., & Amick, H. R. (2012). Behavioral counseling after screening for alcohol misuse in primary care: A systematic review and meta-analysis for the U.S. Preventive Services Task Force. *Annals of Internal Medicine, 157*(9), 645-654.

43. Moyer, V. A. (2013). Screening and behavioral counseling interventions in primary care to reduce alcohol misuse: U.S. Preventive Services Task Force recommendation statement. *Annals of Internal Medicine, 159*(3), 210-218.

44. Maciosek, M. V., Coffield, A. B., Edwards, N. M., Flottemesch, T. J., Goodman, M. J., & Solberg, L. I. (2006). Priorities among effective clinical preventive services: Results of a systematic review and analysis. *American Journal of Preventive Medicine, 31*(1), 52-61.

45. Solberg, L. I., Maciosek, M. V., & Edwards, N. M. (2008). Primary care intervention to reduce alcohol misuse: Ranking its health impact and cost effectiveness. *American Journal of Preventive Medicine, 34*(2), 143-152.

46. Roy-Byrne, P., Bumgardner, K., Krupski, A., Dunn, C., Ries, R., Donovan, D., . . . Graves, M. C. (2014). Brief intervention for problem drug use in safety-net primary care settings: A randomized clinical trial. *JAMA, 312*(5), 492-501.

47. Saitz, R., Palfai, T. P., Cheng, D. M., Alford, D. P., Bernstein, J. A., Lloyd-Travaglini, C. A., . . . Samet, J. H. (2014). Screening and brief intervention for drug use in primary care: The ASPIRE randomized clinical trial. *JAMA, 312*(5), 502-513.

48. Gelberg, L., Andersen, R. M., Afifi, A. A., Leake, B. D., Arangua, L., Vahidi, M., . . . Fleming, M. F. (2015). Project QUIT (Quit Using Drugs Intervention Trial): A randomized controlled trial of a primary care-based multi-component brief intervention to reduce risky drug use. *Addiction, 110*(11), 1777-1790.

49. Heinzerling, K. G., Ober, A. J., Lamp, K., De Vries, D., & Watkins, K. E. (2016). *SUMMIT: Procedures for medication-assisted treatment of alcohol or opioid dependence in primary care.* Santa Monica, CA: RAND Corporation.

50. Shapiro, B., Coffa, D., & McCance-Katz, E. F. (2013). A primary care approach to substance misuse. *American Family Physician, 88*(2), 113-121.

51. Manchikanti, L., Helm II, S., Fellows, B., Janata, J. W., Pampati, V., Grider, J. S., & Boswell, M. V. (2012). Opioid epidemic in the United States. *Pain Physician, 15*(Suppl 3), ES9-ES38.

52. Weisner, C. M., Campbell, C. I., Ray, G. T., Saunders, K., Merrill, J. O., Banta-Green, C., . . . Boudreau, D. (2009). Trends in prescribed opioid therapy for non-cancer pain for individuals with prior substance use disorders. *Pain, 145*(3), 287-293.

53. Campbell, C. I., Weisner, C., LeResche, L., Ray, G. T., Saunders, K., Sullivan, M. D., . . . Boudreau, D. (2010). Age and gender trends in long-term opioid analgesic use for noncancer pain. *American Journal of Public Health, 100*(12), 2541-2547.

54. Office of the Assistant Secretary for Planning and Evaluation. (2015). *Opioid abuse in the U.S. and HHS actions to address opioid-drug related overdoses and deaths.* Washington, DC: U.S. Department of Health and Human Services.

55. Dowell, D., Haegerich, T. M., & R., C. (2016). CDC guideline for prescribing opioids for chronic pain - United States. *MMWR, 65*(1), 1-49.

56. Office of the Assistant Secretary for Health. (2016). *National pain strategy: A comprehensive population health-level strategy for pain.* Washington, DC: U.S. Department of Health and Human Services.

57. National Heroin Task Force. (2015). *National heroin task force final report and recommendations.* Washington, DC: U.S. Department of Justice and The White House Office of National Drug Control Policy.

58. Muhuri, P. K., Gfroerer, J. C., & Davies, M. C. (2013). Associations of nonmedical pain reliever use and initiation of heroin use in the United States. *CBHSQ Data Review*, 1-17.

59. Cicero, T. J., Ellis, M. S., Surratt, H. L., & Kurtz, S. P. (2014). The changing face of heroin use in the United States: A retrospective analysis of the past 50 years. *JAMA Psychiatry, 71*(7), 821-826.

60. Substance Abuse and Mental Health Services Administration. (2013). *SAMHSA Opioid overdose prevention toolkit.* (HHS Publication No. (SMA) 13-4742). Rockville, MD: Substance Abuse and Mental Health Services Administration.

61. Mueller, S. R., Walley, A. Y., Calcaterra, S. L., Glanz, J. M., & Binswanger, I. A. (2015). A review of opioid overdose prevention and naloxone prescribing: Implications for translating community programming into clinical practice. *Substance Abuse, 36*(2), 240-253.

62. Binswanger, I. A., Koester, S., Mueller, S. R., Gardner, E. M., Goddard, K., & Glanz, J. M. (2015). Overdose education and naloxone for patients prescribed opioids in primary care: A qualitative study of primary care staff. *Journal of General Internal Medicine, 30*(12), 1837-1844.

63. Compton, W. M., Blanco, C., & Wargo, E. M. (2015). Integrating addiction services into general medicine. *JAMA, 314*(22), 2401-2402.

64. Mertens, J. R., Lu, Y. W., Parthasarathy, S., Moore, C., & Weisner, C. M. (2003). Medical and psychiatric conditions of alcohol and drug treatment patients in an HMO: Comparison with matched controls. *Archives of Internal Medicine, 163*(20), 2511-2517.

65. Grant, B. F., & Dawson, D. A. (1999). Alcohol and drug use, abuse, and dependence: classification, prevalence, and comorbidity. In B. S. McCrady & E. E. Epstein (Eds.), *Addictions: A comprehensive guidebook.* (pp. 9-29). New York, NY: Oxford University Press.

66. Weisner, C., Mertens, J., Parthasarathy, S., Moore, C., & Lu, Y. (2001). Integrating primary medical care with addiction treatment: A randomized controlled trial. *JAMA, 286*(14), 1715-1723.

67. Stein, M. D. (1999). Medical consequences of substance abuse. *Psychiatric Clinics of North America, 22*(2), 351-370.

68. Wachino, V. (2015). *Re: New service delivery opportunities for individuals with a substance use disorder.* (SMD # 15-003). Baltimore, MD: U.S. Department of Health and Human Services, Centers for Medicare and Medicaid Services. Retrieved from https://www.medicaid.gov/federal-policy-guidance/downloads/SMD15003.pdf. Accessed on April 6, 2016.

69. Mertens, J. R., Weisner, C., Ray, G. T., Fireman, B., & Walsh, K. (2005). Hazardous drinkers and drug users in HMO primary care: Prevalence, medical conditions, and costs. *Alcoholism: Clinical and Experimental Research, 29*(6), 989-998.

70. Lange, R. A., & Hillis, L. D. (2001). Cardiovascular complications of cocaine use. *New England Journal of Medicine, 345*(5), 351-358.

71. Rubin, R. B., & Neugarten, J. (1992). Medical complications of cocaine: Changes in pattern of use and spectrum of complications. *Journal of Toxicology: Clinical Toxicology, 30*(1), 1-12.

72. Ashton, C. H. (2001). Pharmacology and effects of cannabis: A brief review. *British Journal of Psychiatry, 178,* 101-106.

73. Hall, W., & Solowij, N. (1998). Adverse effects of cannabis. *The Lancet, 352*(9140), 1611-1616.

74. Volkow, N. D., Baler, R. D., Compton, W. M., & Weiss, S. R. B. (2014). Adverse health effects of marijuana use. *New England Journal of Medicine, 370*(23), 2219-2227.

75. Rehm, J., Mathers, C., Popova, S., Thavorncharoensap, M., Teerawattananon, Y., & Patra, J. (2009). Global burden of disease and injury and economic cost attributable to alcohol use and alcohol-use disorders. *The Lancet, 373*(9682), 2223-2233.

76. Middleton Fillmore, K., Chikritzhs, T., Stockwell, T., Bostrom, A., & Pascal, R. (2009). Alcohol use and prostate cancer: A meta-analysis. *Molecular Nutrition & Food Research, 53*(2), 240-255.

77. Bagnardi, V., Rota, M., Botteri, E., Tramacere, I., Islami, F., Fedirko, V., . . . Pasquali, E. (2015). Alcohol consumption and site-specific cancer risk: A comprehensive dose–response meta-analysis. *British Journal of Cancer, 112*(3), 580-593.

78. Jung, S., Wang, M., Anderson, K., Baglietto, L., Bergkvist, L., Bernstein, L., . . . Eliassen, A. H. (2015). Alcohol consumption and breast cancer risk by estrogen receptor status: In a pooled analysis of 20 studies. *International Journal of Epidemiology*.

79. May, P. A., Gossage, J. P., Kalberg, W. O., Robinson, L. K., Buckley, D., Manning, M., & Hoyme, H. E. (2009). Prevalence and epidemiologic characteristics of FASD from various research methods with an emphasis on recent in-school studies. *Developmental Disabilities Research Review, 15*(3), 176-192.

80. May, P. A., Baete, A., Russo, J., Elliott, A. J., Blankenship, J., Kalberg, W. O., . . . Hoyme, H. E. (2014). Prevalence and characteristics of fetal alcohol spectrum disorders. *Pediatrics, 134*(5), 855-866.

81. U.S. National Library of Medicine. (2015). Neonatal abstinence syndrome. Retrieved from https://www.nlm.nih.gov/medlineplus/ency/article/007313.htm. Accessed on July 5, 2016.

82. Patrick, S., Davis, M., Lehmann, C., & Cooper, W. (2015). Increasing incidence and geographic distribution of neonatal abstinence syndrome: United States 2009 to 2012. *Journal of Perinatology, 35*(8), 650-655.

83. National Institute on Drug Abuse. (2015). Dramatic increases in maternal opioid use and neonatal abstinence syndrome. Retrieved from https://www.drugabuse.gov/related-topics/trends-statistics/infographics/dramatic-increases-in-maternal-opioid-use-neonatal-abstinence-syndrome. Accessed on July 5, 2016.

84. Floyd, R. L., Jack, B. W., Cefalo, R., Atrash, H., Mahoney, J., Herron, A., . . . Sokol, R. J. (2008). The clinical content of preconception care: Alcohol, tobacco, and illicit drug exposures. *American Journal of Obstetrics and Gynecology, 199*(6), S333-S339.

85. Aarons, G. A., Brown, S. A., Coe, M. T., Myers, M. G., Garland, A. F., Ezzet-Lofstram, R., . . . Hough, R. L. (1999). Adolescent alcohol and drug abuse and health. *Journal of Adolescent Health, 24*(6), 412-421.

86. Arria, A. M., Dohey, M. A., Mezzich, A. C., Bukstein, O. G., & Van Thiel, D. H. (1995). Self-reported health problems and physical symptomatology in adolescent alcohol abusers. *Journal of Adolescent Health, 16*(3), 226-231.

87. Clark, D. B., Lynch, K. G., Donovan, J. E., & Block, G. D. (2001). Health problems in adolescents with alcohol use disorders: Self-report, liver injury, and physical examination findings and correlates. *Alcoholism: Clinical and Experimental Research, 25*(9), 1350-1359.

88. Wachino, V., & Hyde, P. S. (2015). *Coverage of behavioral health services for youth with substance use disorders.* Joint CMCS and SAMHSA Informational Bulletin. Rockville & Baltimore, MD: Substance Abuse and Mental Health Services Administration, Center for Medicaid and CHIP Services.

89. Shrier, L. A., Harris, S. K., Sternberg, M., & Beardslee, W. R. (2001). Associations of depression, self-esteem, and substance use with sexual risk among adolescents. *Preventive Medicine, 33*(3), 179-189.

90. Schwartz, R. H., Luxenberg, M. G., & Hoffmann, N. G. (1991). "Crack" use by American middle-class adolescent polydrug abusers. *Journal of Pediatrics, 118*(1), 150-155.

91. Mertens, J. R., Flisher, A. J., Fleming, M. F., & Weisner, C. M. (2007). Medical conditions of adolescents in alcohol and drug treatment: Comparison with matched controls. *Journal of Adolescent Health, 40*(2), 173-179.

92. Grella, C. E., Hser, Y. I., Joshi, V., & Rounds-Bryant, J. (2001). Drug treatment outcomes for adolescents with comorbid mental and substance use disorders. *Journal of Nervous and Mental Disease, 189*(6), 384-392.

93. Sterling, S., & Weisner, C. (2005). Chemical dependency and psychiatric services for adolescents in private managed care: Implications for outcomes. *Alcoholism: Clinical and Experimental Research, 29*(5), 801-809.

94. Dunne, E. M., Hearn, L. E., Rose, J. J., & Latimer, W. W. (2014). ADHD as a risk factor for early onset and heightened adult problem severity of illicit substance use: An accelerated gateway model. *Addictive Behaviors, 39*(12), 1755-1758.

95. Groenman, A. P., Oosterlaan, J., Rommelse, N., Franke, B., Roeyers, H., Oades, R. D., . . . Faraone, S. V. (2013). Substance use disorders in adolescents with attention deficit hyperactivity disorder: A 4-year follow-up study. *Addiction, 108*(8), 1503-1511.

96. Levy, S., Katusic, S. K., Colligan, R. C., Weaver, A. L., Killian, J. M., Voigt, R. G., & Barbaresi, W. J. (2014). Childhood ADHD and risk for substance dependence in adulthood: A longitudinal, population-based study. *PLOS One, 9*(8), 1-9.

97. Wilens, T. E., & Spencer, T. J. (2010). Understanding attention-deficit/hyperactivity disorder from childhood to adulthood. *Postgraduate Medicine, 122*(5), 97-109.

98. Zulauf, C. A., Sprich, S. E., Safren, S. A., & Wilens, T. E. (2014). The complicated relationship between attention deficit/hyperactivity disorder and substance use disorders. *Current Psychiatry Reports, 16*(3), 436-453.

99. Elkins, I. J., McGue, M., & Iacono, W. G. (2007). Prospective effects of attention-deficit/hyperactivity disorder, conduct disorder, and sex on adolescent substance use and abuse. *Archives of General Psychiatry, 64*(10), 1145-1152.

100. Degenhardt, L., Coffey, C., Romaniuk, H., Swift, W., Carlin, J. B., Hall, W. D., & Patton, G. C. (2013). The persistence of the association between adolescent cannabis use and common mental disorders into young adulthood. *Addiction, 108*(1), 124-133.

101. Armstrong, T. D., & Costello, E. J. (2002). Community studies on adolescent substance use, abuse, or dependence and psychiatric comorbidity. *Journal of Consulting and Clinical Psychology, 70*(6), 1224-1239.

102. Maslowsky, J., Schulenberg, J. E., & Zucker, R. A. (2014). Influence of conduct problems and depressive symptomatology on adolescent substance use: Developmentally proximal versus distal effects. *Developmental Psychology, 50*(4), 1179-1189.

103. Conway, K. P., Compton, W., Stinson, F. S., & Grant, B. F. (2006). Lifetime comorbidity of DSM-IV mood and anxiety disorders and specific drug use disorders: Results from the National Epidemiologic Survey on Alcohol and Related Conditions. *The Journal of Clinical Psychiatry, 67*(2), 247-258.

104. Ammon, L., Sterling, S., Mertens, J., & Weisner, C. (2005). Adolescents in private chemical dependency programs: Who are most at risk for HIV? *Journal of Substance Abuse Treatment, 29*(1), 39-45.

105. Madan, A., Beech, D. J., & Flint, L. (2001). Drugs, guns, and kids: The association between substance use and injury caused by interpersonal violence. *Journal of Pediatric Surgery, 36*(3), 440-442.

106. Williams, A. F., & Tefft, B. C. (2014). Characteristics of teens-with-teens fatal crashes in the United States, 2005-2010. *Journal of Safety Research, 48*, 37-42.

107. Fals-Stewart, W., Golden, J., & Schumacher, J. A. (2003). Intimate partner violence and substance use: A longitudinal day-to-day examination. *Addictive Behaviors, 28*(9), 1555-1574.

108. Hingson, R., Heeren, T., Levenson, S., Jamanka, A., & Voas, R. (2002). Age of drinking onset, driving after drinking, and involvement in alcohol related motor-vehicle crashes. *Accident Analysis & Prevention, 34*(1), 85-92.

109. Hingson, R. W., & Zha, W. (2009). Age of drinking onset, alcohol use disorders, frequent heavy drinking, and unintentionally injuring oneself and others after drinking. *Pediatrics, 123*(6), 1477-1484.

110. Whiteford, H. A., Degenhardt, L., Rehm, J., Baxter, A. J., Ferrari, A. J., Erskine, H. E., . . . Vos, T. (2013). Global burden of disease attributable to mental and substance use disorders: Findings from the Global Burden of Disease Study 2010. *The Lancet, 382*(9904), 1575-1586.

111. McLellan, A. T., Starrels, J. L., Tai, B., Gordon, A. J., Brown, R., Ghitza, U., . . . Horton, T. (2014). Can substance use disorders be managed using the chronic care model? Review and recommendations from a NIDA Consensus Group. *Public Health Reviews, 35*(2), 1-14.

112. Chi, F. W., Parthasarathy, S., Mertens, J. R., & Weisner, C. M. (2011). Continuing care and long-term substance use outcomes in managed care: Early evidence for a primary care based model. *Psychiatric Services, 62*(10), 1194–2000.

113. Parthasarathy, S., Chi, F. W., Mertens, J. R., & Weisner, C. (2012). The role of continuing care on 9-year cost trajectories of patients with intakes into an outpatient alcohol and drug treatment program. *Medical Care, 50*(6), 540–546.

114. Saitz, R., Horton, N. J., Larson, M. J., Winter, M., & Samet, J. H. (2005). Primary medical care and reductions in addiction severity: A prospective cohort study. *Addiction, 100*(1), 70-78.

115. Samet, J. H., Friedmann, P., & Saitz, R. (2001). Benefits of linking primary medical care and substance abuse services: Patient, provider, and societal perspectives. *Archives of Internal Medicine, 161*(1), 85-91.

116. Saitz, R., Cheng, D. M., Winter, M., Kim, T. W., Meli, S. M., Allensworth-Davies, D., . . . Samet, J. H. (2013). Chronic care management for dependence on alcohol and other drugs: The AHEAD randomized trial. *JAMA, 310*(11), 1156-1167.

117. Samet, J. H., Larson, M. J., Horton, N. J., Doyle, K., Winter, M., & Saitz, R. (2003). Linking alcohol-and drug-dependent adults to primary medical care: A randomized controlled trial of a multi-disciplinary health intervention in a detoxification unit. *Addiction, 98*(4), 509-516.

118. Watkins, K., Pincus, H. A., Tanielian, T. L., & Lloyd, J. (2003). Using the chronic care model to improve treatment of alcohol use disorders in primary care settings. *Journal of Studies on Alcohol, 64*(2), 209-218.

119. Park, T. W., Cheng, D. M., Samet, J. H., Winter, M. R., & Saitz, R. (2015). Chronic care management for substance dependence in primary care among patients with co-occurring disorders. *Psychiatric Services, 66*(1), 72-79.

120. Mertens, J. R., Flisher, A. J., Satre, D. D., & Weisner, C. M. (2008). The role of medical conditions and primary care services in 5-year substance use outcomes among chemical dependency treatment patients. *Drug and Alcohol Dependence, 98*(1-2), 45-53.

121. Willenbring, M. L., & Olson, D. H. (1999). A randomized trial of integrated outpatient treatment for medically ill alcoholic men. *Archives of Internal Medicine, 159*(16), 1946-1952.

122. O'Donnell, A., Anderson, P., Newbury-Birch, D., Schulte, B., Schmidt, C., Reimer, J., & Kaner, E. (2014). The impact of brief alcohol interventions in primary healthcare: A systematic review of reviews. *Alcohol and Alcoholism, 49*(1), 66-78.

123. Bien, T. H., Miller, W. R., & Tonigan, J. S. (1993). Brief interventions for alcohol problems: A review. *Addiction, 88*(3), 315-336.

124. Fleming, M. F., Barry, K. L., Manwell, L. B., Johnson, K., & London, R. (1997). Brief physician advice for problem alcohol drinkers: A randomized controlled trial in community-based primary care practices. *JAMA, 277*(13), 1030-1045.

125. Rose, H. L., Miller, P. M., Nemeth, L. S., Jenkins, R. G., Nietert, P. J., Wessell, A. M., & Ornstein, S. (2008). Alcohol screening and brief counseling in a primary care hypertensive population: A quality improvement intervention. *Addiction, 103*(8), 1271-1280.

126. Oslin, D. W., Lynch, K. G., Maisto, S. A., Lantinga, L. J., McKay, J. R., Possemato, K., . . . Wierzbicki, M. (2014). A randomized clinical trial of alcohol care management delivered in Department of Veterans Affairs primary care clinics versus specialty addiction treatment. *Journal of General Internal Medicine, 29*(1), 162-168.

127. England, M. J., Butler, A. S., & Gonzalez, M. L. (2015). *Psychosocial interventions for mental and substance use disorders: A framework for establishing evidence-based standards.* Washington, DC: National Academies Press.

128. Arthur, M. W., & Blitz, C. (2000). Bridging the gap between science and practice in drug abuse prevention through needs assessment and strategic community planning. *Journal of Community Psychology, 28*(3), 241-255.

129. Arthur, M. W., Briney, J. S., Hawkins, J. D., Abbott, R. D., Brooke-Weiss, B. L., & Catalano, R. F. (2007). Measuring risk and protection in communities using the Communities That Care youth survey. *Evaluation and Program Planning, 30*(2), 197-211.

130. Mrazek, P. B., Biglan, A., & Hawkins, J. D. (2004). *Community-monitoring systems: Tracking and improving the well-being of America's children and adolescents.* Fairfax, VA: Society for Prevention Research.

131. McLellan, A. T., Kemp, J., Brooks, A., & Carise, D. (2008). Improving public addiction treatment through performance contracting: The Delaware experiment. *Health Policy, 87*(3), 296-308.

132. Vandrey, R., Stitzer, M. L., Acquavita, S. P., & Quinn-Stabile, P. (2011). Pay-for-performance in a community substance abuse clinic. *Journal of Substance Abuse Treatment, 41*(2), 193-200.

133. Center for Substance Abuse Treatment. (2005). *Substance abuse treatment for persons with co-occurring disorders. Treatment improvement protocol (TIP) series, No. 42.* (DHHS Publication No. (SMA) 05-3992). Rockville, MD: Substance Abuse and Mental Health Services Administration.

134. Friedmann, P. D., D'Aunno, T. A., Jin, L., & Alexander, J. A. (2000). Medical and psychosocial services in drug abuse treatment: Do stronger linkages promote client utilization? *Health Services Research, 35*(2), 443-465.

135. Asarnow, J. R., Rozenman, M., Wiblin, J., & Zeltzer, L. (2015). Integrated medical-behavioral care compared with usual primary care for child and adolescent behavioral health: A meta-analysis. *JAMA, 169*(10), 929-937.

136. Heath, B., Wise Romero, P., & Reynolds, K. A. (2013). *A standard framework for levels of integrated healthcare.* Washington, DC: SAMHSA-HRSA Center for Integrated Health Solutions.

137. Lo, C. C., & Cheng, T. C. (2011). Racial/ethnic differences in access to substance abuse treatment. *Journal of Health Care for the Poor and Underserved, 22*(2), 621-637.

138. Saloner, B., & Le Cook, B. (2013). Blacks and Hispanics are less likely than whites to complete addiction treatment, largely due to socioeconomic factors. *Health Affairs, 32*(1), 135-145.

139. Satre, D. D., Campbell, C. I., Gordon, N. P., & Weisner, C. (2010). Ethnic disparities in accessing treatment for depression and substance use disorders in an integrated health plan. *The International Journal of Psychiatry in Medicine, 40*(1), 57-76.

140. Mulia, N., Tam, T. W., & Schmidt, L. A. (2014). Disparities in the use and quality of alcohol treatment services and some proposed solutions to narrow the gap. *Psychiatric Services, 65*(5), 626-633.

141. Wen, H., Druss, B. G., & Cummings, J. R. (2015). Effect of Medicaid expansions on health insurance coverage and access to care among low-income adults with behavioral health conditions. *Health Services Research, 50*(6), 1787-1809.

142. Artiga, S., Damico, A., & Garfield, R. (2015). *Estimates of eligibility for ACA coverage among the uninsured by race and ethnicity.* Washington, DC: The Henry J. Kaiser Family Foundation.

143. Vestal, C. (2015). States gear up to help Medicaid enrollees beat addictions. Retrieved from http://www.pewtrusts.org/en/research-and-analysis/blogs/stateline/2015/1/13/states-gear-up-to-help-medicaid-enrollees-beat-addictions. Accessed on March 17, 2016.

144. Substance Abuse and Mental Health Services Administration. (2013). *Behavioral health treatment needs assessment toolkit for states.* (HHS Publication No. SMA13-4757). (HHS Publication No. SMA13-4757). Rockville, MD: Substance Abuse and Mental Health Services Administration.

145. Floyd, R. L., Sobell, M., Velasquez, M. M., Ingersoll, K., Nettleman, M., Sobell, L., . . . Nagaraja, J. (2007). Preventing alcohol-exposed pregnancies: A randomized controlled trial. *American Journal of Preventive Medicine, 32*(1), 1-10.

146. Hanson, J. D., & Pourier, S. (2015). The Oglala Sioux Tribe CHOICES program: Modifying an existing alcohol-exposed pregnancy intervention for use in an American Indian community. *International Journal of Environmental Research and Public Health, 13*(1), 1-10.

147. Nayak, M. B., Korcha, R. A., Kaskutas, L. A., & Avalos, L. A. (2014). Feasibility and acceptability of a novel, computerized screening and brief intervention (SBI) for alcohol and sweetened beverage use in pregnancy. *BMC Pregnancy & Childbirth, 14*(379).

148. Lee, C. S., López, S. R., Colby, S. M., Rohsenow, D., Hernández, L., Borrelli, B., & Caetano, R. (2013). Culturally adapted motivational interviewing for Latino heavy drinkers: Results from a randomized clinical trial. *Journal of Ethnicity in Substance Abuse, 12*(4), 356-373.

149. Chan, Y.-F., Lu, S.-E., Howe, B., Tieben, H., Hoeft, T., & Unützer, J. (2016). Screening and follow-up monitoring for substance use in primary care: An exploration of rural–urban variations. *Journal of General Internal Medicine, 31*(2), 215-222.

150. Campbell, C. I., Chi, F., Sterling, S., Kohn, C., & Weisner, C. (2009). Self-initiated tobacco cessation and substance use outcomes among adolescents entering substance use treatment in a managed care organization. *Addictive Behaviors, 34*(2), 171-179.

151. Sterling, S., Chi, F., Campbell, C., & Weisner, C. (2009). Three-year chemical dependency and mental health treatment outcomes among adolescents: The role of continuing care. *Alcoholism: Clinical and Experimental Research, 33*(8), 1417-1429.

152. Chi, F. W., Kaskutas, L. A., Sterling, S., Campbell, C. I., & Weisner, C. (2009). Twelve-step affiliation and 3-year substance use outcomes among adolescents: Social support and religious service attendance as potential mediators. *Addiction, 104*(6), 927-939.

153. Evans, E., Spear, S. E., Huang, Y.-C., & Hser, Y.-I. (2006). Outcomes of drug and alcohol treatment programs among American Indians in California. *American journal of public health, 96*(5), 889-896.

154. Dickerson, D. L., Spear, S., Marinelli-Casey, P., Rawson, R., Li, L., & Hser, Y.-I. (2010). American Indians/Alaska Natives and substance abuse treatment outcomes: Positive signs and continuing challenges. *Journal of Addictive Diseases, 30*(1), 63-74.

155. Satre, D. D., Chi, F. W., Mertens, J. R., & Weisner, C. M. (2012). Effects of age and life transitions on alcohol and drug treatment outcome over nine years. *Journal of Studies on Alcohol and Drugs, 73*(3), 459-468.

156. Field, C., & Caetano, R. (2010). The role of ethnic matching between patient and provider on the effectiveness of brief alcohol interventions with Hispanics. *Alcoholism: Clinical and Experimental Research, 34*(2), 262-271.

157. Ruglass, L. M., Hien, D. A., Hu, M.-C., Campbell, A. N., Caldeira, N. A., Miele, G. M., & Chang, D. F. (2014). Racial/ethnic match and treatment outcomes for women with PTSD and substance use disorders receiving community-based treatment. *Community Mental Health Journal, 50*(7), 811-822.

158. Doty, M. M. (2003). *Hispanic patients' double burden: Lack of health insurance and limited English.* (592). New York, NY: The Commonwealth Fund.

159. Petry, N. M. (2003). A comparison of African American and non-Hispanic Caucasian cocaine-abusing outpatients. *Drug and Alcohol Dependence, 69*(1), 43-49.

160. Bay Area Addiction and Research and Treatment, Inc., 179 F.3d 725 (9th Cir. 1999).

161. Ondersma, S. J., Beatty, J. R., Svikis, D. S., Strickler, R. C., Tzilos, G. K., Chang, G., . . . Sokol, R. J. (2015). Computer-delivered screening and brief intervention for alcohol use in pregnancy: A pilot randomized trial. *Alcoholism: Clinical and Experimental Research, 39*(7), 1219-1226.

162. Belenko, S., Patapis, P., & French, M. T. (2005). Economic benefits of drug treatment: A critical review of the evidence for policy makers. Retrieved from http://www.fccmh.org/resources/docs/EconomicBenefits_of_Drug_Trx_02.05_.pdf. Accessed on October 14, 2015.

163. Cartwright, W. S. (1998). Cost-benefit and cost-effectiveness analysis of drug abuse treatment services. *Evaluation Review, 22*(5), 609-636.

164. Cartwright, W. S. (2000). Cost-benefit analysis of drug treatment services: Review of the literature. *Journal of Mental Health Policy and Economics, 3*(1), 11-26.

165. Harwood, H. J., Malhotra, D., Villarivera, C., Liu, C., Chong, U., & Gilani, J. (2002). *Cost effectiveness and cost benefit analysis of substance abuse treatment: A literature review*. Rockville, MD: U.S. Department of Health and Human Services, Substance Abuse and Mental Health Services Administration, Center for Substance Abuse Treatment.

166. Levit, K. R., Kassed, C. A., Coffey, R. M., Mark, T. L., McKusick, D. R., King, E., . . . Stranges, E. (2008). *Projections of national expenditures for mental health services and substance abuse treatment, 2004–2014*. (SAMHSA Publication No. SMA 08-4326). Rockville, MD: Substance Abuse and Mental Health Services Administration.

167. Substance Abuse and Mental Health Services Administration. (2016). *Behavioral health spending and use accounts, 1986–2014*. (HHS Publication No. SMA-16-4975). Rockville, MD: Substance Abuse and Mental Health Services Administration.

168. Sacks, J. J., Gonzales, K. R., Bouchery, E. E., Tomedi, L. E., & Brewer, R. D. (2015). 2010 national and state costs of excessive alcohol consumption. *American Journal of Preventive Medicine, 49*(5), e73-e79.

169. National Drug Intelligence Center. (2011). *National drug threat assessment*. Washington, DC: U.S. Department of Justice.

170. Ettner, S. L., Huang, D., Evans, E., Ash, D. R., Hardy, M., Jourabchi, M., & Hser, Y. I. (2006). Benefit-cost in the California treatment outcome project: Does substance abuse treatment "pay for itself"? *Health Services Research, 41*(1), 192-213.

171. Godfrey, C., Stewart, D., & Gossop, M. (2004). Economic analysis of costs and consequences of the treatment of drug misuse: 2-year outcome data from the National Treatment Outcome Research Study (NTORS). *Addiction, 99*(6), 697-707.

172. Humphreys, K., Wagner, T. H., & Gage, M. (2011). If substance use disorder treatment more than offsets its costs, why don't more medical centers want to provide it? *Journal of Substance Abuse Treatment, 41*(3), 243-251.

173. National Council for Behavioral Health. (2014). The business case for effective substance use disorder treatment. Retrieved from http://www.thenationalcouncil.org/wp-content/uploads/2015/01/14_Business-Case_Substance-Use.pdf. Accessed on June 27, 2016.

174. Basu, A., Paltiel, A. D., & Pollack, H. A. (2008). Social costs of robbery and the cost-effectiveness of substance abuse treatment. *Health Economics, 17*(8), 927-946.

175. Fleming, M. F., Mundt, M. P., French, M. T., Manwell, L. B., Stauffacher, E. A., & Barry, K. L. (2002). Brief physician advice for problem drinkers: Long-term efficacy and benefit-cost analysis. *Alcoholism: Clinical and Experimental Research, 26*(1), 36-43.

176. Maheswaran, R., Beevers, M., & Beevers, D. G. (1992). Effectiveness of advice to reduce alcohol consumption in hypertensive patients. *Hypertension, 19*(1), 79-84.

177. Parthasarathy, S., Mertens, J., Moore, C., & Weisner, C. (2003). Utilization and cost impact of integrating substance abuse treatment and primary care. *Medical Care, 41*(3), 357-367.

178. Stewart, S. H., Latham, P. K., Miller, P. M., Randall, P., & Anton, R. F. (2008). Blood pressure reduction during treatment for alcohol dependence: Results from the Combining Medications and Behavioral Interventions for Alcoholism (COMBINE) study. *Addiction, 103*(10), 1622-1628.

179. National Institute on Drug Abuse. (2012). *Principles of drug addiction treatment: A research-based guide.* (NIH Publication No. 12–4180). Rockville, MD: National Institutes of Health, U.S. Department of Health and Human Services.

180. Peters, R. H., Wexler, H. K., & Lurigio, A. J. (2015). Co-occurring substance use and mental disorders in the criminal justice system: A new frontier of clinical practice and research. *Psychiatric Rehabilitation Journal, 38*(1), 1-6.

181. Zarkin, G. A., Cowell, A. J., Hicks, K. A., Mills, M. J., Belenko, S., Dunlap, L. J., & Keyes, V. (2015). Lifetime benefits and costs of diverting substance-abusing offenders from state prison. *Crime & Delinquency, 61*(6), 829-850.

182. McCollister, K. E., French, M. T., Prendergast, M., Wexler, H., Sacks, S., & Hall, E. (2003). Is in-prison treatment enough? A cost-effectiveness analysis of prison-based treatment and aftercare services for substance-abusing offenders. *Law & Policy, 25*(1), 63-82.

183. Traube, D. E. (2012). The missing link to child safety, permanency, and well-being: Addressing substance misuse in child welfare. *Social Work Research, 36*(2), 83-87.

184. Berger, L. M., Slack, K. S., Waldfogel, J., & Bruch, S. K. (2010). Caseworker-perceived caregiver substance abuse and child protective services outcomes. *Child Maltreatment, 15*(3), 199-210.

185. Aarons, G. A., Brown, S. A., Hough, R. L., Garland, A. F., & Wood, P. A. (2001). Prevalence of adolescent substance use disorders across five sectors of care. *Journal of the American Academy of Child & Adolescent Psychiatry, 40*(4), 419-426.

186. Institute of Medicine. (2013). *Substance use disorders in the U.S. armed forces.* Washington, DC: The National Academies Press.

187. Harwood, H. J., Zhang, Y., Dall, T. M., Olaiya, S. T., & Fagan, N. K. (2009). Economic implications of reduced binge drinking among the military health system's TRICARE Prime plan beneficiaries. *Military Medicine, 174*(7), 728-736.

188. Estee, S., & Nordlund, D. J. (2003). *Washington State supplemental security income (SSI) cost offset pilot project: 2002 progress report.* Olympia, WA: Washington State Department of Social and Health Services.

189. Wickizer, T. M., Krupski, A., Stark, K. D., Mancuso, D., & Campbell, K. (2006). The effect of substance abuse treatment on Medicaid expenditures among general assistance welfare clients in Washington State. *Milbank Quarterly, 84*(3), 555-576.

190. Wickizer, T. M., Mancuso, D., & Huber, A. (2012). Evaluation of an innovative Medicaid health policy initiative to expand substance abuse treatment in Washington State. *Medical Care Research and Review, 69*(5), 540-559.

191. Zarkin, G. A., Dunlap, L. J., & Homsi, G. (2004). The substance abuse services cost analysis program (SASCAP): A new method for estimating drug treatment services costs. *Evaluation and Program Planning, 27*(1), 35-43.

192. Flynn, P. M., Broome, K. M., Beaston-Blaakman, A., Knight, D. K., Horgan, C. M., & Donald, S. S. (2009). Treatment cost analysis tool (TCAT) for estimating costs of outpatient treatment services. *Drug and Alcohol Dependence, 100*(1-2), 47-53.

193. Bray, J. W., Zarkin, G. A., Hinde, J. M., & Mills, M. J. (2012). Costs of alcohol screening and brief intervention in medical settings: A review of the literature. *Journal of Studies on Alcohol and Drugs, 73*(6), 911-919.

194. Zarkin, G., Bray, J., Hinde, J., & Saitz, R. (2015). Costs of screening and brief intervention for illicit drug use in primary care settings. *Journal of Studies on Alcohol and Drugs, 76*(2), 222-228.

195. Hartung, D. M., McCarty, D., Fu, R., Wiest, K., Chalk, M., & Gastfriend, D. R. (2014). Extended-release naltrexone for alcohol and opioid dependence: A meta-analysis of healthcare utilization studies. *Journal of Substance Abuse Treatment, 47*(2), 113-121.

196. Lynch, F. L., McCarty, D., Mertens, J., Perrin, N. A., Green, C. A., Parthasarathy, S., . . . Pating, D. (2014). Costs of care for persons with opioid dependence in commercial integrated health systems. *Addiction Science & Clinical Practice, 9*(16).

197. McCarty, D., Perrin, N. A., Green, C. A., Polen, M. R., Leo, M. C., & Lynch, F. (2010). Methadone maintenance and the cost and utilization of health care among individuals dependent on opioids in a commercial health plan. *Drug and Alcohol Dependence, 111*(3), 235-240.

198. Zarkin, G. A., Bray, J. W., Aldridge, A., Mitra, D., Mills, M. J., Couper, D. J., & Cisler, R. A. (2008). Cost and cost-effectiveness of the COMBINE study in alcohol-dependent patients. *Archives of General Psychiatry, 65*(10), 1214-1221.

199. Drummond, M. F., Sculpher, M. J., Torrance, G. W., O'Brien, B. J., & Stoddart, G. L. (2005). *Methods for the economic evaluation of health care programmes* (3rd ed.). Oxford, UK: Oxford University Press.

200. Alterman, A. I., O'Brien, C. P., McLellan, A. T., August, D. S., Snider, E. C., Droba, M., . . . Schrade, F. X. (1994). Effectiveness and costs of inpatient versus day hospital cocaine rehabilitation. *Journal of Nervous and Mental Disease, 182*(3), 157-163.

201. Daley, M., Love, C. T., Shepard, D. S., Peterson, C. B., White, K. L., & Hall, F. B. (2004). Cost-effectiveness of Connecticut's in-prison substance abuse treatment. *Journal of Offender Rehabilitation, 39*(3), 69-92.

202. Jofre-Bonet, M., Sindelar, J. L., Petrakis, I. L., Nich, C., Frankforter, T., Rounsaville, B. J., & Carroll, K. M. (2004). Cost effectiveness of disulfiram: Treating cocaine use in methadone-maintained patients. *Journal of Substance Abuse Treatment, 26*(3), 225-232.

203. Masson, C. L., Barnett, P. G., Sees, K. L., Delucchi, K. L., Rosen, A., Wong, W., & Hall, S., M. (2004). Cost and cost-effectiveness of standard methadone maintenance treatment compared to enriched 180-day methadone detoxification. *Addiction, 99*(6), 718-726.

204. McCollister, K. E., French, M. T., Pendergast, M. L., Hall, E., & Sacks, S. (2004). Long-term cost effectiveness of addiction treatment for criminal offenders: Evaluating treatment history and reincarceration five years post-parole. *Justice Quarterly, 21*(3), 659-679.

205. Mojtabai, R., & Zivin, J. G. (2003). Effectiveness and cost-effectiveness of four treatment modalities for substance disorders: A propensity score analysis. *Health Services Research, 38*(1 Pt 1), 233-259.

206. Pettinati, H. M., Meyers, K., Evans, B. D., Ruetsch, C. R., Kaplan, F. N., Jensen, J. M., & Hadley, T. R. (1999). Inpatient alcohol treatment in a private healthcare setting: Which patients benefit and at what cost? *The American Journal on Addictions, 8*(3), 220-233.

207. Schinka, J. A., Francis, E., Hughes, P., LaLone, L., & Flynn, C. (1998). Comparative outcomes and costs of inpatient care and supportive housing for substance-dependent veterans. *Psychiatric Services, 49*(7), 946-950.

208. Shepard, D. S., Larson, M. J., & Hoffmann, N. G. (1999). Cost-effectiveness of substance abuse services: Implications for public policy. *Psychiatric Clinics of North America, 22*(2), 385-400.

209. Sindelar, J. L., Jofre-Bonet, M., French, M. T., & McLellan, A. T. (2004). Cost-effectiveness analysis of addiction treatment: Paradoxes of multiple outcomes. *Drug and Alcohol Dependence, 73*(1), 41-50.

210. Drug Rehab Centers. (n.d.). Self pay drug treatment programs. Retrieved from http://www.drugrehabcenters.org/CityCategory/Fort%20Myers/Florida/Self_Pay_Drug_Treatment_Programs.htm. Accessed on March 16, 2016.

211. Mark, T. L., Yee, T., Levit, K. R., Camacho-Cook, J., Cutler, E., & Carroll, C. D. (2016). Insurance financing increased for mental health conditions but not for substance use disorders, 1986–2014. *Health Affairs, 35*(6), 958-965.

212. Smith, J. C., Medalia, C., & U.S. Census Bureau. (2015). *Health insurance coverage in the United States: 2014*. Current population reports. (P60-253). Washington, DC: U.S. Department of Commerce, Economics and Statistics Administration, Bureau of the Census.

213. American Psychiatric Association. (2000). *Diagnostic and statistical manual of mental disorders (DSM-IV)* (4th ed.). Arlington, VA: American Psychiatric Publishing.

214. Woodward, A. (2016). *Special analysis based on 2013 National Survey on Drug Use and Health data*. Rockville, MD: Substance Abuse and Mental Health Services Administration.

215. Jensen, G. A., & Morrisey, M. A. (1991). Employer-sponsored insurance coverage for alcohol and drug abuse treatment, 1988. *Inquiry, 28*(4), 393-402.

216. Rouse, B. A. (1995). *Substance abuse and mental health statistics sourcebook*. Rockville, MD: Substance Abuse and Mental Health Services Administration.

217. Shepard, D., Daley, M., Ritter, G., Hodgkin, D., & Beinecke, R. (2002). Managed care and the quality of substance abuse treatment. *Journal of Mental Health Policy and Economics, 5*(4), 163-174.

218. Rosenbach, M., & Lake, T. (2003). *Mental health and substance abuse parity in Vermont: What did we learn?* (2). Princeton, NJ: Mathematica Policy Research, Inc.

219. Statista. (n.d.). Health insurance status distribution of the total U.S. population in 2014. Retrieved from http://www.statista.com/statistics/238866/health-insurance-status-of-the-total-us-population/ Accessed on June 13, 2016.

220. U.S. Government Accountability Office. (n.d.). Health > 20. State Medicaid sources of funds. Retrieved from http://www.gao.gov/modules/ereport/handler.php?m=1&p=1&path=/ereport/GAO-15-404SP/data_center_savings/Health/20._State_Medicaid_Sources_of_Funds. Accessed on June 12, 2016.

221. The Henry J. Kaiser Family Foundation. (2016). Federal and state share of Medicaid spending. Retrieved from http://kff.org/medicaid/state-indicator/federalstate-share-of-spending/. Accessed on March 20, 2016.

222. Wachino, V. (2015). *Coverage of housing-related activities and services for individuals with disabilities. CMCS Informational Bulletin.* Baltimore, MD: Center for Medicaid and CHIP Services. Retrieved from https://www.medicaid.gov/federal-policy-guidance/downloads/CIB-06-26-2015.pdf. Accessed on

223. Dey, J., Rosenoff, E., West, K., Ali, M. L., S, McClellan, C., Mutter, R., ... Woodward, A. (2016). *ASPE Issue brief: Benefits of Medicaid expansion for behavioral health.* Washington, DC: U.S. Department of Health and Human Services, Office of the Assistant Secretary for Planning and Evaluation.

224. Centers for Medicare & Medicaid Services. (2016). Medicare enrollment dashboard. Retrieved from https://www.cms.gov/Research-Statistics-Data-and-Systems/Statistics-Trends-and-Reports/Dashboard/Medicare-Enrollment/Enrollment%20Dashboard.html. Accessed on June 12, 2016.

225. Bouchery, E. E., Harwood, H. J., Dilonardo, J., & Vandivort-Warren, R. (2012). Type of health insurance and the substance abuse treatment gap. *Journal of Substance Abuse Treatment, 42*(3), 289-300.

226. Center for Behavioral Health Statistics and Quality. (Unpublished Analysis). *Analysis of the 2013 National Survey of Drug Use and Health.* Rockville, MD: Substance Abuse and Mental Health Services Administration.

227. Jackson, H., Mandell, K., Johnson, K., Chatterjee, D., & Vanness, D. J. (2015). Cost effectiveness of injectable extended release naltrexone compared to methadone maintenance and buprenorphine maintenance treatment for opioid dependence. *Substance Abuse, 36*(2), 226-231.

228. Polsky, D., Glick, H. A., Yang, J., Subramaniam, G. A., Poole, S. A., & Woody, G. E. (2010). Cost-effectiveness of extended buprenorphine-naloxone treatment for opioid-dependent youth: Data from a randomized trial. *Addiction, 105*(9), 1616-1624.

229. Schackman, B. R., Leff, J. A., Polsky, D., Moore, B. A., & Fiellin, D. A. (2012). Cost-effectiveness of long-term outpatient buprenorphine-naloxone treatment for opioid dependence in primary care. *Journal of General Internal Medicine, 27*(6), 669-676.

230. Angus, C., Latimer, N., Preston, L., Li, J., & Purshouse, R. (2014). What are the implications for policy makers? A systematic review of the cost-effectiveness of screening and brief interventions for alcohol misuse in primary care. *Frontiers in Psychiatry, 5*(114).

231. Miller, T., & Hendrie, D. (2008). *Substance abuse prevention dollars and cents: A cost-benefit analysis.* (DHHS-Pub. No. (SMA) 07-4298). Rockville, MD: Substance Abuse and Mental Health Services Administration, Center for Substance Abuse Prevention.

232. Washington State Institute for Public Policy. (2015). Benefit-cost results. Retrieved from http://www.wsipp.wa.gov/BenefitCost?topicId=7. Accessed on April 4, 2016.

233. Substance Abuse and Mental Health Services Administration. (2015). Substance abuse and mental health block grants. Retrieved from http://www.samhsa.gov/grants/block-grants. Accessed on October 14, 2015.

234. Office of National Drug Control Policy. (2015). Drug-free communities support program. Retrieved from https://www.whitehouse.gov/ondcp/Drug-Free-Communities-Support-Program. Accessed on October 14, 2015.

235. Lee, S., Aos, S., Drake, E., Pennucci, A., Miller, M., & Anderson, L. (2012). *Return on investment: Evidence-based options to improve statewide outcomes.* (Document No. 12-04-1201). Olympia, WA: Washington State Institute for Public Policy.

236. GrantSpace. (2015). What is a health conversion foundation? How can I learn more about them? *Knowledge Base.* Retrieved from http://grantspace.org/tools/knowledge-base/Funding-Resources/Foundations/health-conversion-foundations. Accessed on October 10, 2015.

237. Isaacs, S. L., Beatrice, D. F., & Carr, W. (1997). Health care conversion foundations: A status report. *Health Affairs, 16*(6), 228-236.

238. Cantor, J., Mikkelsen, L., Simons, B., & Waters, R. (2013). *How can we pay for a healthy population? Innovative new ways to redirect funds to community prevention.* Oakland, CA: Prevention Institute.

239. Lunder, E. K., & Liu, E. C. (2012). *501(c)(3) Hospitals: Proposed IRS rules under § 9007 of the Affordable Care Act* Washington, DC: Congressional Research Service.

240. Rosenbaum, S., Byrnes, M., & Riek, A. M. (2013). Hospital tax-exempt policy: A comparison of schedule H and state community benefit reporting systems. *Frontiers in Public Health Services and Systems Research, 2*(1), Article 3.

241. Durch, J. S., Bailey, L. A., & Stoto, M. A. (Eds.). (1997). *Improving health in a community: A role for performance monitoring.* Washington, DC: Institute of Medicine, National Academies Press.

242. Huang, J., Walton, K., Gerzoff, R. B., King, B. A., Chaloupka, F. J., & Centers for Disease Control and Prevention. (2015). State tobacco control program spending—United States, 2011. *MMWR, 64*(24), 673-678.

243. Mid-America Regional Council & Homelessness Task Force of Greater Kansas City. (2014). *Investment plan to address the needs of at-risk children and youth in greater Kansas City.* Columbia, MO: University of Missouri Institute of Public Policy.

244. Pérez, A. (2008). *Earmarking state taxes.* (1555165486). Denver, CO: National Conference of State Legislatures.

245. Massachusetts Department of Public Health Bureau of Community Health and Prevention. (2015). *The Massachusetts prevention and wellness trust fund 2014 legislative report.* Boston, MA: Massachusetts Department of Public Health.

246. Congressional Budget Office. (2016). *Federal subsidies for health insurance coverage for people under age 65: 2016 to 2026.* Washington, DC: Congressional Budget Office.

247. Humphreys, K., & Frank, R. G. (2014). The Affordable Care Act will revolutionize care for substance use disorders in the United States. *Addiction, 109*(12), 1957-1958.

248. Buck, J. A. (2011). The looming expansion and transformation of public substance abuse treatment under the Affordable Care Act. *Health Affairs, 30*(8), 1402-1410.

249. Horgan, C. M., Stewart, M. T., Reif, S., Garnick, D. W., Hodgkin, D., Merrick, E. L., & Quinn, A. E. (2015). Behavioral health services in the changing landscape of private health plans. *Psychiatric Services*. Retrieved from http://ps.psychiatryonline.org/doi/abs/10.1176/appi.ps.201500235?url_ver=Z39.88-2003&rfr_id=ori%3Arid%3Acrossref.org&rfr_dat=cr_pub%3Dpubmed. Accessed on April 11, 2016.

250. D'Aunno, T., Friedmann, P. D., Chen, Q., & Wilson, D. M. (2015). Integration of substance abuse treatment organizations into accountable care organizations: Results from a national survey. *Journal of Health Politics, Policy and Law, 40*(4), 797-819.

251. Weisner, C. M., Chi, F. W., Lu, Y., Ross, T. B., Wood, S. B., Hinman, A., . . . Sterling, S. A. (2016). Examination of the effects of an intervention aiming to link patients receiving addiction treatment with health care: The LINKAGE clinical trial. *JAMA Psychiatry*, E1-E11.

252. Molfenter, T. D. (2014). Addiction treatment centers' progress in preparing for health care reform. *Journal of Substance Abuse Treatment, 46*(2), 158–164.

253. Andrews, C., Abraham, A., Grogan, C., Pollack, H., Bersamira, C., Humphreys, K., & Friedmann, P. (2015). Despite resources from the ACA, most states do little to help addiction treatment programs implement health care reform. *Health Affairs, 34*(5), 828-835.

254. Molfenter, T., Capoccia, V. A., Boyle, M. G., & Sherbeck, C. K. (2012). The readiness of addiction treatment agencies for health care reform. *Substance Abuse Treatment, Prevention, and Policy, 7*(16).

255. Knudsen, H. K., Ducharme, L. J., & Roman, P. M. (2006). Early adoption of buprenorphine in substance abuse treatment centers: Data from the private and public sectors. *Journal of Substance Abuse Treatment, 30*(4), 363-373.

256. Wachino, V. (2016). *RE: Availability of HITECH administrative matching funds to help professionals and hospitals eligible for Medicaid EHR incentive payments connect to other Medicaid providers.* Baltimore, MD: U.S. Department of Health and Human Services, Centers for Medicare and Medicaid Services.

257. Corredoira, R., & Kimberly, J. (2006). Industry evolution through consolidation: Implications for addiction treatment. *Journal of Substance Abuse Treatment, 31*(3), 255-265.

258. D'Aunno, T. (2006). The role of organization and management in substance abuse treatment: Review and roadmap. *Journal of Substance Abuse Treatment, 31*(3), 221-233.

259. Knott, A. M., Corredoira, R., & Kimberly, J. (2008). Improving consistency and quality of service delivery: Implications for the addiction treatment field. *Journal of Substance Abuse Treatment, 35*(2), 99-108.

260. Mark, T. L., Kassed, C. A., Vandivort-Warren, R., Levit, K. R., & Kranzler, H. R. (2009). Alcohol and opioid dependence medications: Prescription trends, overall and by physician specialty. *Drug and Alcohol Dependence, 99*(1-3), 345-349.

261. Horgan, C. M., Reif, S., Hodgkin, D., Garnick, D. W., & Merrick, E. L. (2008). Availability of addiction medications in private health plans. *Journal of Substance Abuse Treatment, 34*(2), 147-156.

262. National Treatment Center Study. (2011). *Barriers to the adoption of pharmacotherapies in publicly funded substance abuse treatment: Policy barriers and access to physicians.* Lexington, KY and Athens, GA: University of Kentucky and University of Georgia.

263. Knudsen, H. K., Abraham, A. J., & Roman, P. M. (2011). Adoption and implementation of medications in addiction treatment programs. *Journal of Addiction Medicine, 5*(1), 21-27.

264. Knudsen, H. K., Ducharme, L. J., & Roman, P. M. (2007). The adoption of medications in substance abuse treatment: Associations with organizational characteristics and technology clusters. *Drug and Alcohol Dependence, 87*(2), 164-174.

265. Fuller, B. E., Rieckmann, T., McCarty, D., Smith, K. W., & Levine, H. (2005). Adoption of naltrexone to treat alcohol dependence. *Journal of Substance Abuse Treatment, 28*(3), 273-280.

266. Heinrich, C. J., & Hill, C. J. (2008). Role of state policies in the adoption of naltrexone for substance abuse treatment. *Health Services Research, 43*(3), 951-970.

267. Aletraris, L., & Roman, P. (2015). Adoption of injectable naltrexone in U.S. substance use disorder treatment programs. *Journal of Studies on Alcohol and Drugs, 76*(1), 143-151.

268. Andrews, C. M., D'Aunno, T. A., Pollack, H. A., & Friedmann, P. D. (2014). Adoption of evidence-based clinical innovations: The case of buprenorphine use by opioid treatment programs. *Medical Care Research and Review, 71*(1), 43-60.

269. Stein, B. D., Pacula, R. L., Gordon, A. J., Burns, R. M., Leslie, D. L., Sorbero, M. J., . . . Dick, A. W. (2015). Where is buprenorphine dispensed to treat opioid use disorders? The role of private offices, opioid treatment programs, and substance abuse treatment facilities in urban and rural counties. *Milbank Quarterly, 93*(3), 561-583.

270. Medication assisted treatment for opioid use disorders; 81 Fed. Reg. 44712 (July 8, 2016) (to be codified at 42 C.F.R. pt 8).

271. Assistant Secretary for Public Affairs (ASPA). (2010). Preventive services covered under the Affordable Care Act. Retrieved from http://www.hhs.gov/healthcare/facts-and-features/fact-sheets/preventive-services-covered-under-aca/. Accessed on April 5, 2016.

272. Kaner, E., Bland, M., Cassidy, P., Coulton, S., Dale, V., Deluca, P., . . . Drummond, C. (2013). Effectiveness of screening and brief alcohol intervention in primary care (SIPS trial): Pragmatic cluster randomised controlled trial. *BMJ, 346*(e8501).

273. van Beurden, I., Anderson, P., Akkermans, R. P., Grol, R. P., Wensing, M., & Laurant, M. G. (2012). Involvement of general practitioners in managing alcohol problems: A randomized controlled trial of a tailored improvement programme. *Addiction, 107*(9), 1601-1611.

274. Williams, E. C., Johnson, M. L., Lapham, G. T., Caldeiro, R. M., Chew, L., Fletcher, G. S., . . . Bradley, K. A. (2011). Strategies to implement alcohol screening and brief intervention in primary care settings: A structured literature review. *Psychology of Addictive Behaviors, 25*(2), 206-214.

275. Williams, E. C., Rubinsky, A. D., Chavez, L. J., Lapham, G. T., Rittmueller, S. E., Achtmeyer, C. E., & Bradley, K. A. (2014). An early evaluation of implementation of brief intervention for unhealthy alcohol use in the U.S. Veterans Health Administration. *Addiction, 109*(9), 1472-1481.

276. Barry, K. L., Blow, F. C., Willenbring, M., McCormick, R., Brockmann, L. M., & Visnic, S. (2004). Use of alcohol screening and brief interventions in primary care settings: Implementation and barriers. *Substance Abuse, 25*(1), 27-36.

277. Gassman, R. A. (2003). Medical specialization, profession, and mediating beliefs that predict stated likelihood of alcohol screening and brief intervention: Targeting educational interventions. *Substance Abuse, 24*(3), 141-156.

278. Fitzgerald, N., Platt, L., Heywood, S., & McCambridge, J. (2015). Large-scale implementation of alcohol brief interventions in new settings in Scotland: A qualitative interview study of a national programme. *BMC Public Health, 15*(289).

279. Ozer, E. M., Adams, S. H., Gardner, L. R., Mailloux, D. E., Wibbelsman, C. J., & Irwin, C. E., Jr. (2004). Provider self-efficacy and the screening of adolescents for risky health behaviors. *Journal of Adolescent Health, 35*(2), 101-107.

280. McKnight-Eily, L. R., Liu, Y., Brewer, R. D., Kanny, D., Lu, H., Denny, C. H., . . . Centers for Disease Control and Prevention. (2014). Vital signs: Communication between health professionals and their patients about alcohol use - 44 states and the District of Columbia, 2011. *MMWR, 63*(1), 16-22.

281. Garnick, D. W., Horgan, C. M., Merrick, E. L., & Hoyt, A. (2007). Identification and treatment of mental and substance use conditions: Health plans strategies. *Medical Care, 45*(11), 1060-1067.

282. Sterling, S. A., Kline-Simon, A. H., Wibbelsman, C. J., Wong, A. O., & Weisner, C. M. (2012). Screening for adolescent alcohol and drug use in pediatric health-care settings: Predictors and implications for practice and policy. *Addiction Science and Clinical Practice, 7*(13).

283. Moyer, V. A. (2014). Primary care behavioral interventions to reduce illicit drug and nonmedical pharmaceutical use in children and adolescents: U.S. Preventive Services Task Force recommendation statement. *Annals of Internal Medicine, 160*(9), 634-639.

284. Levy, S. J., Williams, J. F., & Committee on Substance Use and Prevention. (2016). Substance use screening, brief intervention, and referral to treatment. *Pediatrics, 138*(1).

285. Substance Abuse and Mental Health Administration. (2016). Screening, brief intervention, and referral to treatment (SBIRT). Retrieved from http://www.samhsa.gov/sbirt. Accessed on June 27, 2016.

286. National Research Council and Institute of Medicine. (2009). *Preventing mental, emotional, and behavioral disorders among young people: Progress and possibilities*. Washington, DC: National Academies Press.

287. American Academy of Pediatrics Division of Child Health Research. (1998). 45% of fellows routinely screen for alcohol use. *AAP News, 14*(10), 1-2.

288. Bethell, C., Klein, J., & Peck, C. (2001). Assessing health system provision of adolescent preventive services: The Young Adult Health Care Survey. *Medical Care, 39*(5), 478-490.

289. Hassan, A., Harris, S. K., Sherritt, L., Van Hook, S., Brooks, T., Carey, P., . . . Knight, J. R. (2009). Primary care follow-up plans for adolescents with substance use problems. *Pediatrics, 124*(1), 144-150.

290. Wilson, C. R., Sherritt, L., Gates, E., & Knight, J. R. (2004). Are clinical impressions of adolescent substance use accurate? *Pediatrics, 114*(5), e536-e540.

291. Sterling, S., Kline-Simon, A. H., Satre, D. D., Jones, A., Mertens, J., Wong, A., & Weisner, C. (2015). Implementation of screening, brief intervention, and referral to treatment for adolescents in pediatric primary care: A cluster randomized trial. *JAMA Pediatrics, 169*(11).

292. Madras, B. K., Compton, W. M., Avula, D., Stegbauer, T., Stein, J. B., & Clark, H. W. (2009). Screening, brief interventions, referral to treatment (SBIRT) for illicit drug and alcohol use at multiple healthcare sites: Comparison at intake and 6 months later. *Drug and Alcohol Dependence, 99*(1), 280-295.

293. Babor, T. E., Higgins-Biddle, J., Dauser, D., Higgins, P., & Burleson, J. A. (2005). Alcohol screening and brief intervention in primary care settings: Implementation models and predictors. *Journal of Studies on Alcohol and Drugs, 66*(3), 361-368.

294. Babor, T. F., Higgins-Biddle, J. C., Dauser, D., Burleson, J. A., Zarkin, G. A., & Bray, J. (2006). Brief interventions for at-risk drinking: Patient outcomes and cost-effectiveness in managed care organizations. *Alcohol and Alcoholism, 41*(6), 624-631.

295. Cutrona, S. L., Choudhry, N. K., Stedman, M., Servi, A., Liberman, J. N., Brennan, T., . . . Shrank, W. H. (2010). Physician effectiveness in interventions to improve cardiovascular medication adherence: A systematic review. *Journal of General Internal Medicine, 25*(10), 1090-1096.

296. Georgeu, D., Colvin, C. J., Lewin, S., Fairall, L., Bachmann, M. O., Uebel, K., . . . Bateman, E. D. (2012). Implementing nurse-initiated and managed antiretroviral treatment (NIMART) in South Africa: A qualitative process evaluation of the STRETCH trial. *Implementation Science, 7*(66).

297. Rahm, A. K., Boggs, J. M., Martin, C., Price, D. W., Beck, A., Backer, T. E., & Dearing, J. W. (2015). Facilitators and barriers to implementing screening, brief intervention, and referral to treatment (SBIRT) in primary care in integrated health care settings. *Substance Abuse, 36*(3), 281-288.

298. Substance Abuse and Mental Health Services Administration. (2013). *Systems-level implementation of screening, brief intervention, and referral to treatment. Technical Assistance Publication (TAP) Series, No. 33.* (HHS Publication No. (SMA) 13-4741). Rockville, MD: Substance Abuse and Mental Health Services Administration.

299. Bradley, K. A., Williams, E. C., Achtmeyer, C. E., Volpp, B., Collins, B. J., & Kivlahan, D. R. (2006). Implementation of evidence-based alcohol screening in the Veterans Health Administration. *The American Journal of Managed Care, 12*(10), 597-606.

300. Lapham, G. T., Achtmeyer, C. E., Williams, E. C., Hawkins, E. J., Kivlahan, D. R., & Bradley, K. A. (2012). Increased documented brief alcohol interventions with a performance measure and electronic decision support. *Medical Care, 50*(2), 179-187.

301. Mertens, J. R., Chi, F. W., Weisner, C. M., Satre, D. D., Ross, T. B., Allen, S., . . . Sterling, S. A. (2015). Physician versus non-physician delivery of alcohol screening, brief intervention and referral to treatment in adult primary care: The ADVISe cluster randomized controlled implementation trial. *Addiction Science & Clinical Practice, 10*(1), 1-17.

302. Williams, E. C., Lapham, G., Achtmeyer, C. E., Volpp, B., Kivlahan, D. R., & Bradley, K. A. (2010). Use of an electronic clinical reminder for brief alcohol counseling is associated with resolution of unhealthy alcohol use at follow-up screening. *Journal of General Internal Medicine, 25*(Suppl 1), 11-17.

303. Seale, J. P., Johnson, J. A., Clark, D. C., Shellenberger, S., Pusser, A. T., Dhabliwala, J., . . . Clemow, D. (2015). A multisite initiative to increase the use of alcohol screening and brief intervention through resident training and clinic systems changes. *Academic Medicine, 90*(12), 1701-1712.

304. Seale, J. P., Shellenberger, S., Tillery, W. K., Boltri, J., Vogel, R., Barton, B., & McCauley, M. (2005). Implementing alcohol screening and intervention in a family medicine residency clinic. *Substance Abuse, 26*(1), 23-31.

305. Williams, E. C., Achtmeyer, C. E., Young, J. P., Rittmueller, S. E., Ludman, E. J., Lapham, G. T., . . . Bradley, K. A. (2016). Local implementation of alcohol screening and brief intervention at five Veterans Health Administration primary care clinics: Perspectives of clinical and administrative staff. *Journal of Substance Abuse Treatment, 60*, 27-35.

306. Hoge, M. A., Stuart, G. W., Morris, J., Flaherty, M. T., Paris, M., Jr., & Goplerud, E. (2013). Mental health and addiction workforce development: Federal leadership is needed to address the growing crisis. *Health Affairs, 32*(11), 2005-2012.

307. Substance Abuse and Mental Health Services Administration. (2013). *Report to Congress on the nation's substance abuse and mental health workforce issues.* Rockville, MD: Substance Abuse and Mental Health Services Administration.

308. Bureau of Labor Statistics. (n.d.). Occupational outlook handbook 2010-11 Retrieved from http://bls.gov/oco/. Accessed on April 6, 2016.

309. Health Resources and Services Administration. (n.d.). Shortage areas. Retrieved from http://datawarehouse.hrsa.gov/topics/shortageAreas.aspx. Accessed on July 9, 2016.

310. Corwin, E. (2016). Shortage of addiction counselors further strained by opioid epidemic. *Shots: Health news from NPR.* Retrieved from http://www.npr.org/sections/health-shots/2016/02/24/467143265/shortage-of-addiction-counselors-further-strained-by-opioid-epidemic. Accessed on March 16, 2016.

311. Eby, L. T., Burk, H., & Maher, C. P. (2010). How serious of a problem is staff turnover in substance abuse treatment? A longitudinal study of actual turnover. *Journal of Substance Abuse Treatment, 39*(3), 264-271.

312. Peikes, D. N., Reid, R. J., Day, T. J., Cornwell, D. D., Dale, S. B., Baron, R. J., . . . Shapiro, R. J. (2014). Staffing patterns of primary care practices in the comprehensive primary care initiative. *The Annals of Family Medicine, 12*(2), 142-149.

313. Hall, J., Cohen, D. J., Davis, M., Gunn, R., Blount, A., Pollack, D. A., . . . Miller, B. F. (2015). Preparing the workforce for behavioral health and primary care integration. *Journal of the American Board of Family Medicine, 28* (Suppl 1), S41-S51.

314. Miller, B. F., Brown Levey, S. M., Payne-Murphy, J. C., & Kwan, B. M. (2014). Outlining the scope of behavioral health practice in integrated primary care: Dispelling the myth of the one-trick mental health pony. *Families, Systems, & Health, 32*(3), 338-343.

315. Urada, D., Schaper, E., Alvarez, L., Reilly, C., Dawar, M., Field, R., . . . Rawson, R. A. (2012). Perceptions of mental health and substance use disorder services integration among the workforce in primary care settings. *Journal of Psychoactive Drugs, 44*(4), 292-298.

316. Haack, M. R., & Adger, J. H. (Eds.). (2002). *Strategic plan for interdisciplinary faculty development: Arming the nation's health professional workforce for a new approach to substance use disorders.* Providence, RI: Association for Medical Education and Research in Substance Abuse (AMERSA).

317. Isaacson, J. H., Fleming, M., Kraus, M., Kahn, R., & Mundt, M. (2000). A national survey of training in substance use disorders in residency programs. *Journal of Studies on Alcohol and Drugs, 61*(6), 912-915.

318. The Annapolis Coalition on the Behavioral Health Workforce. (2007). *An action plan for behavioral health workforce development: A framework for discussion.* Cincinnati, OH: The Annapolis Coalition.

319. Kerwin, M. E., Walker-Smith, K., & Kirby, K. C. (2006). Comparative analysis of state requirements for the training of substance abuse and mental health counselors. *Journal of Substance Abuse Treatment, 30*(3), 173-181.

320. Dilonardo, J. (2011). *Workforce issues related to: Bi-directional physical and behavioral healthcare integration specifically substance use disorders and primary care. Issue Brief #4.* Rockville, MD: Substance Abuse and Mental Health Services Administration, Center for Integrated Health Solutions.

321. Dilonardo, J. (2011, August 3). *Workforce issues related to: Physical and behavioral healthcare integration: Specifically substance use disorders and primary care.* Paper presented at the Workforce Issues: Integrating Substance Use Services into Primary Care Conference, Washington, DC.

322. International Certification & Reciprocity Consortium. (n.d.). Prevention specialist (PS): A credential for your career & your community. Retrieved from http://www.internationalcredentialing.org/creds/ps. Accessed on November 14, 2015.

323. National Association of State Alcohol and Drug Abuse Directors (NASADAD), & Northrop Grumman Information Technology. (2005). *A national review of state alcohol and drug treatment programs and certification standards for substance abuse counselors and prevention professionals.* (DHHS Publication No. 05-3994). Rockville, MD: Substance Abuse and Mental Health Services Administration.

324. Health Resources and Services Administration (HRSA). (2015). *FY 2016 annual performance report.* Rockville, MD: Health Resources and Services Administration.

325. HealthIT.gov. (2016). Standards and certification regulations: 2015 edition final rule. Retrieved from https://www.healthit.gov/policy-researchers-implementers/2015-edition-final-rule. Accessed on August 30, 2016.

326. Clark, T., Eadie, J., Kreiner, P., & Strickler, G. (2012). *Prescription drug monitoring programs: An assessment of the evidence for best practices.* Prescription Drug Monitoring Program Center of Excellence Waltham, MA: Brandeis University for the Pew Charitable Trusts.

327. U.S. Department of Justice Drug Enforcement Administration Office of Diversion Control. (2011). State prescription drug monitoring programs. Retrieved from http://www.deadiversion.usdoj.gov/faq/rx_monitor.htm. Accessed on October 10, 2010.

328. Substance Abuse and Mental Health Services Administration. (2013). *Medicaid handbook: Interface with behavioral health services.* (HHS Publication No. SMA-13-4773). Rockville, MD: Substance Abuse and Mental Health Services Administration.

329. Medicaid.gov. (n.d.). Benefits. Retrieved from http://www.medicaid.gov/medicaid-chip-program-information/by-topics/benefits/medicaid-benefits.html. Accessed on October 15, 2015.

330. Mann, C. (2012). *Policy considerations for integrated care models* Baltimore, MD: Centers for Medicare & Medicaid Services.

331. Centers for Medicare & Medicaid Services. (n.d.). Medicaid innovation accelerator program (IAP). Retrieved from https://www.medicaid.gov/state-resource-center/innovation-accelerator-program/innovation-accelerator-program.html. Accessed on April 6, 2016.

332. Centers for Medicare & Medicaid Services. (2012). *Health homes (Section 2703) frequently asked questions.* Baltimore, MD: Centers for Medicare and Medicaid Services.

333. Nardone, M., & Paradise, J. (2014). *Medicaid health homes: A profile of newer programs. Issue Brief.* Washington, DC: The Kaiser Commission on Medicaid and the Uninsured.

334. Health Home Information Resource Center. (2015). Medicaid health homes: SPA overview. Baltimore, MD: Centers for Medicare & Medicaid Services.

335. Centers for Medicare & Medicaid Services. (2015). State innovation models initiative: General information. *CMS.gov*. Retrieved from http://innovation.cms.gov/initiatives/state-innovations/. Accessed on October 12, 2015.

336. Ormond, B., Richardson, E., Spillman, B., & Feder, J. (2014). *Health homes in Medicaid: The promise and the challenge*. Washington, DC: Urban Institute.

337. Spillman, B. C., Ormond, B. A., & Richardson, E. (2012). *Evaluation of the Medicaid health home option for beneficiaries with chronic conditions: Final annual report - base year*. Washington, DC: Office of The Assistant Secretary for Planning and Evaluation (ASPE).

338. Phillips, R. L., Jr., Han, M., Petterson, S. M., Makaroff, L. A., & Liaw, W. R. (2014). Cost, utilization, and quality of care: An evaluation of Illinois' Medicaid primary care case management program. *Annals of Family Medicine, 12*(5), 408-416.

339. Baird, M., Blount, A., Brungardt, S., Dickinson, P., Dietrich, A., Epperly, T., . . . Korsen, N. (2014). Joint principles: Integrating behavioral health care into the patient-centered medical home. *The Annals of Family Medicine, 12*(2), 183-185.

340. Substance Abuse and Mental Health Services Administration. (2014). *Advancing behavioral health integration within NCQA recognized patient-centered medical homes*. Rockville, MD: SAMHSA-HRSA Center for Integrated Health Solutions (CIHS).

341. Andrews, C., Grogan, C., Brennan, M., & Pollack, H. A. (2015). Lessons From Medicaid's divergent paths on mental health and addiction services. *Health Affairs, 34*(7), 1131-1138.

342. Berwick, D. M., Nolan, T. W., & Whittington, J. (2008). The triple aim: Care, health, and cost. *Health Affairs 27*(3), 759-769.

343. Hacker, K., & Walker, D. K. (2013). Achieving population health in accountable care organizations. *American Journal of Public Health, 103*(7), 1163-1167.

344. Alley, D. E., Asomugha, C. N., Conway, P. H., & Sanghavi, D. M. (2016). Accountable health communities — Addressing social needs through Medicare and Medicaid. *New England Journal of Medicine, 374*(1), 8-11.

345. National Academy for State Health Policy (NASHP). (2012). State 'accountable care' activity map. Retrieved from http://www.nashp.org/state-accountable-care-activity-map/. Accessed on April 11, 2016.

346. Purington, K., Gauthier, A., Patel, S., & Miller, C. (2011). *On the road to better value: State roles in promoting accountable care organizations*. (Publication No. 1479). Portland, ME: National Academy for State Health Policy (NASHP).

347. Rodin, D., & Silow-Carroll, S. (2013). *Medicaid payment and delivery reform in Colorado: ACOs at the regional level*. (Publication No. 1666). New York, NY: The Commonwealth Fund.

348. Schoenherr, K. E., Van Citters, A. D., Carluzzo, K. L., Bergquist, S., Fisher, E. S., & Lewis, V. A. (2013). *Establishing a coalition to pursue accountable care in the safety net: A case study of the FQHC urban health network*. (1710). New York, NY: The Commonwealth Fund.

349. Association of State and Territorial Health Officials. (2015). *Community-clinical linkages to improve hypertension identification, management, and control*. Issue Brief. Arlington, VA: Association of State and Territorial Health Officials.

350. Institute of Medicine, Roundtable on Population Health Improvement, & Board on Population Health and Public Health Practice. (2014). *Population health implications of the Affordable Care Act: Workshop summary.* Washington, DC: National Academies Press.

351. Oregon Health Authority Office of Health Analytics. (2015). *Oregon's health system transformation: 2014 final report* Salem, OR: Oregon Health Authority.

352. Health Resources and Services Administration. (n.d.). What is a health center? Retrieved from http://bphc.hrsa.gov/about/what-is-a-health-center/index.html. Accessed on July 9, 2016.

353. Health Resources and Services Administration (HRSA). (2016). HHS awards $94 million to health centers to help treat the prescription opioid abuse and heroin epidemic in America [Press release]. Retrieved from http://www.hhs.gov/about/news/2016/03/11/hhs-awards-94-million-to-health-centers.html. Accessed on April 12, 2016.

354. Haddad, M. S., Zelenev, A., & Altice, F. L. (2013). Integrating buprenorphine maintenance therapy into federally qualified health centers: Real-world substance abuse treatment outcomes. *Drug and Alcohol Dependence, 131*(1), 127-135.

355. Centers for Medicare & Medicaid Services. (2016). April 2016 EHR incentive program. Retrieved from https://www.cms.gov/Regulations-and-Guidance/Legislation/EHRIncentivePrograms/Downloads/April_2016_Summary_Report.pdf. Accessed on June 13, 2016.

356. Heisey-Grove, D., & Patel, V. (2015). *Any, certified, and basic: Quantifying physician EHR adoption through 2014.* (ONC Data Brief 28). Washington, DC: Office of the National Coordinator for Health Information Technology.

357. Leveille, S. G., Huang, A., Tsai, S. B., Allen, M., Weingart, S. N., & Iezzoni, L. I. (2009). Health coaching via an internet portal for primary care patients with chronic conditions: A randomized controlled trial. *Medical Care, 47*(1), 41-47.

358. Health Resources and Services Administration. (2012). Affordable Care Act helps expand the use of health information technology. Retrieved from http://www.hrsa.gov/about/news/pressreleases/121220healthcenternetworks.html. Accessed on July 9, 2016.

359. Centers for Medicare & Medicaid Services. (2014). *Eligible professional meaningful use table of contents core and menu set objectives.* Baltimore, MD: Centers for Medicare & Medicaid Services.

360. Office of the National Coordinator for Health Information Technology. (2013). Meaningful use. *HealthIT.gov.* Retrieved from http://www.healthit.gov/policy-researchers-implementers/meaningful-use. Accessed on October 31, 2015.

361. Terry, N. P. (2013). Meaningful adoption: What we know or think we know about the financing, effectiveness, quality, and safety of electronic medical records. *Journal of Legal Medicine, 34*(1), 7-42.

362. Centers for Medicare & Medicaid Services. (2015). Fact sheet: Electronic health record incentive program and health IT certification program final rule. Retrieved from https://www.cms.gov/Newsroom/MediaReleaseDatabase/Fact-sheets/2015-Fact-sheets-items/2015-10-06.html. Accessed on April 5, 2016.

363. Ghitza, U. E., & Tai, B. (2014). Challenges and opportunities for integrating preventive substance-use-care services in primary care through the Affordable Care Act. *Journal of Health Care for the Poor and Underserved, 25*(10), 36-45.

364. National Institute on Alcohol Abuse and Alcoholism. (2005). Helping patients who drink too much: A clinician's guide. Retrieved from http://pubs.niaaa.nih.gov/publications/Practitioner/CliniciansGuide2005/clinicians_guide.htm. Accessed on March 20, 2015.

365. Shimada, S. L., Brandt, C. A., Feng, H., McInnes, D. K., Rao, S. R., Rothendler, J. A., . . . Houston, T. K. (2014). Personal health record reach in the Veterans Health Administration: A cross-sectional analysis. *Journal of Medical Internet Research, 16*(12).

366. Goldzweig, C. L., Orshansky, G., Paige, N. M., Towfigh, A. A., Haggstrom, D. A., Miake-Lye, I., . . . Shekelle, P. G. (2013). Electronic patient portals: evidence on health outcomes, satisfaction, efficiency, and attitudes: A systematic review. *Annals of Internal Medicine, 159*(10), 677-687.

367. Weingart, S. N., Rind, D., Tofias, Z., & Sands, D. Z. (2006). Who uses the patient internet portal? The PatientSite experience. *Journal of the American Medical Informatics Association, 13*(1), 91-95.

368. Ancker, J. S., Barrón, Y., Rockoff, M. L., Hauser, D., Pichardo, M., Szerencsy, A., & Calman, N. (2011). Use of an electronic patient portal among disadvantaged populations. *Journal of General Internal Medicine, 26*(10), 1117-1123.

369. Ghitza, U. E., Gore-Langton, R. E., Lindblad, R., Shide, D., Subramaniam, G., & Tai, B. (2013). Common data elements for substance use disorders in electronic health records: The NIDA clinical trials network experience. *Addiction, 108*(1), 3-8.

370. Tai, B., & McLellan, A. T. (2012). Integrating information on substance use disorders into electronic health record systems. *Journal of Substance Abuse Treatment, 43*(1), 12-19.

371. Ray, G. T., Bahorik, A., Weisner, C., Wakim, P., VanHelhuisen, P., & Campbell, C. I. (Under review). Development of a prescription opioid registry in an integrated health system: Characteristics of prescription opioid use.

372. Campbell, C. I., Kline-Simon, A. H., Von Korff, M., Saunders, K. W., & Weisner, C. (Under review). Alcohol and drug use and aberrant drug-related behavior among patients on chronic opioid therapy.

373. Minnesota Department of Human Services. (2012). *Minnesota state substance abuse strategy*. (DHS-6543-ENG). St. Paul, MO: Minnesota Department of Human Services.

374. Agency Medical Directors' Group (AMDG). (2015). Interagency guideline on prescribing opioids for pain. Retrieved from http://www.agencymeddirectors.wa.gov/Files/2015AMDGOpioidGuideline.pdf. Accessed on October 13, 2015.

375. Session Law 2013-23, Bill No. 20, General Assembly of North Carolina (2013).

376. Humphreys, K. (2015). An overdose antidote goes mainstream. *Health Affairs, 34*(10), 1624-1627.

377. Join Together Staff. (2015). CVS will sell naloxone without prescription in 14 states. Retrieved from http://www.drugfree.org/join-together/cvs-will-sell-naloxone-without-prescription-14-states/. Accessed on April 5, 2016.

378. Davis, C. (2015). *Addressing legal barriers to naloxone access*. Paper presented at the FDA Meeting on Exploring Naloxone Uptake and Use, Silver Spring, MD. Retrieved from http://www.fda.gov/downloads/Drugs/NewsEvents/UCM454758.pdf. Accessed on April 13, 2016.

379. American Pharmacists Association. (2013). Collaborative practice agreements vary among the states. Retrieved from http://www.pharmacist.com/collaborative-practice-agreements-vary-among-states. Accessed on July 9, 2016.

380. Centers for Disease Control Prevention. (2013). Acetyl fentanyl overdose fatalities—Rhode Island, March-May 2013. *MMWR, 62*(34), 703-704.

381. State of Rhode Island and Providence Plantations Department of Health. (2014). *Rules and regulations pertaining to opioid overdose prevention* (R23-1-OPOID).

382. Wheeler, E., Jones, T. S., Gilbert, M. K., Davidson, P. J., & Centers for Disease Control and Prevention. (2015). Opioid overdose prevention programs providing naloxone to laypersons—United States, 2014. *MMWR, 64*(23), 631-635.

383. Vermont Agency of Human Services. (2012). Integrated treatment continuum for substance use dependence "Hub/Spoke" Initiative—Phase 1: Opiate dependence. Retrieved from http://www.healthvermont.gov/adap/documents/HUBSPOKEBriefingDocV122112.pdf. Accessed on July 26, 2016.

384. American Association for the Treatment of Opioid Dependence, Inc.,. (n.d.). F3 VT's Hub and Spoke model for opioid addiction. Retrieved from http://www.aatod.org/f3-vts-hub-and-spoke-model-for-opioid-addiction/. Accessed on July 26, 2016.

CHAPTER 7.
VISION FOR THE FUTURE: A PUBLIC HEALTH APPROACH

Substance misuse and substance use disorders directly affect millions of Americans every year, causing motor vehicle crashes, crimes, injuries, reduced quality of life, impaired health, and far too many deaths. Throughout this *Report*, we have summarized the research demonstrating that:

- The problems caused by substance misuse are not limited to substance use disorders, but include many other possible health and safety problems that can result from substance misuse even in the absence of a disorder;

- Substance use has complex biological and social determinants, and substance use disorders are medical conditions involving disruption of key brain circuits;

- Prevention programs and policies that are based on sound evidence-based principles have been shown to reduce substance misuse and related harms significantly;

- Evidence-based behavioral and medication-assisted treatments (MAT) applied using a chronic-illness-management approach have been shown to facilitate recovery from substance use disorders, prevent relapse, and improve other outcomes, such as reducing criminal behavior and the spread of infectious diseases;

- A chronic-illness-management approach may be needed to treat the most severe substance use disorders; and

- Access to recovery support services can help former substance users achieve and sustain long-term wellness.

Embedding prevention, treatment, and recovery services into the larger health care system will increase access to care, improve quality of services, and produce improved outcomes for countless Americans.

VISION FOR THE FUTURE

Time for a Change

It is time to change how we as a society address alcohol and drug misuse and substance use disorders. A national opioid overdose epidemic has captured the attention of the public as well as federal, state, local, and tribal leaders across the country. Ongoing efforts to reform health care and criminal justice systems are creating new opportunities to increase access to prevention and treatment services. Health care reform and parity laws are providing significant opportunities and incentives to address substance misuse and related disorders more effectively in diverse health care settings. At the same time, many states are making changes to drug policies, ranging from mandating use of prescription drug monitoring programs (PDMPs) to eliminating mandatory minimum drug sentences. These changes represent new opportunities to create policies and practices that are more evidence-informed to address health and social problems related to substance misuse.

The moral obligation to address substance misuse and substance use disorders effectively for all Americans also aligns with a strong economic imperative. Substance misuse and substance use disorders are estimated to cost society $442 billion each year in health care costs, lost productivity, and criminal justice costs.[1,2] However, numerous evidence-based prevention and treatment policies and programs can be implemented to reduce these costs while improving health and wellness. More than 10 million full-time workers in our nation have a substance use disorder—a leading cause of disability[3]—and studies have demonstrated that prevention and treatment programs for employees with substance use disorders are cost effective in improving worker productivity.[4,5] Prevention and treatment also reduce criminal justice-related costs, and they are much less expensive than alternatives such as incarceration. Implementation of evidence-based interventions (EBIs) can have a benefit of more than $58 for every dollar spent; and studies show that every dollar spent on substance use disorder treatment saves $4 in health care costs and $7 in criminal justice costs.[6] Yet, effective prevention interventions are highly underused. For example, only 8 to 10 percent of school administrators report using EBIs to prevent substance misuse,[7,8] and only about 11 percent of youth (aged 12 to 17) report participating in a substance use prevention program outside of school.[9] Further, only 10.4 percent of individuals with a substance use disorder receive treatment,[9] and only about a third of those individuals receives treatment that meets minimal standards of care.[10]

The public health-based approach called for in this *Report* aims to address the broad individual, environmental, and societal factors that influence substance misuse and its consequences, to improve the health, safety, and well-being of the entire population. It aims to understand and address the wide range of interacting factors that influence substance misuse and substance use disorders in different communities and coordinates efforts across diverse stakeholders to achieve reductions in both.

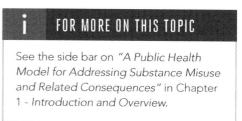

FOR MORE ON THIS TOPIC

See the side bar on *"A Public Health Model for Addressing Substance Misuse and Related Consequences"* in Chapter 1 - *Introduction and Overview*.

The following five general messages described within the *Report* have important implications for policy and practice. These are followed by specific evidence-based suggestions for the roles individuals, families, organizations, and communities can play in more effectively addressing this major health issue.

1. Both substance misuse and substance use disorders harm the health and well-being of individuals and communities. Addressing them requires implementation of effective strategies.

Substance misuse is the use of alcohol or illicit or prescription drugs in a manner that may cause harm to users or to those around them. Harms can include overdoses, interpersonal violence, motor vehicle crashes, as well as injuries, homicides, and suicides—the leading causes of death in adolescents and young adults (aged 12 to 25).[11] In 2015, 47.7 million Americans used an illicit drug or misused a prescription medication in the past year, 66.7 million binge drank in the past month, and 27.9 million self-reported driving under the influence (DUI) in the past year.[9]

Substance use disorders are medical illnesses that develop in some individuals who misuse substances—more than 20 million individuals in 2015.[9] These disorders involve impaired control over substance use that results from disruption of specific brain circuits. Substance use disorders occur along a continuum from mild to severe; severe substance use disorders are also called *addictions*. Because substances have particularly powerful effects on the developing adolescent brain, young adults who misuse substances are at increased risk of developing a substance use disorder at some point in their lives.

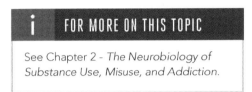

FOR MORE ON THIS TOPIC

See Chapter 2 - *The Neurobiology of Substance Use, Misuse, and Addiction.*

Implications for Policy and Practice

Expanding access to effective, evidence-based treatments for those with addiction and also less severe substance use disorders is critical, but broader prevention programs and policies are also essential to reduce substance misuse and the pervasive health and social problems caused by it. Although they cannot address the chronic, severe impairments common among individuals with substance use disorders, education, regular monitoring, and even modest legal sanctions may significantly reduce substance misuse in the wider population. Additionally, these measures are cost-effective. Many policies at the federal, state, local, and tribal levels that aim to reduce the harms associated with substance use have proven very effective in preventing and reducing alcohol misuse (e.g., binge drinking) and its consequences. More than 300,000 deaths have been avoided over the past decade simply from the implementation and enforcement of effective policies to reduce underage drinking and DUI.[12] Needle/syringe exchange programs also represent effective and cost-effective prevention strategies that have been shown to reduce the transmission of HIV in communities implementing them, without increasing rates of injection drug use. These programs also provide the opportunity to engage people who inject drugs in treatment. These types of effective prevention policies can and should be adapted and extended to reduce the injuries, disabilities, and deaths caused by substance misuse.[13]

2. Highly effective community-based prevention programs and policies exist and should be widely implemented.

This *Report* describes the significant advances in prevention science over the past two decades, including the identification of major risk and protective factors and the development of more than four dozen research-tested prevention interventions that can be delivered in households, schools, clinical settings, and community centers. Three key findings from the *Report* are especially important in this regard. First, science has shown that adolescence and young adulthood are major "at risk" periods for substance misuse and related harms. Second, most of the major genetic, social, and environmental risk factors that predict substance misuse also predict many other serious adverse outcomes and risks. Third, several community-delivered prevention programs and policies have been shown to significantly reduce rates of substance-use initiation and misuse-related harms.

Prevention programs and interventions can have a strong impact and be cost-effective, but only if evidence-based components are used and if those components are delivered in a coordinated and consistent fashion throughout the at-risk period. Parents, schools, health care systems, faith communities, and social service organizations should be involved in delivering comprehensive, evidence-based community prevention programs that are sustained over time.

Additionally, research has demonstrated that policies and environmental strategies are highly effective in reducing alcohol-related problems by focusing on the social, political, and economic contexts in which these problems occur. These evidence-based policies include regulating alcohol outlet density, restricting hours and days of sale, and policies to increase the price of alcohol at the federal, state, or local level.

Implications for Policy and Practice

To be effective, prevention programs and policies should be designed to address the common risk and protective factors that influence the most common health threats affecting young people. They should be tested through research and should be delivered continuously throughout the entire at-risk period by those who have been properly trained and supervised to use them. Federal and state funding incentives could increase the number of properly organized community coalitions using effective prevention practices that adhere to commonly defined standards. The research reviewed in this *Report* suggests that such coordinated efforts could significantly improve the impact of existing prevention funding, programs, and policies, enhancing quality of life for American families and communities.

3. Full integration of the continuum of services for substance use disorders with the rest of health care could significantly improve the quality, effectiveness, and safety of all health care.

Individuals with substance use disorders at all levels of severity can benefit from treatment, and research shows that integrating substance use disorder treatment into mainstream health care can improve the quality of treatment services. Historically, however, only individuals with the most severe substance use disorders have received treatment, and only in independent "addiction treatment programs" that were originally designed in the early 1960s to treat addictions as personality or character disorders. Moreover, although 45 percent of patients seeking treatment for substance use disorders have a co-occurring mental disorder,[14] most specialty substance use disorder treatment programs are not part of, or even affiliated with, mental or physical health care organizations. Similarly, most general health care organizations—even teaching hospitals—do not provide screening, diagnosis, or treatment for substance use disorders.

This separation of substance use disorder treatment from the rest of health care has contributed to the lack of understanding of the medical nature of these conditions, lack of awareness among affected individuals that they have a significant health problem, and slow adoption of scientifically supported medical treatments by addiction treatment providers. Additionally, mainstream health care has been inadequately prepared to address the prevalent substance misuse–related problems of patients in many clinical settings. This has contributed to incorrect diagnoses, inappropriate treatment plans, poor adherence to treatment plans by patients, and high rates of emergency department and hospital admissions.

The goals of substance use disorder treatment are very similar to the treatment goals for other chronic illnesses: to eliminate or reduce the primary symptoms (substance use), improve general health and function, and increase the motivation and skills of patients and their families to manage threats of relapse. Even serious substance use disorders can be treated effectively, with recurrence rates equivalent to those of other chronic illnesses such as diabetes, asthma, or hypertension.[15] With comprehensive continuing care, recovery is an achievable outcome: More than 25 million individuals with a previous substance use disorder are estimated to be in remission.[16] Integrated treatment can dramatically improve patient health and quality of life, reduce fatalities, address health disparities, and reduce societal costs that result from unrecognized, unaddressed substance use disorders among patients in the general health care system. However, most existing substance use disorder treatment programs lack the needed training, personnel, and infrastructure to provide treatment for co-occurring physical and mental illnesses. Similarly, most physicians, nurses, and other health care professionals working in general health care settings have not received training in screening, diagnosing, or addressing substance use disorders.

Implications for Policy and Practice

Policy changes, particularly at the state level, are needed to better integrate care for substance use disorders with the rest of health care. States have substantial power to shape the nature of care within these programs. State licensing and financing policies should be designed to better incentivize programs that offer the full continuum of care (residential, outpatient, continuing care, and recovery supports); offer a full range of evidence-based behavioral treatments and medications; and maintain working affiliations with general and mental health care professionals to integrate care. Within general health care, federal and state grants and development programs should make eligibility contingent on integrating care for mental and substance use disorders or provide incentives for organizations that support this type of integration.

But integration of mental health and substance use disorder care into general health care will not be possible without a workforce that is competently cross-educated and trained in all these areas. Currently, only 8 percent of American medical schools offer a separate, required course on addiction medicine and 36 percent have an elective course; minimal or no professional education on substance use disorders is available for other health professionals.[17-19] Federal and state policies should require or incentivize medical, nursing, dental, pharmacy, and other clinical professional schools to provide mandatory courses to properly equip young health care professionals to address substance misuse and related health consequences. Similarly, associations of clinical professionals should continue to provide continuing education and training courses for those already in practice.

4. Coordination and implementation of recent health reform and parity laws will help ensure increased access to services for people with substance use disorders.

The Paul Wellstone and Pete Domenici Mental Health Parity and Addiction Equity Act of 2008 (MHPAEA) and the 2010 Affordable Care Act increased access to coverage for mental health and substance use disorder treatment services for more than 161 million Americans. Even so, just 10.4 percent of people with substance use disorders who need treatment are accessing care.[9] These pieces of legislation, besides promoting equity, make good long-term economic sense: Research reviewed in **Chapter 6 - Health Care Systems and Substance Use Disorders** highlights the extraordinary costs to society from unaddressed substance misuse and from untreated or inappropriately treated substance use disorders—more than $422 billion annually (including more than $120 billion in health care costs). However, there remains great uncertainty on the part of affected individuals and their families, as well as among many health care professionals, about the nature and range of health care benefits and covered services available for prevention, early intervention, and treatment of substance use disorders.

Implications for Policy and Practice

Enhanced federal communication will help increase public understanding about individuals' rights to appropriate care and services for substance use disorders. This communication could help eliminate confusion among patients, providers, and insurers. But, more will be needed to extend the reach of treatment and thereby reduce the prevalence, severity, and costs associated with substance use disorders. Within health care organizations, active screening for substance misuse and substance use disorders combined with effective communication around the availability of treatment programs could do much to engage untreated individuals in care. Screening and treatment must incorporate brief interventions for mildly affected individuals as well as the full range of evidence-based behavioral therapies and medications for more severe disorders, and must be provided by a fully trained complement of health care professionals.

5. A large body of research has clarified the biological, psychological, and social underpinnings of substance misuse and related disorders and described effective prevention, treatment, and recovery support services. Future research is needed to guide the new public health approach to substance misuse and substance use disorders.

Five decades ago, basic, pharmacological, epidemiological, clinical, and implementation research played important roles in informing a skeptical public about the harms of cigarette smoking and creating new and better prevention and treatment options. Similarly, research reviewed in this *Report* should eliminate many of the long-held, but incorrect, stereotypes about substance misuse and substance use disorders, such as that alcohol and drug problems are the product of faulty character or willful rejection of social norms.

Thanks to scientific research over the past two decades, we know far more about alcohol and drugs and their effects on health than we knew about the effects of smoking when the first *Surgeon General's Report on Smoking and Health* was released in 1964. For instance, we now know that repeated substance misuse carries the greatest threat of developing into a substance use disorder when substance use begins in adolescence. We also know that substance use disorders involve persistent changes in specific brain circuits that control the perceived value of a substance as well as reward, stress, and executive functions, like decision making and self-control.

However, although this body of knowledge provides a firm foundation for developing effective prevention, early intervention, treatment, and recovery strategies, achieving the vision of this *Report* will require redoubled research efforts. We still do not fully understand how the brain changes involved in substance use disorders occur, how individual biological and environmental risk factors contribute to those changes, or the extent to which these brain changes reverse after long periods of abstinence from alcohol or drug use.

Implications for Policy and Practice

Future research should build upon our existing knowledge base to inform the development of prevention and treatment strategies that more directly target brain circuit abnormalities that underlie substance use disorders; identify which prevention and treatment interventions are most effective for which patients (personalizing medicine); clarify how the brain and body regain function and recover after chronic drug exposure; and inform the development of evidence-based strategies for supporting recovery. Also critically needed are long-term prospective studies of youth (particularly those deemed most at risk) that will concurrently study changes in personal and environmental risks; the nature, amount, and frequency of substance use; and changes in brain structure and function.

To guide the important system-wide changes recommended in this *Report*, research to optimize strategies for broadly and sustainably implementing evidence-based prevention, treatment, and recovery interventions across the community is necessary. Within traditional substance use disorder treatment programs, research is needed on how to use new insurance benefits and financing models to enhance service delivery most effectively, how to form working alliances with general physical and mental health providers, and how to integrate new technologies and information systems to enhance care without compromising patient confidentiality.

Specific Suggestions for Key Stakeholders

Current health reform efforts and recent advances in technology are playing a crucial role in moving toward an effective public health-based model for addressing substance misuse and its consequences. But the health care system cannot address all of the major determinants of health related to substance misuse without the help of the wider community. This *Report* calls on a range of stakeholder groups to do their part to change the culture, attitudes, and practices around substance use and to keep the conversation going until this goal is met. Prejudice and discrimination have created many of the challenges that plague

VISION FOR THE FUTURE

the substance use disorder treatment field. These factors can have a profound influence on individuals' willingness to talk to their health care professional about their substance use concerns; to seek or access treatment services; and to be open with friends, family, and coworkers about their treatment and recovery needs. Changing the culture is an essential piece of lasting reforms, creating a society in which:

- People who need help feel comfortable seeking it;
- There is "no wrong door" for accessing health services;
- Communities are willing to invest in prevention services, knowing that such investment pays off over the long term, with wide-ranging benefits for everyone;
- Health care professionals treat substance use disorders with the same level of compassion and care as they would any other chronic disease, such as diabetes or heart disease;
- People are celebrated for their efforts to get well and for their steps in recovery; and
- Everyone knows that their care and support can make a meaningful difference in someone's recovery.

In addition to facilitating such a mindset, community leaders can work together to mobilize the capacities of health care organizations, social service organizations, educational systems, community-based organizations, government health agencies, religious institutions, law enforcement, local businesses, researchers, and other public, private, and voluntary entities that impact public health. *Everyone has a role to play in addressing substance misuse and substance use disorders and in changing the conversation around substance use, to improve the health, safety, and well-being of individuals and communities across our nation.*

Individuals and Families

Reach out, if you think you have a problem.

In the past, many individuals and families have kept silent about substance-related issues because of shame, guilt, or fear of exposure or recrimination. Breaking the silence and isolation around such issues is crucial, so that individuals and families confronting substance misuse and its consequences know that they are not alone and can openly seek treatment. As with other chronic illnesses, the earlier treatment begins, the better the outcomes are likely to be.

Be supportive (not judgmental) if a loved one has a problem.

Recognizing that substance use disorders are medical conditions and not moral failings can help remove negative attitudes and promote open and healthy discussion between individuals with substance use disorders and their loved ones, as well as with their health care professionals. Overcoming the powerful drive to continue substance use can be difficult, and making the lifestyle changes necessary for successful treatment—such as changing relationships, jobs, or living environments—can be daunting. Providing sensitivity and support can ease this transition.

This can be challenging for partners, parents, siblings, and other loved ones of people with substance use disorders; many of the behaviors associated with substance misuse can be damaging to relationships. Being compassionate and caring does not mean that you do not hold the person accountable for their actions. It means that you see the person's behaviors in the light of a medical illness. Love and support can be offered while maintaining the boundaries that are important for your health and the health of everyone around you.

Show support toward people in recovery.

As a community, we typically show empathy when someone we know is ill, and we celebrate when people we know overcome an illness. Extending these kindnesses to people with substance use disorders and those in recovery can provide added encouragement to help them realize and maintain their recovery. It also will encourage others to seek out treatment when they need it.

Advocate for the changes needed in your community.

As discussed throughout this *Report*, many challenges need to be addressed to support a public health-based approach to substance misuse and related disorders. Everyone can play an important role in advocating for their needs, the needs of their loved ones, and the needs of their community. It is important that all voices are heard as we come together to address these challenges.

Parents, talk to your children about alcohol and drugs.

Parents have more influence over their children's behavior, including substance use, than they often think. For instance, according to one study, young adults who reported that their parents monitored their behavior and showed concern about them were less likely to report misusing substances.[20] Talking to your children about alcohol and drug use is not always easy, but it is crucial. Become informed, from reliable sources, about substances to which your children could be exposed, and about substance use disorders, and talk openly with your children about the risks. Some tips to keep in mind:

- Be a good listener;
- Set clear expectations about alcohol and drug use, including real consequences for not following family rules;
- Help your child deal with peer pressure;
- Get to know your child's friends and their parents;
- Talk to your child early and often; and
- Support your school district's efforts to implement evidence-based prevention interventions and treatment and recovery support.

Educators and Academic Institutions

Implement evidence-based prevention interventions.

Schools represent one of the most effective channels for influencing youth substance use. Many highly effective evidence-based programs are available that provide a strong return on investment, both in the well-being of the children they reach and in reducing long-term societal costs. Prevention programs for adolescents should target improving academic as well as social and emotional learning to address risk factors for substance misuse, such as early aggression, academic failure, and school dropout.

VISION FOR THE FUTURE

When combined with family-based and community programs that present consistent messages, these programs are even more powerful. Interventions that target youth who have already initiated use of alcohol or drugs should also be implemented to prevent escalation of use. Colleges, too, should implement EBIs to reduce student alcohol misuse.

Provide treatment and recovery supports.

Many students lack regular access to the health care system. For students with substance use problems, schools—ranging from primary school through university—can provide an entry into treatment and support for ongoing recovery. School counselors and school health care programs can provide enrolled students with screening, brief counseling, and referral to more comprehensive treatment services. Schools can also help create a supportive environment that fosters recovery. Many institutions of higher learning incorporate collegiate recovery programs that can make a profound difference for young people trying to maintain recovery in an environment with high rates of substance misuse.

Teach accurate, up-to-date scientific information about alcohol and drugs and about substance use disorders as medical conditions.

Teachers, professors, and school counselors play an obvious and central role as youth influencers, teaching students about the health consequences of substance use and misuse and about substance use disorders as medical conditions, as well as facilitating open dialogue. They can also play an active role in educating parents and community members on these topics and the role they can play in preventing youth substance use. For example, they can educate businesses near schools about the positive impact of strong enforcement of underage drinking laws and about the potential harms of synthetic drugs (such as K2 and bath salts), to discourage their sale. They can also promote non-shaming language that underscores the medical nature of addiction—for instance avoiding terms like "abuser" or "addict" when describing people with substance use disorders.[21]

Enhance training of health care professionals.

As substance use treatment becomes more integrated with the health care delivery system, there is a need for advanced education and training for providers in all health care roles and disciplines, including primary care doctors, nurses, specialty treatment providers, and prevention and recovery specialists. It is essential that professional schools of social work, psychology, public health, nursing, medicine, dentistry, and pharmacy incorporate curricula that reflect the current science of prevention, treatment, and recovery. Health care professionals must also be alert for the possibility of adverse drug reactions (e.g., co-prescribing of drugs with similar effects, drug overdoses), and co-occurring psychiatric conditions and infectious diseases, and should be trained on how to address these issues. These topics should also be covered in formal post-graduate training programs (e.g., physician residencies and psychology internships) as well as in board certification and continuing education requirements for professionals in these fields. Continuing education should include not only subject matter knowledge but the professional skills necessary to provide integrated care within cross-disciplinary health care teams that address substance-related health issues.

Health Care Professionals and Professional Associations

Address substance use-related health issues with the same sensitivity and care as any other chronic health condition.

All health care professionals—including physicians, physician assistants, nurses, nurse practitioners, dentists, social workers, therapists, and pharmacists—can play a role in addressing substance misuse and substance use disorders, not only by directly providing health care services, but also by promoting prevention strategies and supporting the infrastructure changes needed to better integrate care for substance use disorders into general health care and other treatment settings.

Support high-quality care for substance use disorders.

Professional associations can be instrumental in setting workforce guidelines, advocating for curriculum changes in professional schools, promoting professional continuing education training, and developing evidence-based guidelines that outline best practices for prevention, screening and assessment, brief interventions, diagnosis, and treatment of substance-related health issues. For example, to help address the current prescription opioid crisis and overdose epidemic, associations should raise awareness of the most recent guidelines for opioid prescribing and commend the use of PDMPs by providers. Associations also should raise awareness of the benefits of making naloxone more readily available without a prescription and providing legal protection to physician-prescribers and bystanders ("Good Samaritans") who administer naloxone when encountering an overdose situation.

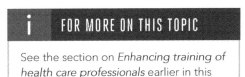

FOR MORE ON THIS TOPIC

See the section on *Enhancing training of health care professionals* earlier in this chapter.

Health Care Systems

Promote primary prevention.

Health care systems can help prevent prescription drug misuse and related substance use disorders by holding staff accountable for safe prescribing of controlled substances, training staff on alternative ways of managing pain and anxiety, and increasing use of PDMPs by pharmacists, physicians, and other providers.

Promote use of evidence-based treatments.

Substance use disorders cannot be effectively addressed without much wider adoption and implementation of scientifically tested and proven effective behavioral and pharmacological treatments. The full spectrum of evidence-based treatments should be available across all contexts of care, and treatment plans should be tailored to meet the specific needs of individual patients. Health care systems should take every step to educate health care professionals and the public about the value of MAT for alcohol and opioid use disorders, correcting misconceptions that have barred their wider adoption in the past.

VISION FOR THE FUTURE

Promote effective integration of prevention and treatment services.

Effective integration of behavioral health and general health care is essential for identifying patients in need of treatment, engaging them in the appropriate level of care, and ensuring ongoing monitoring of patients with substance use disorders to reduce their risk of relapse. Implementation of systems to support this type of integration requires care and foresight and should include educating and training the relevant workforces; developing new workflows to support universal screening, appropriate follow-up, coordination of care across providers, and ongoing recovery management; and linking patients and families to available support services. Quality measurement and improvement processes should also be incorporated to ensure that the services provided are effectively addressing the needs of the patient population and improving outcomes.

Work with payors to develop and implement comprehensive billing models.

Consideration of how payors can develop and implement comprehensive billing models is crucial to enabling health care systems to sustainably implement integrated services to address substance use disorders. Coverage policies will need to be updated to support implementation of prevention measures, screening, brief counseling, and recovery support services within the general health care system, and to support coordination of care between specialty substance use disorder treatment programs, mental health organizations, and the general health care system.

Implement health information technologies to promote efficiency and high-quality care.

Health information technology—ranging from electronic health records to patient registries, computer-based educational systems, and mobile applications—has the power to increase efficiency, improve clinical decision making, supplement patient services, extend the reach of the workforce, improve quality measurement, and support a "learning health care system." Health care systems should explore how these and other technologies can be used to support substance use disorder prevention, treatment, and recovery.

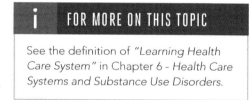

FOR MORE ON THIS TOPIC

See the definition of *"Learning Health Care System"* in Chapter 6 - *Health Care Systems and Substance Use Disorders.*

Communities

Build awareness of substance use as a public health problem.

Civic and advocacy groups, neighborhood associations, and community-based organizations can all play a major role in communication, education, and advocacy efforts that seek to address substance use-related health issues. These organizations provide community leadership and communicate urgent and emerging issues to specific audiences and constituencies. Communication vehicles such as newsletters, blogs, op-ed articles, and storytelling can be used to raise awareness and underscore the importance of placing substance use-related health issues in a public health framework. Community groups and organizations can host community forums, town hall meetings, listening sessions, and education and awareness days. These events foster public discourse, create venues in which diverse voices can be heard, and provide opportunities to educate the community. In addition, they can promote an awareness of the medical nature of addiction, to encourage acceptance of opioid treatment programs and other substance use disorder treatment services embedded in the community. Communities also can sponsor prevention and recovery campaigns, health fairs, marches, and rallies that emphasize wellness activities that bring attention to substance use-related health issues.

Invest in evidence-based prevention interventions and recovery supports.

Prevention research has developed effective community-based prevention programs that reduce substance use and delinquent behavior among youth. Although the process of getting these programs implemented in communities has been slow, resources are available to help individual communities identify the risk factors for future substance use among youth that are most prevalent within their community and choose evidence-based prevention strategies to address them. Research shows that for each dollar invested in research-based prevention programs, up to $10 is saved in treatment for alcohol or other substance misuse-related costs.[22-25]

Implement interventions to reduce harms associated with alcohol and drug misuse.

An essential part of a comprehensive public health approach to addressing substance misuse is wider use of strategies to reduce individual and societal harms, such as overdoses, motor vehicle crashes, and the spread of infectious diseases. Communities across the country are implementing programs to distribute naloxone to first responders, opioid users, and potential bystanders, preventing thousands of deaths.[26] Others have implemented needle/syringe exchange programs, successfully reducing the spread of HIV and Hepatitis C without seeing an increase in injection drug use. These and other evidence-based strategies can have a profound impact on the overall health and well-being of the community.

Private Sector: Industry and Commerce

Promote only responsible, safe use of legal substances, by adults.

Companies that manufacture and sell alcohol and legal drugs, as well as products related to use of these substances, can demonstrate social responsibility by taking measures to discourage and prevent the misuse of their products. Companies can take steps to ensure that the public is aware of the risks associated with substance use, including the use of medications with addictive potential alone and in combination with alcohol or other drugs.

Support youth substance use prevention.

Manufacturers and sellers of alcohol, legal drugs, and related products have a role in reducing and preventing youth substance use. They can discourage the sale and promotion of alcohol and other substances to minors and support evidence based programs to prevent and reduce youth substance use.

Continue to collaborate with the federal initiative to reduce prescription opioid- and heroin-related overdose, death, and dependence.

Pharmaceutical companies and pharmacies can continue to collaborate with the U.S. Department of Health and Human Services to identify and implement evidence-informed solutions to the current opioid crisis. This collaboration may include examining and revising product labeling, funding continuing medical education for providers on the appropriate use of opioid medications, developing abuse-deterrent formulations of opioids, prioritizing development of non-opioid alternatives for pain relief, and conducting studies to determine the appropriate dosing of opioids in children and safe prescribing practices for both children and adults.[27]

Federal, State, Local, and Tribal Governments

Provide leadership, guidance, and vision in supporting a science-based approach to addressing substance use-related health issues.

Coordinated federal, state, local, and tribal efforts are needed to promote a public health approach to addressing substance use, misuse, and related disorders. As discussed throughout this *Report*, widespread cultural and systemic issues need to be addressed to reduce the prevalence of substance misuse and related public health consequences. Government agencies have a major role to play in:

- Improving public education and awareness;
- Conducting research and evaluations;
- Monitoring public health trends;
- Providing incentives, funding, and assistance to promote implementation of effective prevention, treatment, and recovery practices, policies, and programs;
- Addressing legislative and regulatory barriers;
- Improving coordination between health care, criminal justice, and social service organizations; and
- Fostering collaborative initiatives with the private sector.

For example, federal and state agencies can implement policies to integrate current best practices—such as the Centers for Disease Control and Prevention (CDC) *Guideline for Prescribing Opioids for Chronic Pain*[29] or mandatory use of PDMPs—among federal and state supported service providers.

Improve coordination between social service systems and the health care system to address the social and environmental factors that contribute to the risk for substance use disorders.

Social service systems serve individuals, families, and communities in a variety of capacities, often in tandem with the health care system. Social workers can play a significant role in helping patients with substance use disorders with the wrap-around services that are vital for successful treatment, including finding stable housing, obtaining job training or employment opportunities, and accessing recovery supports and other resources available in the community. In addition, they can coordinate care across providers, offer support for families, and help implement prevention programs. Child and family welfare systems also should implement trauma-informed, recovery-oriented, and public health approaches for parents who are misusing substances, while maintaining a strong focus on the safety and welfare of children.

Implement criminal justice reforms to transition to a less punitive and more health-focused approach.

The criminal justice and juvenile justice systems can play pivotal roles in addressing substance use-related health issues across the community. These systems are engaged with a population at high-risk for substance use disorders and often at a teachable moment—when individuals are more open to prevention messaging or to accepting the need for treatment. Less punitive, health-focused initiatives can have a critical impact on long-term outcomes. Sheriff's offices, police departments, and county jails should work closely with citizens' groups, prevention initiatives, treatment agencies, and recovery community organizations to create alternatives to arrest and lockup for nonviolent and substance use-related offenses. For example, drug courts have been a very successful model for diverting people with substance use disorders away from incarceration and into treatment.[30] It is essential that these programs promote the delivery of evidence-based treatment services, including MAT.

Many prisoners have access to regular health care services only when they are incarcerated. Significant research supports the value of integrating prevention and treatment into criminal justice settings.[31,32] In addition, community re-entry is a particularly high-risk time for relapse and overdose. Criminal justice systems can reduce these risks and reduce recidivism by coordinating with community health settings to ensure that patients with substance use disorders have continuing access to care upon release.

Facilitate research on Schedule I substances

Some researchers indicate that the process for conducting studies on Schedule I substances, such as marijuana, can be burdensome and act as disincentives. It is clear that more research is needed to understand how use of these substances affect the brain and body in order to help inform effective treatments for overdose, withdrawal management, and addiction, as well as explore potential therapeutic uses. To help ease administrative burdens, federal agencies should continue to enhance efforts and partnerships to facilitate research. Some of these efforts have already borne positive outcomes. For example, a recent policy change will foster research by expanding the number of U.S. Drug Enforcement Administration (DEA) registered marijuana growers. Making marijuana available from new sources could both speed the pace of research and afford medication developers and researchers more options for formulating marijuana-derived investigational products.

Researchers

Conduct research that focuses on implementable, sustainable solutions to address high-priority substance use issues.

Scientific research should be informed by ongoing public health needs. This includes research on the basic genetic and epigenetic contributors to substance use disorders and the environmental and social factors that influence risk; basic neuroscience research on substance use-related effects and brain recovery; studies adapting existing prevention programs to different populations and audiences; and trials of new and improved treatment approaches. Focused research is also needed to help address the significant research-to-practice gap in the implementation of evidence-based prevention and treatment interventions. Closing the gap between research discovery and clinical and community practice is both a complex challenge and an absolute necessity if we are to ensure that all populations benefit from the nation's investments in scientific discoveries. Research is needed to better understand the barriers to successful and sustainable implementation of evidence-based interventions and to develop implementation strategies that effectively overcome these barriers.

Researchers should collaborate with health care professionals, payors, educators, people in treatment and recovery, community coalitions, and others to ensure that real-world barriers, such as workforce issues and billing limitations, are taken into consideration. These collaborations should also help researchers prioritize efforts to address critical ongoing barriers to effective prevention and treatment of substance use disorders.

Consider how scientific research can inform public policy.

Effective communication is critical for ensuring that the policies and programs that are implemented reflect the state of the science and have the greatest chance for improving outcomes. Scientific findings are often misrepresented in public policy debates. Scientific experts have a significant role to play in ensuring that the science is accurately represented in policies and program.

Promote rigorous evaluation of programs and policies.

Many programs and policies are often implemented without a sufficient evidence base or with limited fidelity to the evidence base; this may have unintended consequences when they are broadly implemented. Rigorous evaluation is needed to determine whether programs and policies are having their intended effect and to guide necessary changes when they are not.

Conclusion

This *Report* is a call to all Americans to change the way we address substance misuse and substance use disorders in our society. Past approaches to these issues have been rooted in misconceptions and prejudice and have resulted in a lack of preventive care; diagnoses that are made too late or never; and poor access to treatment and recovery support services, which exacerbated health disparities and deprived countless individuals, families, and communities of healthy outcomes and quality of life. Now is the time to acknowledge that these disorders must be addressed with compassion and as preventable and treatable medical conditions.

By adopting an evidence-based public health approach, we have the opportunity as a nation to take effective steps to prevent and treat substance use-related issues. Such an approach can prevent the initiation of substance use or escalation from use to a disorder, and thus it can reduce the number of people affected by these conditions; it can shorten the duration of illness for individuals who already have a disorder; and it can reduce the number of substance use-related deaths. A public health approach will also reduce collateral damage created by substance misuse, such as infectious disease transmission and motor vehicle crashes. Thus, promoting much wider adoption of appropriate evidence-based prevention, treatment, and recovery strategies needs to be a top public health priority.

Making this change will require a major cultural shift in the way Americans think about, talk about, look at, and act toward people with substance use disorders. Negative public attitudes about substance misuse and use disorders can be entrenched, but it *is* possible to change social viewpoints. This has been done many times in the past: For example, cancer and HIV used to be surrounded by fear and judgment, but they are now regarded by most Americans as medical conditions like many others. This has helped to make people comfortable talking about their concerns with their health care professionals, widening access to prevention and treatment. We can similarly change our attitudes toward substance use disorders if we come together as a society with the resolve to do so. With the moral case so strongly aligned with the economic case, and supported by all the available science, now is the time to make this change for the health and well-being of all Americans.

References

1. Sacks, J. J., Gonzales, K. R., Bouchery, E. E., Tomedi, L. E., & Brewer, R. D. (2015). 2010 national and state costs of excessive alcohol consumption. *American Journal of Preventive Medicine, 49*(5), e73-e79.

2. National Drug Intelligence Center. (2011). *National drug threat assessment.* Washington, DC: U.S. Department of Justice.

3. National Council for Behavioral Health. (2014). The business case for effective substance use disorder treatment. Retrieved from http://www.thenationalcouncil.org/wp-content/uploads/2015/01/14_Business-Case_Substance-Use.pdf. Accessed on June 27, 2016.

4. Jordan, N., Grissom, G., Alonzo, G., Dietzen, L., & Sangsland, S. (2008). Economic benefit of chemical dependency treatment to employers. *Journal of Substance Abuse Treatment, 34*(3), 311-319.

5. Slaymaker, V. J., & Owen, P. L. (2006). Employed men and women substance abusers: Job troubles and treatment outcomes. *Journal of Substance Abuse Treatment, 31*(4), 347-354.

6. Ettner, S. L., Huang, D., Evans, E., Ash, D. R., Hardy, M., Jourabchi, M., & Hser, Y. I. (2006). Benefit-cost in the California treatment outcome project: Does substance abuse treatment "pay for itself"? *Health Services Research, 41*(1), 192-213.

7. Ringwalt, C., Hanley, S., Vincus, A. A., Ennett, S. T., Rohrbach, L. A., & Bowling, J. M. (2008). The prevalence of effective substance use prevention curricula in the Nation's high schools. *The Journal of Primary Prevention, 29*(6), 479-488.

8. Crosse, S., Williams, B., Hagen, C. A., Harmon, M., Ristow, L., DiGaetano, R., . . . Derzon, J. H. (2011). *Prevalence and implementation fidelity of research-based prevention programs in public schools: Final report.* Washington, DC: U.S. Department of Education, Office of Planning, Evaluation and Policy Development, Policy and Program Studies Service.

9. Center for Behavioral Health Statistics and Quality. (2016). *Results from the 2015 National Survey on Drug Use and Health: Detailed tables.* Rockville, MD: Substance Abuse and Mental Health Services Administration.

10. Substance Abuse and Mental Health Services Administration. (2013). *Behavioral health, United States, 2012.* (HHS Publication No. (SMA) 13-4797). Rockville, MD: Substance Abuse and Mental Health Services Administration.

11. Blum, R. W., & Qureshi, F. (2011). *Morbidity and mortality among adolescents and young adults in the United States.* AstraZeneca Fact Sheet 2011. Baltimore, MD: Johns Hopkins Bloomberg School of Public Health, Department of Population, Family and Reproductive Health.

12. Fell, J. C., & Voas, R. B. (2006). Mothers Against Drunk Driving (MADD): The first 25 years. *Traffic Injury Prevention, 7*(3), 195-212.

13. Aspinall, E. J., Nambiar, D., Goldberg, D. J., Hickman, M., Weir, A., Van Velzen, E., . . . Hutchinson, S. J. (2014). Are needle and syringe programmes associated with a reduction in HIV transmission among people who inject drugs: A systematic review and meta-analysis. *International Journal of Epidemiology, 43*(1), 235-248.

14. Substance Abuse and Mental Health Services Administration. (2015). Behavioral health treatments and services. Retrieved from http://www.samhsa.gov/treatment. Accessed on January 25, 2016.

15. McLellan, A. T., Lewis, D. C., O'Brien, C. P., & Kleber, H. D. (2000). Drug dependence, a chronic medical illness: Implications for treatment, insurance, and outcomes evaluation. *JAMA, 284*(13), 1689-1695.

16. White, W. L. (2012). *Recovery/remission from substance use disorders: An analysis of reported outcomes in 415 scientific reports, 1868-2011.* Philadelphia, PA: Philadelphia Department of Behavioral Health and Intellectual Disability Services.

17. Institute of Medicine, & Committee on Crossing the Quality Chasm. (2006). *Improving the quality of health care for mental and substance-use conditions.* Washington, DC: National Academies Press.

18. Haack, M. R., & Adger, J. H. (Eds.). (2002). *Strategic plan for interdisciplinary faculty development: Arming the nation's health professional workforce for a new approach to substance use disorders.* Providence, RI: Association for Medical Education and Research in Substance Abuse (AMERSA).

19. Parish, C. L., Pereyra, M. R., Pollack, H. A., Cardenas, G., Castellon, P. C., Abel, S. N., . . . Metsch, L. R. (2015). Screening for substance misuse in the dental care setting: Findings from a nationally representative survey of dentists. *Addiction, 110*(9), 1516-1523.

20. MetLife Foundation, & The Partnership at Drugfree.org. (2013). *2012 Partnership attitude tracking study: Teens and parents.* Retrieved from: http://www.drugfree.org/wp-content/uploads/2013/04/PATS-2012-FULL-REPORT2.pdf. Accessed on July 28, 2016.

21. Kelly, J. F., Saitz, R., & Wakeman, S. (2016). Language, substance use disorders, and policy: The need to reach consensus on an "addiction-ary". *Alcoholism Treatment Quarterly, 34*(1), 116-123.

22. Hawkins, J. D., Catalano, R. F., Kosterman, R., Abbott, R., & Hill, K. G. (1999). Preventing adolescent health-risk behaviors by strengthening protection during childhood. *Archives of Pediatrics and Adolescent Medicine, 153*(3), 226-234.

23. Spoth, R. L., Redmond, C., Trudeau, L., & Shin, C. (2002). Longitudinal substance initiation outcomes for a universal preventive intervention combining family and school programs. *Psychology of Addictive Behaviors, 16*(2), 129-134.

24. Aos, S., Phipps, P., Barnoski, R., & Lieb, R. (2001). *The comparative costs and benefits of programs to reduce crime. Version 4.0.* Olympia, WA: Washington State Institute for Public Policy.

25. Pentz, M. A. (1998). Costs, benefits, and cost-effectiveness of comprehensive drug abuse prevention. In W. J. Bukoski & R. I. Evans (Eds.), *Cost-benefit/cost-effectiveness research of drug abuse prevention: Implications for programming and policy. NIDA Research Monograph No. 176.* (pp. 111-129). Washington, DC: U.S. Government Printing Office.

26. Wheeler, E., Davidson, P. J., Jones, T. S., & Irwin, K. S. (2012). Community-based opioid overdose prevention programs providing naloxone—United States, 2010. *MMWR, 61*(6), 101-105.

27. Califf, R. M., Woodcock, J., & Ostroff, S. (2016). A proactive response to prescription opioid abuse. *New England Journal of Medicine, 374*(15), 1480-1485.

28. Evans, J. M., Krainsky, E., Fentonmiller, K., Brady, C., Yoeli, E., & Jaroszewicz, A. (2014). *Self-regulation in the alcohol industry: Report of the Federal Trade Commission.* Washington, DC: U.S. Federal Trade Commission.

29. Substance Abuse and Mental Health Services Administration. (2015). *Federal guidelines for opioid treatment programs.* (HHS Publication No. (SMA) PEP15-FEDGUIDEOTP). Rockville, MD: Substance Abuse and Mental Health Services Administration.

30. Wilson, D. B., Mitchell, O., & MacKenzie, D. L. (2006). A systematic review of drug court effects on recidivism. *Journal of Experimental Criminology, 2*(4), 459-487.

31. Belenko, S., Hiller, M., & Hamilton, L. (2013). Treating substance use disorders in the criminal justice system. *Current Psychiatry Reports, 15*(11), 1-11.

32. Fletcher, B. W., & Wexler, H. K. (2005). *National Criminal Justice Drug Abuse Treatment Studies (CJ-DATS): Update and progress.* Justice Research and Statistics Association Forum.

GLOSSARY OF TERMS

Term	Definition
12-Step Program	A group providing mutual support and fellowship for people recovering from addictive behaviors. The first 12-step program was Alcoholics Anonymous (AA), founded in 1935; an array of 12-step groups following a similar model have since emerged and are the most widely used mutual aid groups and steps for maintaining recovery recovery from alcohol and drug use disorders. It is not a form of treatment, and it is not to be confused with the treatment modality called Twelve-Step Facilitation.
Abstinence	Not using alcohol or drugs.
Addiction	The most severe form of *substance use disorder*, associated with compulsive or uncontrolled use of one or more substances. Addiction is a chronic brain disease that has the potential for both recurrence (relapse) and recovery.
Agonist	A chemical substance that binds to and activates certain receptors on cells, causing a biological response. Fentanyl and methadone are examples of opioid receptor agonists.
Antagonist	A chemical substance that binds to and blocks the activation of certain receptors on cells, preventing a biological response. Naloxone is an example of an opioid receptor antagonist.
Binge Drinking	For men, drinking 5 or more standard alcoholic drinks, and for women, 4 or more standard alcoholic drinks on the same occasion on at least 1 day in the past 30 days.
Case Management	A coordinated approach to delivering health care, substance use disorder treatment, mental health care, and social services. This approach links clients with appropriate services to address specific needs and goals.
Clinical Decision Support	A system that provides health care professionals, staff, patients, or other individuals with knowledge and person-specific information, intelligently filtered or presented at appropriate times, to enhance health and health care.
Clinical Trial	Any research study that prospectively assigns human participants or groups of participants to one or more health-related interventions to evaluate the effects on health outcomes.
Compulsivity	Repetitive behaviors in the face of adverse consequences, as well as repetitive behaviors that are inappropriate to a particular situation. People suffering from compulsions often recognize that the behaviors are harmful, but they nonetheless feel emotionally compelled to perform them. Doing so reduces tension, stress, or anxiety.

GLOSSARY

Term	Definition
Continuum of Care	An integrated system of care that guides and tracks a person over time through a comprehensive array of health services appropriate to the individual's need. A continuum of care may include prevention, early intervention, treatment, continuing care, and recovery support.
Cost-Benefit Study	A study that determines the economic worth of an intervention by quantifying its costs in monetary terms and comparing them with the benefits, also expressed in monetary terms. Total benefits divided by total costs is called a cost-benefit ratio. If the ratio is greater than 1, the benefits outweigh the costs.
Cost-Effectiveness Study	A comparative analysis of two or more interventions against their health and economic outcomes. These outcomes could be lives saved, illnesses prevented, or years of life gained.
Dependence	A state in which an organism only functions normally in the presence of a substance, experiencing physical disturbance when the substance is removed. A person can be dependent on a substance without being addicted, but dependence sometimes leads to addiction
Dissemination	The active distribution of evidence-based interventions (EBIs) to specific audiences, with the goal of increasing their adoption.
Drug Diversion	A medical and legal concept involving the transfer of any legally prescribed controlled substance from the person for whom it was prescribed to another person for any illicit use.
Fidelity	The extent to which an intervention is delivered as it was designed and intended to be delivered.
Gender	The social, cultural, or community designations of masculinity or femininity.
Health Care System	The World Health Organization defines a health care system as (1) all the activities whose primary purpose is to promote, restore, and/or maintain health, and (2) the people, institutions, and resources, arranged together in accordance with established policies, to improve the health of the population they serve. The health care system is made up of diverse health care organizations ranging from primary care, specialty substance use disorder treatment (including residential and outpatient settings), mental health care, infectious disease clinics, school clinics, community health centers, hospitals, emergency departments, and others.
Health Disparities	Preventable differences in the burden of disease or opportunities to achieve optimal health that are experienced by socially disadvantaged populations, defined by factors such as race or ethnicity, gender, education or income, disability, geographic location (e.g., rural or urban), or sexual orientation.
Heavy Drinking	Defined by the Centers for Disease Control and Prevention (CDC) as consuming 8 or more drinks per week for women, and 15 or more drinks per week for men, and by the Substance Abuse and Mental Health Services Administration (SAMHSA), for research purposes, as binge drinking on 5 or more days in the past 30 days.
Implementation	A specified set of activities designed to put policies and programs into practice.
Impulsivity	Inability to resist urges, deficits in delaying gratification, and unreflective decision-making. Impulsivity is a tendency to act without foresight or regard for consequences and to prioritize immediate rewards over long-term goals.
Inpatient Treatment	Intensive, 24-hour-a-day services delivered in a hospital setting.
Integration	The systematic coordination of general and behavioral health care. Integrating services for primary care, mental health, and substance use use-related problems together produces the best outcomes and provides the most effective approach for supporting whole-person health and wellness.

GLOSSARY

Term	Definition
Intervention	A professionally delivered program, service, or policy designed to prevent substance misuse (prevention intervention) or treat a substance use disorder (treatment intervention).
Learning Health Care System	As described by the IOM, a learning health care system is "designed to generate and apply the best evidence for the collaborative healthcare choices of each patient and provider; to drive the process of discovery as a natural outgrowth of patient care; and to ensure innovation, quality, safety, and value in health care."
Longitudinal Study	A type of study in which data on a particular group of people are gathered repeatedly over a period of years or even decades.
Meaningful Use	Using certified EHR technology to improve quality, safety, efficiency, and reduce health disparities; engage patients and family; improve care coordination and population and public health; and maintain privacy and security of patient health information.
Negative Reinforcement	The process by which removal of a stimulus such as negative feelings or emotions increases the probability of a response like drug taking.
Net Economic Benefit	The value of total benefits minus total costs.
Neurobiology	The study of the anatomy, function, and diseases of the brain and nervous system.
Opioid Treatment Program (OTP)	SAMHSA-certified program, usually comprising a facility, staff, administration, patients, and services, that engages in supervised assessment and treatment, using methadone, buprenorphine, or naltrexone, of individuals who have opioid use disorders. An OTP can exist in a number of settings, including but not limited to intensive outpatient, residential, and hospital settings. Services may include medically supervised withdrawal and/or maintenance treatment, along with various levels of medical, psychiatric, psychosocial, and other types of supportive care.
Pharmacokinetics	What the body does to a drug after it has been taken, including how rapidly the drug is absorbed, broken down, and processed by the body.
Positive Reinforcement	The process by which presentation of a stimulus such as a drug increases the probability of a response like drug taking.
Prescription Drug Misuse	Use of a drug in any way a doctor did not direct an individual to use it.
Prevalence	The proportion of a population who have (or had) a specific characteristic—for example, an illness, condition, behavior, or risk factor— in a given time period.
Protective Factors	Factors that directly decrease the likelihood of substance use and behavioral health problems or reduce the impact of risk factors on behavioral health problems.
Public Health System	Defined as "all public, private, and voluntary entities that contribute to the delivery of essential public health services within a jurisdiction" and includes state and local public health agencies, public safety agencies, health care providers, human service and charity organizations, recreation and arts-related organizations, economic and philanthropic organizations, education and youth development organizations, and education and youth development organizations.
Quality-Adjusted Life Year (QALY)	A measure of the burden of disease used in economic evaluations of the value of health care interventions that accounts for both the years of life lived and the quality of life experienced during those years, relative to quality associated with perfect health.
Randomized Controlled Trial (RCT)	A clinical trial of an intervention in which people are randomly assigned either to a group receiving the intervention being studied or to a *control group* receiving a standard intervention, a placebo (a medicine with no therapeutic effect), or no intervention. At the end of the study, the results from the different groups are compared.

Term	Definition
Recovery	A process of change through which individuals improve their health and wellness, live a self-directed life, and strive to reach their full potential. Even individuals with severe and chronic substance use disorders can, with help, overcome their substance use disorder and regain health and social function. This is called remission. When those positive changes and values become part of a voluntarily adopted lifestyle, that is called "being in recovery". Although abstinence from all substance misuse is a cardinal feature of a recovery lifestyle, it is not the only healthy, pro-social feature.
Relapse	The return to alcohol or drug use after a significant period of abstinence.
Remission	A medical term meaning that major disease symptoms are eliminated or diminished below a pre-determined, harmful level.
Residential Treatment	Intensive, 24-hour a day services delivered in settings other than a hospital.
Risk Factors	Factors that increase the likelihood of beginning substance use, of regular and harmful use, and of other behavioral health problems associated with use.
Sex	The biological and physiological characteristics that define human beings as female or male.
Standard Drink	Based on the 2015-2020 Dietary Guidelines for Americans, a standard drink is defined as 12 fl. oz. of regular beer, 8-9 fl. oz. of malt liquor, 5 fl. oz. of table wine, or 1.5 fl. oz. of 80-proof distilled spirits. All of these drinks contain 14 grams (0.6 ounces) of pure alcohol.
Substance	A psychoactive compound with the potential to cause health and social problems, including substance use disorders (and their most severe manifestation, addiction).
Substance Misuse	The use of any substance in a manner, situation, amount or frequency that can cause harm to users or to those around them. For some substances or individuals, any use would constitute as misuse (e.g., under-age drinking, injection drug use).
Substance Misuse Problems or Consequences	Any health or social problem that results from substance misuse. Substance misuse problems or consequences may affect the substance user or those around them, and they may be acute (e.g., an argument or fight, a motor vehicle crash, an overdose) or chronic (e.g., a long-term substance-related medical, family, or employment problem, or chronic medical condition, such as various cancers, heart disease, and liver disease). These problems may occur at any age and are more likely to occur with greater frequency of substance misuse.
Substance Use	The use—even one time—of any substance.
Substance Use Disorders	A medical illness caused by repeated misuse of a substance or substances. According to the Fifth Edition of the *Diagnostic and Statistical Manual of Mental Disorders* (DSM-5), substance use disorders are characterized by clinically significant impairments in health, social function, and impaired control over substance use and are diagnosed through assessing cognitive, behavioral, and psychological symptoms. Substance use disorders range from mild to severe and from temporary to chronic. They typically develop gradually over time with repeated misuse, leading to changes in brain circuits governing incentive salience (the ability of substance-associated cues to trigger substance seeking), reward, stress, and executive functions like decision making and self-control. Note: Severe substance use disorders are commonly called *addictions*.
Substance Use Disorder Treatment	A service or set of services that may include medication, counseling, and other supportive services designed to enable an individual to reduce or eliminate alcohol and/or other drug use, address associated physical or mental health problems, and restore the patient to maximum functional ability.
Telehealth	The use of digital technologies such as electronic health records, mobile applications, telemedicine, and web-based tools to support the delivery of health care, health-related education, or other health-related services and functions.
Telemedicine	Two-way, real-time interactive communication between a patient and a physician or other health care professional at a distant site. Telemedicine is a subcategory of *telehealth*.

Term	Definition
Tolerance	Alteration of the body's responsiveness to alcohol or a drug such that higher doses are required to produce the same effect achieved during initial use.
Withdrawal	A set of symptoms that are experienced when discontinuing use of a substance to which a person has become dependent or addicted, which can include negative emotions such as stress, anxiety, or depression, as well as physical effects such as nausea, vomiting, muscle aches, and cramping, among others. Withdrawal symptoms often lead a person to use the substance again.
Wrap-Around Services	Wrap-around services are non-clinical services that facilitate patient engagement and retention in treatment as well as their ongoing recovery. This can include services to address patient needs related to transportation, employment, childcare, housing, legal and financial problems, among others.

LIST OF ABBREVIATIONS

Abbreviation	Definition
AA	Alcoholics Anonymous
ACC	Accountable Care Community
ACO	Accountable Care Organization
AIDS	Acquired Immune Deficiency Syndrome
ASAM	American Society of Addiction Medicine
ASI	Addiction Severity Index
AUDIT	Alcohol Use Disorders Identification Test
BAC	Blood Alcohol Content
BASICS	Brief Alcohol Screening and Intervention for College Students
BNST	Bed Nucleus of the Stria Terminalis
BRAIN	Brain Research through Advancing Innovative Neurotechnologies
CADCA	Community Anti-Drug Coalitions of America
CARA	Comprehensive Addiction and Recovery Act
CARPS	Computerized Alcohol-Related Problems Survey
CBT	Cognitive Behavioral Therapy
CCO	Coordinated Care Organization
CDC	Centers for Disease Control and Prevention
CeA	Central Nucleus of the Amygdala
CHIP	Children's Health Insurance Program
CIDI	Composite International Diagnostic Interview
CMCA	Communities Mobilizing for Change on Alcohol
CMS	Centers for Medicare & Medicaid Services
CRF	Corticotropin-Releasing Factor
CSA	Controlled Substances Act
CTC	Communities That Care
DEA	Drug Enforcement Administration

ABBREVIATIONS

Abbreviation	Definition
DSM-IV	Diagnostic and Statistical Manual of Mental Disorders, Fourth Edition
DSM-5	Diagnostic and Statistical Manual of Mental Disorders, Fifth Edition
DUI	Driving Under the Influence
DS	Dorsal Striatum
EBI	Evidence-Based Interventions
EHR	Electronic Health Record
FASD	Fetal Alcohol Spectrum Disorder
FBT	Family Behavior Therapy
FDA	Food and Drug Administration
FQHC	Federally Qualified Health Center
GABA	Gamma-Aminobutyric Acid
HEDIS	Healthcare Effectiveness Data and Information Set
HHS	U.S. Department of Health and Human Services
HIPAA	Health Insurance Portability and Accountability Act
HIV	Human Immunodeficiency Virus
HRSA	Health Resources and Services Administration
ICCPUD	Interagency Coordinating Committee on the Prevention of Underage Drinking
IOM	Institute of Medicine, now known as the Health and Medicine Division of the National Academies of Science, Engineering, and Medicine
LGBT	Lesbian, Gay, Bisexual, and Transgender
LST	Life Skills Training
MADD	Mothers Against Drunk Driving
MET	Motivational Enhancement Therapy
MHPAEA	Paul Wellstone and Pete Domenici Mental Health Parity and Addiction Equity Act of 2008
MLDA	Minimum Legal Drinking Age
MRI	Magnetic Resonance Imaging
NA	Narcotics Anonymous
NAc	Nucleus Accumbens
NASPER	National All Schedules Prescription Electronic Reporting Act
NFP	Nurse-Family Partnership Program
NHTSA	National Highway Traffic Safety Administration
NIAAA	National Institute on National Institute on Alcohol Abuse and Alcoholism
NIDA	National Institute on Drug Abuse
NIH	National Institutes of Health
NREPP	National Registry of Evidence-based Programs and Practices
NSDUH	National Survey on Drug Use and Health
OTP	Opioid Treatment Program
PDMP	Prescription Drug Monitoring Program
PET	Positron Emission Tomography
PFC	Prefrontal Cortex
PRISM	Psychiatric Research Interview for Substance and Mental Disorders
PROSPER	PROmoting School-community-university Partnerships to Enhance Resilience

Abbreviation	Definition
PTSD	Post-Traumatic Stress Disorder
QALY	Quality-Adjusted Life Year
RHC	Raising Healthy Children
RMC	Recovery Management Check-up
RSS	Recovery Support Services
SAMHSA	Substance Abuse and Mental Health Services Administration
SBI	Screening and Brief Intervention
SBIRT	Screening, Brief Intervention, and Referral to Treatment
SFP	Strengthening Families Program
SIM	State Innovation Models
SPA	State Plan Amendment
THC	Δ^9-tetrahydrocannabinol
USPSTF	U.S. Preventive Services Task Force
VTA	Ventral Tegmental Area

LIST OF TABLES AND FIGURES

CHAPTER 1. INTRODUCTION AND OVERVIEW OF THE REPORT

Figure 1.1	Past Month Rates of Substance Use Among People Aged 12 or Older: Percentages, 2002-2014, 2014 National Survey on Drug Use and Health (NSDUH)	1-2
Table 1.1	Categories and Examples of Substances	1-5
Table 1.2	Past Year Substance Use, Past Year Initiation of Substance Use, and Met Diagnostic Criteria for a Substance Use Disorder in the Past Year Among Persons Aged 12 Years or Older for Specific Substances: Numbers in Millions and Percentages, 2015 National Survey on Drug Use and Health (NSDUH)	1-9
Figure 1.2	Trends in Binge Drinking and Past 30-Day Use of Illicit Drugs among Persons Aged 12 Years or Older, 2014 National Survey on Drug Use and Health (NSDUH)	1-10
Table 1.3	Past Year Alcohol Use, Past Month Binge Alcohol Use, and Met Diagnostic Criteria for a Substance Use Disorder in the Past Year Among Persons Aged 12 Years or Older: Numbers in Millions and Percentages, 2015 National Survey on Drug Use and Health (NSDUH)	1-11
Table 1.4	Past Year Substance Use, Past 30-Day Illicit Drug Use, and Met Diagnostic Criteria for a Substance Use Disorder in the Past Year Among Persons Aged 12 Years or Older: Numbers in Millions and Percentages, 2015 National Survey on Drug Use and Health (NSDUH)	1-11
Table 1.5	Criteria for Diagnosing Substance Use Disorders	1-17

CHAPTER 2. THE NEUROBIOLOGY OF SUBSTANCE USE, MISUSE, AND ADDICTION

Figure 2.1	A Neuron and its Parts	2-4
Figure 2.2	Areas of the Human Brain that Are Especially Important in Addiction	2-5
Figure 2.3	The Three Stages of the Addiction Cycle and the Brain Regions Associated with Them	2-7

LIST OF TABLES AND FIGURES

Figure 2.4	The Binge/Intoxication Stage and the Basal Ganglia	2-9
Figure 2.5	Actions of Addictive Substances on the Brain	2-10
Figure 2.6	Major Neurotransmitter Systems Implicated in the Neuroadaptations Associated with the Binge/Intoxication Stage of Addiction	2-11
Figure 2.7	The Withdrawal/Negative Affect Stage and the Extended Amygdala	2-13
Figure 2.8	Time-Related Decrease in Dopamine Released in the Brain of a Cocaine User	2-14
Figure 2.9	Major Neurotransmitter Systems Implicated in the Neuroadaptations Associated with the Withdrawal/Negative Affect Stage of Addiction	2-15
Figure 2.10	The Preoccupation/Anticipation Stage and the Prefrontal Cortex	2-16
Figure 2.11	Major Neurotransmitter Systems Implicated in the Neuroadaptations Associated with the Preoccupation/Anticipation Stage of Addiction	2-17

CHAPTER 3. PREVENTION PROGRAMS AND POLICIES

Figure 3.1	Past-Month Alcohol Use, Binge Alcohol Use, and Marijuana Use, by Age: Percentages, 2015 National Survey on Drug and Health (NSDUH)	3-3
Table 3.1	Risk Factors for Adolescent and Young Adult Substance Use	3-5
Table 3.2	Protective Factors for Adolescent and Young Adult Substance Use	3-6
Table 3.3	Cost-Benefit of EBIs Reviewed by the Washington State Institute for Public Policy, 2016	3-14
Figure 3.2	Alcohol- Versus Non-alcohol-related Traffic Deaths, Rate per 100,000, All Ages, United States, 1982-2013	3-19
Figure 3.3	Trends in 2-Week Prevalence of 5 or More Drinks in a Row among 12th Graders, 1980-2015	3-21
Table 3.4	Status of Selected Evidence-Based Strategies in States for Preventing Alcohol Misuse and Related Harms	3-24

CHAPTER 4. EARLY INTERVENTION, TREATMENT, AND MANAGEMENT OF SUBSTANCE USE DISORDERS

Figure 4.1	Substance Use Status and Substance Use Care Continuum	4-4
Table 4.1	Evidence-Based Screening Tools for Substance Use	4-7
Table 4.2	Principles of Effective Treatment for Substance Use Disorders	4-14
Table 4.3	Detailed Information on Substance Use Disorder Assessment Tools	4-16
Table 4.4	Pharmacotherapies Used to Treat Alcohol and Opioid Use Disorders	4-19
Table 4.5	Examples of Technology-Assisted Interventions	4-33

LIST OF TABLES AND FIGURES

CHAPTER 6. HEALTH CARE SYSTEMS AND SUBSTANCE USE DISORDERS

Figure 6.1	Substance Use Disorders Services: Past and Future	6-8
Figure 6.2	A Continuum of Collaboration between Health Care and Specialty Services	6-14
Figure 6.3	Eligibility for Affordable Care Act Coverage Among the Nonelderly Uninsured by Race and Ethnicity, as of 2015	6-16
Figure 6.4	Percentage Distribution of Spending on Substance Misuse Treatment by Setting, 1986–2014	6-24

APPENDIX B. EVIDENCE-BASED PREVENTION PROGRAMS AND POLICIES

Table B.1	Evidence-Based Interventions for Children Under Age 10	17
Table B.2	Evidence-Based Interventions for Youth Aged 10 to18	20
Table B.3	Evidence-Based Interventions for Age 18+	27
Table B.4	Evidence-Based Community Implementation Systems/ Coalition Models and Environmental Interventions	29
Table B.5	Community Preventive Services Task Force Recommendations for Preventing Alcohol Misuse	32

APPENDIX A. REVIEW PROCESS FOR PREVENTION PROGRAMS

Sources and Process

The review of published research primarily focused on refereed, professional journals, which were searched using PubMed and PsycINFO. Government reports, annotated bibliographies, and relevant books and book chapters also were reviewed. In addition, programs were searched on SAMHSA's National Registry of Evidence-based Programs and Practices (NREPP) and the Centers for Disease Control and Prevention (CDC) Guide to Community Preventive Services. From these collective sources, a set of 600 core prevention programs was identified for possible inclusion in this *Report*. Of those, 42 met the evaluation criteria listed below and were included.

Evaluation Criteria

Programs were included only if they met the program criteria of the Blueprints for Healthy Youth Development listed below. All of these programs fit within CDC's well-supported category.

- *Experimental design:* All programs were evaluated using a randomized trial design or a quasi-experimental design that used an adequate comparison group. The prevention effects described compare the group or individuals that got the prevention intervention with those who did not.

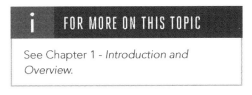

FOR MORE ON THIS TOPIC

See Chapter 1 - *Introduction and Overview.*

- *Sample specification:* The behavioral and social characteristics of the sample for which outcomes were measured must have been specified.
- *Outcome assessments:* These assessments must have included pretest, posttest, and follow-up findings. The need for follow-up findings was considered essential given the frequently observed dissipation of positive posttest results. Follow-up data had to be reported more than

APPENDICES

6 months beyond the time point at which the primary components of the intervention were delivered, in order to examine the duration and stability of intervention effects.

- *Effects:* Independent of whether the prevention intervention began prenatally, in the early years of life, or in adolescence or adulthood, programs were included only if they produced outcomes showing a measurable difference in substance use or substance use-related outcomes between intervention and comparison groups based on statistical significance testing. Level of significance and the size of the effects are reported in **Appendix B - Evidence-Based Prevention Programs and Policies**. Programs that broadly affected other behavioral health problems but did not show reductions in at least one direct measure of substance use were excluded.

- *Additional quality of evidence criteria:* The program provided evidence that seven quality of evidence criteria consistent with those of NREPP[i] were met: (1) reliability of outcome measures, (2) validity of outcome measures, (3) pretest equivalence, (4) intervention fidelity, (5) analysis of missing data, (6) degree and evaluation of sample attrition, and (7) appropriate statistical analyses.

- *Operations Manual:* The program had a written manual that specified the procedures used in the intervention to increase likelihood that the prevention intervention would be replicated with fidelity.

---

i   Substance Abuse and Mental Health Services Administration. National registry of evidence-based programs and practices (NREPP). Retrieved from http://www.samhsa.gov/nrepp. Accessed on March 11, 2016.

APPENDIX B.
EVIDENCE-BASED PREVENTION PROGRAMS AND POLICIES

Table B.1: Evidence-Based Interventions for Children Under Age 10

Intervention	Type (Universal, Selective, Indicated)	Domain/Level (Family, School, Community, Multicomponent)	Sample (at pretest)/ Ethnicity/ Setting Design	Summary Results	Citations: Key Outcome Research/ Program Information Source
Nurse-Family Partnership Program (NFP)	Selective	Family	Study 1: N = 300 rural, poor pregnant White women, first births	Study 1: At 13-year follow-up (age 15), parents in the nurse-visits intervention reported their children had fewer behavioral problems due to use of substances (0.15 vs. 0.34), and youth reported fewer days of alcohol consumption in past 6 months (1.09 vs. 2.49). No effects on binge drinking or illicit drug use at age 19.	Olds, et al. (1998)[1]
			Study 2: N = 743 urban, poor pregnant African American women, first births	Study 2: At 10-year follow-up (age 12), lower 30-day use of cigarettes, alcohol, and marijuana (OR = 0.31).	Eckenrode, et al. (2010)[2] Kitzman, et al. (2010)[3]
			All studies: RCT/NTC		

Intervention	Type (Universal, Selective, Indicated)	Domain/Level (Family, School, Community, Multicomponent)	Sample (at pretest)/ Ethnicity/ Setting Design	Summary Results	Citations: Key Outcome Research/ Program Information Source
Raising Healthy Children (RHC) (Seattle Social Development Project elementary only)	Universal	Family and School	N = 18 urban, multiethnic schools; 810 students in Grades 1-5 QED/NTC RCT/NTC	At 6-year follow-up (age 18), reductions in heavy drinking (15.4% vs. 25.0%); high rates of attrition (quasi–experimental). At ages 21, 24, and 27, no significant effects on any form or drug or alcohol use. At grades 8-10, reduced growth of frequency of alcohol and marijuana use, no effects on initiation of alcohol, marijuana, and cigarettes(d = .40 for alcohol, d = .57 for marijuana).	Hawkins, et al. (1992)[4] and (1999)[5] Hawkins, et al. (2005)[6] and (2008)[7] Brown, et al. (2005)[8]
Good Behavior Game	Universal	School	N = 864 large urban, multiethnic students in Grades 1-2 RCT/NTC	At ages 19 to 21, intervention males with high aggression in 1st grade (about 25% of boys) had lower rates of alcohol and drug abuse and dependence (65.6% vs. 28.1%). No effect for moderately or low aggressive males and no effect for females. Finding was not replicated in second cohort of the same study.	Kellam, et al. (2008)[9] and (2014)[10]
Classroom Centered Intervention	Universal	School	N = 9 urban, multiethnic schools; 576 students in Grades1 and 2 RCT/NTC	At 6-year follow-up (Grade 8), reduced risk of starting to use other illegal drugs (heroin, crack, and cocaine powder; 7% vs. 2.6%). No effects on alcohol initiation or marijuana use.	Ialongo, et al. (2001)[11] Furr-Holden, et al. (2004)[12] Liu, et al. (2013)[13]

APPENDICES

Intervention	Type (Universal, Selective, Indicated)	Domain/Level (Family, School, Community, Multicomponent)	Sample (at pretest)/ Ethnicity/ Setting Design	Summary Results	Citations: Key Outcome Research/ Program Information Source
Linking the Interests of Families and Teachers (LIFT)	Universal	Multicomponent	N = 6 schools; 348 primarily White students in Grade 5, college town RCT/NTC	At 2- and 3-year follow-up, effects on patterned alcohol use (OR = 1.49) across Grades 6-8. Lower risk of initiating alcohol use (7% reduction). Also reduced growth of illicit drug use, particularly for females.	Eddy, et al. (2003)[14] DeGarmo, et al. (2009)[15]
Fast Track	Indicated	Multicomponent	N = 4 urban and rural multiethnic communities; 891 children with behavioral problems selected in kindergarten, Grades 1-10 RCT/TAU	No effects on substance use in Grades 9-12. At 10-year follow-up (age 25), decreased probability of DSM alcohol abuse (OR = 0.69), serious substance use (OR = 0.58). Lower drug crime conviction rate (34.7% reduction). No effect on binge drinking or heavy marijuana use.	Dodge, et al. (2015)[16]
Preventive Treatment Program (Montreal)	Selective	Multicomponent	N = 166 urban French Canadian students in Grades 1-2 with early behavioral problems RCT/TAU	At 7-year follow-up, effects on drinking to the point of being drunk at age 15. At 6- to 8- year follow-up, reduction in alcohol use at age 17 (ES = 0.48), and the slope of the number of drugs used between age 14 and 17 (ES = 0.70).	Tremblay, et al. (1996)[17] Masse, (1996)[18]

Abbreviations: RCT - Randomized Controlled Trial, QED - Quasi-Experimental Design, TAU - Control Group Received Treatment As Usual, NTC - No Treatment Control, ES - Effect Size, OR - Odds Ratio

Table B.2: Evidence-Based Interventions for Youth Aged 10 to18

Intervention	Type (Universal, Selective, Indicated)	Domain/Level (Family, School, Community, Multicomponent)	Sample (at pretest)/ Ethnicity/ Setting/Design	Summary Results	Citations: Key Outcome Research/ Program Information Source
Life Skills Training (LST)	Universal	School	Study 1: N = 56 public schools; 5,954 White, urban students in Grade 7 (1985-1991)	Study 1: 6-year follow-up showed significantly lower incidence of drunkenness (33.5% vs. 40%) but not on rate of monthly, or weekly alcohol use); no effect on marijuana use. 66% reduction in weekly polydrug use (alcohol, marijuana, and tobacco).	Botvin, et al. (1995)[19]
			Study 2: N =29 schools in New York; 3,791 urban youth in Grade 7 (high-risk subsample), primarily African American and Hispanic	Study 2: 1- and 2-year follow-up showed lower rates of alcohol use, binge drinking, and inhalant use.	Botvin, et al. (2001)[20] Griffin, et al. (2003)[21]
			Study 2a: N = 758 high-risk students from Study 2	Study 2a: At 1-year follow-up, high-risk participants (21% of sample) reported less drinking (ES = 0.22), inhalant use (ES = 0.14), and polydrug use (ES = 0.21).	Smith, et al. (2004)[22]
			Study 3: N = 9 rural public schools; 732 White students in Grade 6 (1999-2002)	Study 3: No significant findings.	Spoth, et al. (2005)[23]
			Study 4: N = 36 rural schools; 1,650 primarily White students in Grade 7 (1998-2006) All Studies: RCT/ NTC	Study 4: At 1.5-year follow-up, reduction in substance use for females, which became nonsignificant at 2.5-year follow-up. No significant effects for males.	Spoth, et al. (2008)[25] and (2006)[24]

Intervention	Type (Universal, Selective, Indicated)	Domain/Level (Family, School, Community, Multicomponent)	Sample (at pretest)/ Ethnicity/ Setting/Design	Summary Results	Citations: Key Outcome Research/ Program Information Source
				At 5.5-year follow-up, lower rate of SU initiation, marijuana initiation (23% reduction), drunkenness (10% reduction), polydrug use, and lifetime methamphetamine use (2.4% vs. 7.6%) when combined with the Strengthening Families Program: For Parents and Youth 10–14.	
School Health and Alcohol Harm Reduction Project (SHAHRP)	Universal	School	N = 14 public secondary schools in metropolitan Perth, Australia; 2,300 students aged 12 to 14 (1997-1999) QED/NTC	At 17-month follow-up (after two years of intervention), reduced weekly drinking (5%) and harm from alcohol use.	McBride, et al. (2000)[26] and (2004)[27]
Preventure/ Adventure	Selective (by Personality Risk)	School	Study 1: N = 13 UK secondary schools; 732 youth aged 13 to 16. Wave 2 youth only (N = 364)	Study 1: At 2-year follow-up, reduced initiation of l cocaine (OR = 0.20) and other drugs (OR = 0.50). No effect on marijuana use. Strongest effects on impulsive subsample. Effects on quantity and binge drinking fade after 6 months. A 24 months, still an effect on problem drinking (ES=0.33; Rutgers Scale).	Conrod, et al. (2010)[28] and (2011)[29]
			Study 2: N = 21 UK secondary schools; 1,210 high-risk students in Grade 9. Selected as in Study 1, lower risk sample = 1,433 students	Study 2: At 24-month follow-up, high-risk students had lowered quantity of drinking (29% reduction), binge drinking (43% reduction), and problem drinking (29% reduction). Low risk students had lower quantity of drinking (29% reduction) and lower rates of binge drinking (35% reduction).	Conrod, et al. (2013)[30]
				At 24-month follow-up, effects on marijuana use fade and are unclear. 24-month effects maintained in the sensation-seeking subsample only (OR = 0.25).	Mahu, et al. (2015)[31]

Intervention	Type (Universal, Selective, Indicated)	Domain/Level (Family, School, Community, Multicomponent)	Sample (at pretest)/ Ethnicity/ Setting/Design	Summary Results	Citations: Key Outcome Research/ Program Information Source
			Study 3: N = 15 Schools in The Netherlands; 699 high-risk students aged 13 to 15 All Studies: RCT/NTC	Study 3: At 12-month follow-up, effects were ambiguous. Regression models revealed no significant effects on alcohol use, binge drinking, or problem drinking. Latent growth model showed effect on binge drinking.	Lammers, et al. (2015)[32]
Unplugged	Universal	School	N = 170 schools in 7 European countries; 7,079 students aged 12 to 14	At 18-month follow-up, reductions in any drunkenness (3.8% reduction), frequent drunkenness (2.5% reduction), any cannabis use (2.9% reduction), and frequent cannabis use (2.2% reduction).	Faggiano, et al. (2010)[33]
keepin' It REAL	Universal	School	Study 1: N = 35 public schools in Phoenix, Arizona; 4,235 multiethnic/urban students in Grade 7 (1998-2000)	Study 1: At 19-month follow-up, lower increases in past-month alcohol and marijuana use for the Mexican American and multicultural version of the program. No effects on the Black/White version.	Hecht, et al. (2003)[34] and (2006)[35] Kulis, et al. (2007)[36]
			Study 2: N = 30 public schools in Phoenix, Arizona; 3,038 students in Grade 7 (74.3% were Mexican-American) All Studies: RCT/NTC	Study 2: At 1-year follow-up, no significant difference in alcohol or marijuana use.	Marsiglia, et al. (2012)[37]
ATLAS (Athletes Training and Learning to Avoid Steroids)	Universal	School	N = 31 high school football teams from Portland, Oregon; 3,207 athletes (1994-1996) RCT/NTC	At 1-year follow-up, reduced use of alcohol and illicit drug use, and lower rate of drinking and driving.	Goldberg, et al. (2000)[38]

Intervention	Type (Universal, Selective, Indicated)	Domain/Level (Family, School, Community, Multicomponent)	Sample (at pretest)/ Ethnicity/ Setting/Design	Summary Results	Citations: Key Outcome Research/ Program Information Source
Strengthening Families Program: For Parents and Youth 10-14	Universal	Family and School/ Multicomponent	Study 1: N = 33 Midwestern public schools; 667 primarily White, rural students in Grade 6	Study 1: At 4-year follow-up, lower lifetime alcohol use (50% vs. 68%), drunkenness (26% vs. 44%), marijuana use (7% vs. 17%), and lower rates of amphetamine use (0% vs. 3.2%).	Spoth, et al. (2001)[39]
				At 6-year follow-up, lower rates of substance use initiation (OR = 2.34), lower drunkenness (41% reduction) and lower illicit drug use.	Spoth, et al. (2004)[40]
				At age 21, lower rates of substance use initiation (27.5% vs. 28.3%), drunkenness (19% reduction) and illicit drug use (31% reduction).	Spoth, et al. (2009)[41] and (2012)[42]
			Study 2: N = 36 public schools, 1,650 primarily White students in Grade 7 from rural Iowa (1998-2004) All Studies: RCT/ NTC	Study 2: At 2.5-year follow-up, shows significantly less alcohol initiation (25.7% vs. 36.7%), marijuana initiation (4.1% vs. 7.9%), and slower growth in weekly drunkenness (39% reduction) when combined with Life Skills Training.	Spoth, et al. (2002)[43] and (2005)[23]
				At 5.5-year follow-up, lower rate of SU initiation, marijuana initiation (23% reduction), polydrug use, and lifetime methamphetamine use (2.5% vs. 7.6%) when combined with Life Skills Training.	Spoth, et al. (2008)[25]
				At age 25, lower rates of prescription opioid misuse (6.0% vs. 8.8%) and lifetime prescription drug misuse overall (6.3 vs. 9.4) when combined with Life Skills Training.	Spoth, et al. (2013)[44]

Intervention	Type (Universal, Selective, Indicated)	Domain/Level (Family, School, Community, Multicomponent)	Sample (at pretest)/ Ethnicity/ Setting/Design	Summary Results	Citations: Key Outcome Research/ Program Information Source
Guiding Good Choices	Universal	Family	N =33 rural, Midwestern schools; 883 students in Grade 7 RCT/NTC	Effects on substance use initiation through high school and alcohol-related problems and illicit drug use through early adulthood. No effects on drunkenness. At age 22, lower rate of alcohol misuse for women (6% vs. 16%); no effect for men.	Spoth, et al. (2009)[41] Mason, et al (2009)[45]
Strong African American Families	Universal	Family	N = 667 Southern U.S. rural African American students in Grade 7 RCT/NTC	At 2-year follow-up, slower rate of initiation of alcohol (37% vs. 43%). Effect on growth trajectory of alcohol use through 4.5-year follow-up.	Brody, et al. (2006)[46] and (2010)[47]
SODAS City	Universal	Family	N = 43 community agencies in New York, New Jersey, and Delaware; 514 urban youth (1991-2010) RCT/NTC	At 3-year follow-up, CD-ROM alone and CD-ROM plus parent intervention showed significantly lower past-month alcohol use. At 7-year follow-up, lower past-month alcohol use, heavy drinking, and marijuana use.	Schinke, et al. (2004)[48] Schinke, et al. (2010)[49]
I Hear What You're Saying	Universal (Mother-Daughter)	Family	Study 1: N = 591 adolescent girls and their mothers Study 2: N = 108 Asian American girls and their mothers (2007-2010) All studies: RCT/NTC	Study 1: At 1-year follow-up, reductions in use of alcohol, marijuana, and prescription drugs. Study 2: At 2-year follow-up, reductions in use of alcohol, marijuana, and prescription drugs.	Schinke, et al. (2009)[50] Fang & Schinke (2013)[51]

Intervention	Type (Universal, Selective, Indicated)	Domain/Level (Family, School, Community, Multicomponent)	Sample (at pretest)/ Ethnicity/ Setting/Design	Summary Results	Citations: Key Outcome Research/ Program Information Source
Familias Unidas	Universal/ Brief Version Selective	Family	Study 1: N = 160 Hispanic students in Grade 8 Study 2: N = 213 Hispanic students in Grade 8 with behavior problems All studies. RCT/ TAU	Study 1: At 2-year follow-up, lower substance use initiation (28.6% vs. 65.2%) and substance use initiation (30.4% vs. 64.0%) among girls. Study 2: Significantly lower past 30-day substance use at 18-month (ES = 0.25) and 30-month follow-ups (25% vs. 34%).	Estrada, et al. (2015)[52] Pantin, et al. (2009)[53]
Bicultural Competence Skills Program (BCSP)	Universal	Clinic/School	N = 27 public and tribal schools; 1,396 students from an American Indian Reservation in the Midwest (1986-1999) RCT/NTC	At 42-month follow-up, weekly alcohol use (22% vs. 30%) and weekly marijuana use (7 % vs. 15%) was lower in BCSP-only group. Results for a BCSP plus community group were not significant.	Schinke, et al. (2000)[54]
Project Chill	Universal	Primary Care	N = 7 urban health centers; 714 youth with no prior use aged 12 to 18 RCT/NTC	At 12-month follow-up, computer-based participants had lower rates of marijuana use at any point during the year (16.8% vs. 24.2%), but non-significant effect on 12 month use. No effects on alcohol.	Walton, et al. (2014)[55]
Positive Family Support (Family Check Up)	Selective	Family	N = 593 Grade 6-8 urban youth and their parents RCT/TAU	Lower rates of marijuana use through age 23. No effect on adult tobacco or alcohol use. For the 42% of families who engaged in the intervention, CACE analysis showed significantly less growth in tobacco, alcohol, and marijuana use across two years	Véronneau, et al. (in press)[56] Stormshak, et al. (2011)[57]
Keep Safe	Selective	School and Family	N = 100 girls in foster care entering middle school	At 18-month follow-up lower rate of substance use (ES = 0.47).	Kim et al (2011)[58]

Intervention	Type (Universal, Selective, Indicated)	Domain/Level (Family, School, Community, Multicomponent)	Sample (at pretest)/ Ethnicity/ Setting/Design	Summary Results	Citations: Key Outcome Research/ Program Information Source
Coping Power	Selective	School	Study 1: N = 245 high-aggression African American and White students in Grade 5	Study 1: At 1-year follow-up (7th grade), lower self-reported past-month use of substances (ES = 0.58).	Lochman & Wells (2003)[59]
			Study 2: N = 183 high-aggression African American and White students in Grade 5	Study 2: At 1-year follow-up (7th grade), lower parent-reported substance use (ES = 0.31).	Lochman & Wells (2004)[60]
			Study 3: N = 77 Dutch youth All Studies: RCT/TAU	Study 3: At 4-year follow-up, lower use of marijuana (13% vs. 35%), no differences in alcohol use.	Zonnevylle, et al. (2007)[61]
Project Toward No Drug Abuse (TND)	Selective and Indicated	School	Study 1: N = 42 schools in Southern California; 2,468 high school students	Study 1: At 1-year follow-up, reduction in levels of alcohol use among baseline users. At 5-year follow-up, reduced hard drug use.	Sussman, et al. (2002)[62] Sun, et al. (2006)[62]
			Study 2: N = 1,186 alternative high school students All studies: RCT/TAU	Study 2: At 1-year follow-up, reductions in alcohol use (OR = 0.68), drunkenness (OR = 0.67), and hard drug use (OR = 0.68).	Sussman, et al. (2012)[63]

Abbreviations: RCT - Randomized Controlled Trial, QED - Quasi-Experimental Design, TAU - Control Group Received Treatment As Usual, NTC - No Treatment Control, ES - Effect Size, OR - Odds Ratio

Table B.3: Evidence-Based Interventions for Age 18+

Intervention	Type (Universal, Selective, Indicated)	Domain/Level (Family, School, Workplace, Community, Multicomponent)	Sample (at pretest)/ Ethnicity/ Setting/Design	Summary Results	Citations: Key Outcome Research/ Program Information Source
BASICS	Indicated	College	Study 1: N = 508 heavy drinking college freshmen	Study 1: At 1- and 2- year follow-ups, reductions in drinking frequency., At 4 year follow-up, reduction in drinking consequences.	Marlatt, et al. (1998)[64] and Baer, et al. (2001)[65]
			Study 2: N = 159 Fraternity-connected college students (81% White)	Study 2: At 1-year follow-up, reductions in average drinks per week (ES = 0.42) and typical peak BAC levels (ES = 0.38).	Larimer, et al. (2001)[66]
			Study 3: N = 550 heavy drinking college students All studies: RCT/TAU	Study 3: At 1-year follow-up, lower typical drinking (ES = 0.11) and peak drinking (ES = 0.42), and alcohol problem (ES = 0.56) for both volunteer and mandated students.	Terlecki, et al. (2015)[67]
Parent Handbook	Universal	College	Study 1: N = 882 college-bound students (79% White)	Study 1: At 8-month follow-up, females were less likely to transition into heavy drinking status, but males were more likely to do so. No effects on rate of alcohol-related problems.	Ichiyama, et al. (2009)[68]
			Study 2: N = 1,900 college-bound students (87% White)	Study 2: Reduced the odds of continuing to be a heavy drinker for the first two years of college for students who came to campus with prior high-risk drinking habits (OR = 0.05).	Turrisi, et al. (2013)[69]
			Study 3: N = 1,275 college-bound students, high-risk, athletes (80% White) All studies: RCT/NTC	Study 3: At 10-month follow-up, reduced alcohol peak consumption (ES = 0.26) .and alcohol-related consequences (ES = 0.20) for PH and BASICS combined.	Turrisi, et al. (2009)[70]
				At 22 months, reduction in the onset of alcohol consequences (ES = 0.21). No effect for PH alone.	Wood, et al. (2010)[71]

Intervention	Type (Universal, Selective, Indicated)	Domain/Level (Family, School, Workplace, Community, Multicomponent)	Sample (at pretest)/ Ethnicity/ Setting/Design	Summary Results	Citations: Key Outcome Research/ Program Information Source
Yale Work and Family Stress Project	Universal	Workplace	N = 4 job sites; 239 primarily White female secretarial employees from Connecticut-based corporations RTC/NTC	At 22-month follow-up, reduced number of drinks per month.	Snow, et al. (2003)[72]
Brief Motivational Intervention in Emergency Department	Universal and Selective	Community	N = 539 injured patients treated in the ED; mostly males from urban, Southern New England (72% White) RCT/TAU	At 1-year follow-up, patients receiving brief intervention (BI) with booster reduced alcohol-related negative consequences and alcohol-related injuries; no differences were observed for heavy drinking days. No effects of BI without booster.	Longabaugh, et al. (2001)[73]
Team Awareness	Universal	Workplace	N = 235 employees in 28 restaurants RCT/NTC	At 1-year follow-up, the odds of recurring heavy drinking declined by 50%, and the number of work-related problem areas declined by one-third.	Broome and Bennett (2011)[74]
Computerized Alcohol-Related Problems Survey (CARPS)	Universal	Primary Care	N = 771 Primary care patients aged 65 and older RCT/TAU	At 1-year follow-up, participants decreased their harmful drinking 23% and increased their nonhazardous drinking 12%.	Fink, et al. (2008)[75]
Project Share	Selective	Primary Care	N = 1,186 Primary care patients aged 60 or older screened for at-risk drinking patterns RCT/TAU	At 1-year follow-up, and reductions in at-risk drinking (56% vs. 67%), lower rates of alcohol consumption.	Ettner, et al. (2014)[76]

Abbreviations: RCT - Randomized Controlled Trial, QED - Quasi-Experimental Design, TAU - Control Group Received Treatment As Usual, NTC - No Treatment Control, ES - Effect Size, OR - Odds Ratio

Table B.4: Evidence-Based Community Implementation Systems/ Coalition Models and Environmental Interventions

Intervention	Type (Universal, Selective, Indicated)	Domain/Level (Family, School, Community, Multicomponent)	Sample (at pretest)/ Ethnicity/ Setting/Design)	Summary Results	Citations: Key Outcome Research/ Program Information Source
COMMUNITY COALITION MODELS					
Communities That Care (CTC)	Universal	Multi-component	N = 24 communities in 7 States; 4,407 students in Grade 5 (20% Hispanic, 67% White, 3% African American) RCT/TAU	By Grade 10, students in CTC communities were less likely to initiate alcohol (OR = 0.62). At 10th grade there were no differences rates of binge drinking or in past-month alcohol, marijuana, prescription, or other illicit drug use.	Hawkins, et al. (2012)[77]
				By Grade 12, fewer CTC students had initiated any drug (OR = 0.71), alcohol (OR = 0.70), or cigarette (OR = 0.80) use. There were no differences in past-month or past-year alcohol, marijuana, or other illicit drug use, with the exception of higher rate of ecstasy use in the CTC condition.	Hawkins, et al. (2014)[78]
PROmoting School-community-university Partnerships to Enhance Resilience (PROSPER)	Universal	Multi-component	N = 28 rural and small town communities in Pennsylvania and Iowa;10,849 primarily White students in Grade 6 RCT/TAU	At 3.5-year and 4.5-year follow-up (Grades 11 and 12) youth in PROSPER communities showed lower past-year marijuana (13.5% reduction) and methamphetamine use (30.9% reduction). At Grade 12 only, PROSPER youth showed lower past-year inhalant use (28.3% reduction). Six-year growth curve effects lower for marijuana, amphetamine use, and drunkenness.	Spoth, et al. (2013a)[79] and(2013b)[44]
				By Grade 12, lower lifetime rates of prescription opioid misuse (22.1% vs. 27.8%) and lifetime prescription drug misuse overall (23.1% vs. 29.0%).	Spoth, et al. (2013a)[79]

Intervention	Type (Universal, Selective, Indicated)	Domain/Level (Family, School, Community, Multicomponent)	Sample (at pretest)/ Ethnicity/ Setting/Design)	Summary Results	Citations: Key Outcome Research/ Program Information Source
Project Northland	Universal	Multi-component	N = 24 multiethnic urban, rural, and tribal school districts in Northern Minnesota RCT/TAU	The Phase 1 intervention was conducted when the targeted cohort was in Grade 6 to Grade 8. At 2.5 years past baseline, lower past-month and past-week alcohol use. The Phase 2 intervention was conducted when the cohort was in Grade 11 toGrade 12. At 6.5 years past baseline, reductions in binge drinking.	Phase 1: Perry, et al. (1996)[80] and Klepp, et al. (1995)[81] Phase 2: Perry, et al. (2002)[82]
Project Star (Midwestern Prevention Project)	Universal	School and Community/ Multicomponent	N = 42 urban public middle and junior high schools in Kansas City, Missouri and Indianapolis, Indiana; 3,412 White and African American students RCT/TAU	At 1-year follow-up, lower proportion of students reporting past-week and past-month use of alcohol. Secondary prevention effects on baseline users were observed up to 1.5 years past baseline, not at 2.5 and 3.5 years past baseline. Reductions in growth of amphetamine use through age 28.	Report 1: Pentz, et al. (1989)[83] Report 2: Pentz & Valente (1993)[84] Report 3: Pentz, et al. (1990)[85] Report 4: Chou, et al. (1998)[86] Report 5: Riggs, et al. (2009)[87]
ENVIRONMENTAL INTERVENTIONS					
Reducing Underage Drinking Through State Coalitions	Universal	Community	N = National data from the Monitoring the Future Survey of students in Grades 8, 10, and 12 in ten states compared to all others QED	At posttest, significant effects in the proportion of Grade 8 and Grade 12 students reporting past month drunkenness (ES = 1.36; ES = 1.29) and in Grade 12 students reporting binge drinking (ES = 2.18) and past year drinking (ES = 0.75).	Wagenaar, et al. (2006)[88]
Safer California Universities	Universal	Community	N=14 California universities; 19,791 students (49% White) RCT/TAU	At posttest, significant effects in the proportion of students reporting intoxication (ORs = 0.76 to 0.81).	Saltz, et al. (2010)[89]

Intervention	Type (Universal, Selective, Indicated)	Domain/Level (Family, School, Community, Multicomponent)	Sample (at pretest)/ Ethnicity/ Setting/Design	Summary Results	Citations: Key Outcome Research/ Program Information Source
Saving Lives	Universal	Community	N = 6 Massachusetts communities compared to all others in the state; 15,188 surveys of adults and youth aged 16 to 19 (90% White) QED	At posttest, a 42% reduction in fatal alcohol-related motor vehicle crashes and a 40% reduction in self-reported DUI among 16- to 19-year-olds.	Hingson, et al. (1996)[90]
Communities Mobilizing for Change on Alcohol	Universal	Community	Report 1: N = 15 Minnesota & Wisconsin communities	Report 1: At posttest, a 17% reduction in the proportion reporting that they provided alcohol to minors.	Wagenaar, et al. (2000)[91]
			Report 2: N = 1,721-3,095 surveys of 18-20 year-olds (96% White) RCT/TAU	Report 2: At posttest, a reduction in the number of arrests for DUI.	Wagenaar, et al. (2000)[92]
Study to Prevent Alcohol Related Consequences (SPARC)	Universal	Community	N = 10 colleges/ universities in North Carolina; 3,811 students (80% White) RCT/TAU	At posttest, signification reductions in student reports of alcohol-related personal harms and causing injuries to others.	Wolfson, et al. (2012)[93]
Sacramento Neighborhood Alcohol Prevention Project (SNAPP)	Selective	Community	N = 2 low-income communities compared to all others in the city (35% Hispanic, 18% African American) QED	At posttest, fewer arrests for assaults (ES = 0.48), Emergency Medical Services (EMS) calls for assaults (ES = 0.57), and car accidents (ES = 0.55).	Treno, et al. (2007)[94]

Abbreviations: RCT - Randomized Controlled Trial, QED - Quasi-Experimental Design, TAU - Control Group Received Treatment As Usual, NTC - No Treatment Control, ES - Effect Size, OR - Odds Ratio

Table B.5: Community Preventive Services Task Force Recommendations for Preventing Alcohol Misuse

Policy Interventions
Increase Alcohol Taxes
Regulate Alcohol Outlet Density
Dram Shop (Commercial Host) Liability
Avoid Further Privatization of Alcohol Sales
Maintain Limits on Days of Sale
Maintain Limits on Hours of Sale
Enhanced Enforcement of Laws Prohibiting Sales to Minors
Electronic Screening and Brief Intervention (e-SBI)

Source: Community Preventive Services Task Force, (2016).[95]

References

1. Olds, D., Henderson Jr, C. R., Cole, R., Eckenrode, J., Kitzman, H., Luckey, D., . . . Powers, J. (1998). Long-term effects of nurse home visitation on children's criminal and antisocial behavior: 15-year follow-up of a randomized controlled trial. *Journal of the American Medical Association, 280*(14), 1238-1244.

2. Eckenrode, J., Campa, M., Luckey, D. W., Henderson, C. R., Cole, R., Kitzman, H., . . . Olds, D. (2010). Long-term effects of prenatal and infancy nurse home visitation on the life course of youths: 19-year follow-up of a randomized trial. *Archives of Pediatrics and Adolescent Medicine, 164*(1), 9-15.

3. Kitzman, H. J., Olds, D. L., Cole, R. E., Hanks, C. A., Anson, E. A., Arcoleo, K. J., . . . Holmberg, J. R. (2010). Enduring effects of prenatal and infancy home visiting by nurses on children: follow-up of a randomized trial among children at age 12 years. *Archives of pediatrics & adolescent medicine, 164*(5), 412-418.

4. Hawkins, J. D., Catalano, R. F., Morrison, D. M., O'Donnell, J., Abbott, R. D., & Day, L. E. (1992). The Seattle Social Development Project: Effects of the first four years on protective factors and problem behaviors. In J. McCord & R. E. Tremblay (Eds.), *Preventing antisocial behavior: Interventions from birth through adolescence.* (pp. 139-161). New York: Guilford Press.

5. Hawkins, J. D., Catalano, R. F., Kosterman, R., Abbott, R., & Hill, K. G. (1999). Preventing adolescent health-risk behaviors by strengthening protection during childhood. *Archives of Pediatrics and Adolescent Medicine, 153*(3), 226-234.

6. Hawkins, J. D., Kosterman, R., Catalano, R. F., Hill, K. G., & Abbott, R. D. (2005). Promoting positive adult functioning through social development intervention in childhood: Long-term effects from the Seattle Social Development Project. *Archives of Pediatrics & Adolescent Medicine, 159*(1), 25-31.

7. Hawkins, J. D., Kosterman, R., Catalano, R. F., Hill, K. G., & Abbott, R. D. (2008). Effects of social development intervention in childhood 15 years later. *Archives of Pediatrics and Adolescent Medicine, 162*(12), 1133-1141.

8. Brown, E. C., Catalano, R. F., Fleming, C. B., Haggerty, K. P., & Abbott, R. D. (2005). Adolescent substance use outcomes in the Raising Healthy Children project: A two-part latent growth curve analysis. *Journal of Consulting and Clinical Psychology, 73*(4), 699-710.

9. Kellam, S. G., Brown, C. H., Poduska, J. M., Ialongo, N. S., Wang, W., Toyinbo, P., . . . Wilcox, H. C. (2008). Effects of a universal classroom behavior management program in first and second grades on young adult behavioral, psychiatric, and social outcomes. *Drug and Alcohol Dependence, 95*(Suppl 1), S5-S28.

10. Kellam, S. G., Wang, W., Mackenzie, A. C. L., Brown, C. H., Ompad, D. C., Or, F., . . . Windham, A. (2014). The impact of the Good Behavior Game, a universal classroom-based preventive intervention in first and second grades, on high-risk sexual behaviors and drug abuse and dependence disorders into young adulthood. *Prevention Science, 15*(1), S6-S18.

11. Ialongo, N., Poduska, J., Werthamer, L., & Kellam, S. (2001). The distal impact of two first-grade preventive interventions on conduct problems and disorder in early adolescence. *Journal of Emotional and Behavioral Disorders, 9*(3), 146-160.

12. Furr-Holden, C. D. M., Ialongo, N. S., Anthony, J. C., Petras, H., & Kellam, S. G. (2004). Developmentally inspired drug prevention: Middle school outcomes in a school-based randomized prevention trial. *Drug and Alcohol Dependence, 73*(2), 149-158.

13. Liu, W., Lynne-Landsman, S. D., Petras, H., Masyn, K., & Ialongo, N. (2013). The evaluation of two first-grade preventive interventions on childhood aggression and adolescent marijuana use: A latent transition longitudinal mixture model. *Prevention Science, 14*(3), 206-217.

14. Eddy, J. M., Reid, J. B., Stoolmiller, M., & Fetrow, R. A. (2003). Outcomes during middle school for an elementary school-based preventive intervention for conduct problems: Follow-up results from a randomized trial. *Behavior Therapy, 34*(4), 535-552.

15. DeGarmo, D. S., Eddy, J. M., Reid, J. B., & Fetrow, R. A. (2009). Evaluating mediators of the impact of the Linking the Interests of Families and Teachers (LIFT) multimodal preventive intervention on substance use initiation and growth across adolescence. *Prevention Science, 10*(3), 208-220.

16. Dodge, K. A., Bierman, K. L., Coie, J. D., Greenberg, M. T., Lochman, J. E., McMahon, R. J., & Pinderhughes, E. E. (2014). Impact of early intervention on psychopathology, crime, and well-being at age 25. *American Journal of Psychiatry, 172*(1), 59-70.

17. Tremblay, R. E., Masse, L. C., Pagani, L., & Vitaro, F. (1996). From childhood physical aggression to adolescent maladjustment: The Montreal Prevention Experiment. In R. D. Peters & R. J. McMahon (Eds.), *Preventing childhood disorders, substance abuse, and delinquency.* (Vol. 3, pp. 268-298). Thousand Oaks, CA: Sage Publications.

18. Masse, L. C. (1996). From childhood physical aggression to adolescent maladjustment. Preventing childhood disorders, substance abuse, and delinquency, 3, 268..

19. Botvin, G. J., Baker, E., Dusenbury, L., Botvin, E. M., & Diaz, T. (1995). Long-term follow-up results of a randomized drug abuse prevention trial in a white middle-class population. *JAMA, 273*(14), 1106-1112.

20. Botvin, G. J., Griffin, K. W., Diaz, T., & Ifill-Williams, M. (2001). Preventing binge drinking during early adolescence: One-and two-year follow-up of a school-based preventive intervention. *Psychology of Addictive Behaviors, 15*(4), 360-365.

21. Griffin, K. W., Botvin, G. J., Nichols, T. R., & Doyle, M. M. (2003). Effectiveness of a universal drug abuse prevention approach for youth at high risk for substance use initiation. *Preventive Medicine, 36*(1), 1-7.

22. Smith, E. A., Swisher, J. D., Vicary, J. R., Bechtel, L. J., Minner, D., Henry, K. L., & Palmer, R. (2004). Evaluation of Life Skills Training and Infused-Life Skills Training in a rural setting: Outcomes at two years. *Journal of Alcohol and Drug Education, 48*(1), 51-70.

23. Spoth, R., Randall, G. K., Shin, C., & Redmond, C. (2005). Randomized study of combined universal family and school preventive interventions: Patterns of long-term effects on initiation, regular use, and weekly drunkenness. *Psychology of Addictive Behaviors, 19*(4), 372-381.

24. Spoth, R. L., Clair, S., Shin, C., & Redmond, C. (2006). Long-term effects of universal preventive interventions on methamphetamine use among adolescents. *Archives of Pediatrics and Adolescent Medicine, 160*(9), 876-882.

25. Spoth, R. L., Randall, G. K., Trudeau, L., Shin, C., & Redmond, C. (2008). Substance use outcomes 5½ years past baseline for partnership-based, family-school preventive interventions. *Drug and Alcohol Dependence, 96*(1-2), 57-68.

26. McBride, N., Midford, R., Farringdon, F., & Phillips, M. (2000). Early results from a school alcohol harm minimization study: The School Health and Alcohol Harm Reduction Project. *Addiction, 95*(7), 1021-1042.

27. McBride, N., Farringdon, F., Midford, R., Meuleners, L., & Phillips, M. (2004). Harm minimization in school drug education: Final results of the School Health and Alcohol Harm Reduction Project (SHAHRP). *Addiction, 99*(3), 278-291.

28. Conrod, P. J., Castellanos-Ryan, N., & Strang, J. (2010). Brief, personality-targeted coping skills interventions and survival as a non–drug user over a 2-year period during adolescence. *Archives of General Psychiatry, 67*(1), 85-93.

29. Conrod, P. J., Castellanos-Ryan, N., & Mackie, C. (2011). Long-term effects of a personality-targeted intervention to reduce alcohol use in adolescents. *Journal of Consulting and Clinical Psychology, 79*(3), 296-306.

30. Conrod, P. J., O'Leary-Barrett, M., Newton, N., Topper, L., Castellanos-Ryan, N., Mackie, C., & Girard, A. (2013). Effectiveness of a selective, personality-targeted prevention program for adolescent alcohol use and misuse: A cluster randomized controlled trial. *JAMA Psychiatry, 70*(3), 334-342.

31. Mahu, I. T., Doucet, C., O'Leary-Barrett, M., & Conrod, P. J. (2015). Can cannabis use be prevented by targeting personality risk in schools? 24-month outcome of the adventure trial on cannabis use: A cluster randomized controlled trial. *Addiction, 110*(10), 1625-1633.

32. Lammers, J., Goossens, F., Conrod, P., Engels, R., Wiers, R. W., & Kleinjan, M. (2015). Effectiveness of a selective intervention program targeting personality risk factors for alcohol misuse among young adolescents: Results of a cluster randomized controlled trial. *Addiction, 110*(7), 1101-1109.

33. Faggiano, F., Vigna-Taglianti, F., Burkhart, G., Bohrn, K., Cuomo, L., Gregori, D., . . . Varona, L. (2010). The effectiveness of a school-based substance abuse prevention program: 18-month follow-up of the EU-Dap cluster randomized controlled trial. *Drug and Alcohol Dependence, 108*(1-2), 56-64.

34. Hecht, M. L., Marsiglia, F. F., Elek, E., Wagstaff, D. A., Kulis, S., Dustman, P., & Miller-Day, M. (2003). Culturally grounded substance use prevention: An evaluation of the keepin'it REAL curriculum. *Prevention Science, 4*(4), 233-248.

35. Hecht, M. L., Graham, J. W., & Elek, E. (2006). The drug resistance strategies intervention: Program effects on substance use. *Health Communication, 20*(3), 267-276.

36. Kulis, S., Marsiglia, F. F., Sicotte, D., & Nieri, T. (2007). Neighborhood effects on youth substance use in a southwestern city. *Sociological Perspectives, 50*(2), 273-301.

37. Marsiglia, F. F., Ayers, S., Gance-Cleveland, B., Mettler, K., & Booth, J. (2012). Beyond primary prevention of alcohol use: A culturally specific secondary prevention program for Mexican heritage adolescents. *Prevention Science, 13*(3), 241-251.

38. Goldberg, L., MacKinnon, D. P., Elliot, D. L., Moe, E. L., Clarke, G., & Cheong, J. (2000). The adolescents training and learning to avoid steroids program: Preventing drug use and promoting health behaviors. *Archives of Pediatrics and Adolescent Medicine, 154*(4), 332-338.

39. Spoth, R. L., Redmond, C., & Shin, C. (2001). Randomized trial of brief family interventions for general populations: Adolescent substance use outcomes 4 years following baseline. *Journal of Consulting and Clinical Psychology, 69*(4), 627-642.

40. Spoth, R., Redmond, C., Shin, C., & Azevedo, K. (2004). Brief family intervention effects on adolescent substance initiation: School-level growth curve analyses 6 years following baseline. *Journal of Consulting and Clinical Psychology, 72*(3), 535-542.

41. Spoth, R., Trudeau, L., Guyll, M., Shin, C., & Redmond, C. (2009). Universal intervention effects on substance use among young adults mediated by delayed adolescent substance initiation. *Journal of Consulting and Clinical Psychology, 77*(4), 620-632.

42. Spoth, R. L., Trudeau, L. S., Guyll, M., & Shin, C. (2012). Benefits of universal intervention effects on a youth protective shield 10 years after baseline. *Journal of Adolescent Health, 50*(4), 414-417.

43. Spoth, R. L., Redmond, C., Trudeau, L., & Shin, C. (2002). Longitudinal substance initiation outcomes for a universal preventive intervention combining family and school programs. *Psychology of Addictive Behaviors, 16*(2), 129-134.

44. Spoth, R., Trudeau, L., Shin, C., Ralston, E., Redmond, C., Greenberg, M., & Feinberg, M. (2013). Longitudinal effects of universal preventive intervention on prescription drug misuse: Three randomized controlled trials with late adolescents and young adults. *American Journal of Public Health, 103*(4), 665-672.

45. Mason, W. A., Kosterman, R., Haggerty, K. P., Hawkins, J. D., Redmond, C., Spoth, R. L., & Shin, C. (2009). Gender moderation and social developmental mediation of the effect of a family-focused substance use preventive intervention on young adult alcohol abuse. *Addictive Behaviors, 34*(6), 599-605.

46. Brody, G. H., Murry, V. M., Kogan, S. M., Gerrard, M., Gibbons, F. X., Molgaard, V., . . . Wills, T. A. (2006). The Strong African American Families Program: A cluster-randomized prevention trial of long-term effects and a mediational model. *Journal of Consulting and Clinical Psychology, 74*(2), 356-366.

47. Brody, G. H., Chen, Y.-F., Kogan, S. M., Murry, V. M., & Brown, A. C. (2010). Long-term effects of the Strong African American Families program on youths' alcohol use. *Journal of Consulting and Clinical Psychology, 78*(2), 281-285.

48. Schinke, S. P., Schwinn, T. M., Di Noia, J., & Cole, K. C. (2004). Reducing the risks of alcohol use among urban youth: Three-year effects of a computer-based intervention with and without parent involvement. *Journal of Studies on Alcohol, 65*(4), 443-449.

49. Schinke, S. P., Schwinn, T. M., & Fang, L. (2010). Longitudinal outcomes of an alcohol abuse prevention program for urban adolescents. *Journal of Adolescent Health, 46*(5), 451-457.

50. Schinke, S. P., Fang, L., & Cole, K. C. (2009). Computer-delivered, parent-involvement intervention to prevent substance use among adolescent girls. *Preventive Medicine, 49*(5), 429-435.

51. Fang, L., & Schinke, S. P. (2013). Two-year outcomes of a randomized, family-based substance use prevention trial for Asian American adolescent girls. *Psychology of Addictive Behaviors, 27*(3), 788-798.

52. Estrada, Y., Rosen, A., Huang, S., Tapia, M., Sutton, M., Willis, L., ... Prado, G. (2015). Efficacy of a brief intervention to reduce substance use and Q1 human immunodeficiency virus infection risk among Latino youth. *Journal of Adolescent Health, 57*(6), 651-657.

53. Pantin, H., Prado, G., Lopez, B., Huang, S., Tapia, M. I., Schwartz, S. J., ... Branchini, J. (2009). A randomized controlled trial of Familias Unidas for Hispanic adolescents with behavior problems. *Psychosomatic Medicine, 71*(9), 987-995.

54. Schinke, S. P., Tepavac, L., & Cole, K. C. (2000). Preventing substance use among Native American youth: Three-year results. *Addictive Behaviors, 25*(3), 387-397.

55. Walton, M. A., Resko, S., Barry, K. L., Chermack, S. T., Zucker, R. A., Zimmerman, M. A., ... Blow, F. C. (2014). A randomized controlled trial testing the efficacy of a brief cannabis universal prevention program among adolescents in primary care. *Addiction, 109*(5), 786-797.

56. Veronneau, M. H., Dishion, T. J., & Connell, A. M. (In press). 10 year ITT effects on marijuana use. *Journal of Consulting and Clinical Psychology*.

57. Stormshak, E. A., Connell, A. M., Véronneau, M. H., Myers, M. W., Dishion, T. J., Kavanagh, K., & Caruthers, A. S. (2011). An ecological approach to promoting early adolescent mental health and social adaptation: Family-centered intervention in public middle schools. *Child Development, 82*(1), 209-225.

58. Kim, H. K., & Leve, L. D. (2011). Substance use and delinquency among middle school girls in foster care: A three-year follow-up of a randomized controlled trial. *Journal of Consulting and Clinical Psychology, 79*(6), 740-750.

59. Lochman, J. E., & Wells, K. C. (2003). Effectiveness of the Coping Power Program and of classroom intervention with aggressive children: Outcomes at a 1-year follow-up. *Behavior Therapy, 34*(4), 493-515.

60. Lochman, J. E., & Wells, K. C. (2004). The coping power program for preadolescent aggressive boys and their parents: Outcome effects at the 1-year follow-up. *Journal of Consulting and Clinical Psychology, 72*(4), 571-578.

61. Zonnevylle-Bender, M. J. S., Matthys, W., & Lochman, J. E. (2007). Preventive effects of treatment of disruptive behavior disorder in middle childhood on substance use and delinquent behavior. *Journal of the American Academy of Child & Adolescent Psychiatry, 46*(1), 33-39.

62. Sun, W., Skara, S., Sun, P., Dent, C. W., & Sussman, S. (2006). Project Towards No Drug Abuse: Long-term substance use outcomes evaluation. *Preventive Medicine, 42*(3), 188-192.

63. Sussman, S., Sun, P., Rohrbach, L. A., & Spruijt-Metz, D. (2012). One-year outcomes of a drug abuse prevention program for older teens and emerging adults: Evaluating a motivational interviewing booster component. *Health Psychology, 31*(4), 476-485.

64. Marlatt, G. A., Baer, J. S., Kivlahan, D. R., Dimeff, L. A., Larimer, M. E., Quigley, L. A., ... Williams, E. (1998). Screening and brief intervention for high-risk college student drinkers: Results from a 2-year follow-up assessment. *Journal of Consulting and Clinical Psychology, 66*(4), 604-615.

65. Baer, J. S., Kivlahan, D. R., Blume, A. W., McKnight, P., & Marlatt, G. A. (2001). Brief intervention for heavy-drinking college students: 4-year follow-up and natural history. *American Journal of Public Health, 91*(8), 1310-1316.

66. Larimer, M. E., Turner, A. P., Anderson, B. K., Fader, J. S., Kilmer, J. R., Palmer, R. S., & Cronce, J. M. (2001). Evaluating a brief alcohol intervention with fraternities. *Journal of Studies on Alcohol, 62*(3), 370-380.

67. Terlecki, M. A., Buckner, J. D., Larimer, M. E., & Copeland, A. L. (2015). Randomized controlled trial of brief alcohol screening and intervention for college students for heavy-drinking mandated and volunteer undergraduates: 12-month outcomes. *Psychology of Addictive Behaviors, 29*(1), 2-16.

68. Ichiyama, M. A., Fairlie, A. M., Wood, M. D., Turrisi, R., Francis, D. P., Ray, A. E., & Stanger, L. A. (2009). A randomized trial of a parent-based intervention on drinking behavior among incoming college freshmen. *Journal of Studies on Alcohol and Drugs Supplement*(16), 67-76.

69. Turrisi, R., Mallett, K. A., Cleveland, M. J., Varvil-Weld, L., Abar, C., Scaglione, N., & Hultgren, B. (2013). Evaluation of timing and dosage of a parent-based intervention to minimize college students' alcohol consumption. *Journal of Studies on Alcohol and Drugs, 74*(1), 30-40.

70. Turrisi, R., Larimer, M. E., Mallett, K. A., Kilmer, J. R., Ray, A. E., Mastroleo, N. R., . . . Montoya, H. (2009). A randomized clinical trial evaluating a combined alcohol intervention for high-risk college students. *Journal of Studies on Alcohol and Drugs, 70*(4), 555-567.

71. Wood, M. D., Fairlie, A. M., Fernandez, A. C., Borsari, B., Capone, C., Laforge, R., & Carmona-Barros, R. (2010). Brief motivational and parent interventions for college students: A randomized factorial study. *Journal of Consulting and Clinical Psychology, 78*(3), 349-361.

72. Snow, D. L., Swan, S. C., & Wilton, L. (2003). A workplace coping-skills intervention to prevent alcohol abuse. In J. B. Bennett & W. E. K. Lehman (Eds.), *Preventing workplace substance abuse: Beyond drug testing to wellness.* (pp. 57-96). Washington, DC: American Psychological Association.

73. Longabaugh, R., Woolard, R. E., Nirenberg, T. D., Minugh, A. P., Becker, B., Clifford, P. R., . . . Gogineni, A. (2001). Evaluating the effects of a brief motivational intervention for injured drinkers in the emergency department. *Journal of Studies on Alcohol, 62*(6), 806-816.

74. Broome, K. M., & Bennett, J. B. (2011). Reducing heavy alcohol consumption in young restaurant workers. *Journal of Studies on Alcohol and Drugs, 72*(1), 117-124.

75. Fink, A., Elliott, M. N., Tsai, M., & Beck, J. C. (2008). An evaluation of an intervention to assist primary care physicians in screening and educating older patients who use alcohol: Erratum. *Journal of the American Geriatrics Society, 56*(6), 1165-1165.

76. Ettner, S. L., Xu, H., Duru, O. K., Ang, A., Tseng, C.-H., Tallen, L., . . . Moore, A. A. (2014). The effect of an educational intervention on alcohol consumption, at-risk drinking, and health care utilization in older adults: The Project SHARE study. *Journal of Studies on Alcohol and Drugs, 75*(3), 447-457.

77. Hawkins, J. D., Oesterle, S., Brown, E. C., Monahan, K. C., Abbott, R. D., Arthur, M. W., & Catalano, R. F. (2012). Sustained decreases in risk exposure and youth problem behaviors after installation of the Communities That Care prevention system in a randomized trial. *Archives of Pediatrics & Adolescent Medicine, 166*(2), 141-148.

78. Hawkins, J. D., Oesterle, S., Brown, E. C., Abbott, R. D., & Catalano, R. F. (2014). Youth problem behaviors 8 years after implementing the Communities That Care prevention system: A community-randomized trial. *JAMA Pediatrics, 168*(2), 122-129.

79. Spoth, R., Redmond, C., Shin, C., Greenberg, M., Feinberg, M., & Schainker, L. (2013). PROSPER community–university partnership delivery system effects on substance misuse through 6 1/2 years past baseline from a cluster randomized controlled intervention trial. *Preventive Medicine, 56*(3), 190-196.

80. Perry, C. L., Williams, C. L., Veblen-Mortenson, S., Toomey, T. L., Komro, K. A., Anstine, P. S., . . . Wagenaar, A. C. (1996). Project Northland: Outcomes of a communitywide alcohol use prevention program during early adolescence. *American Journal of Public Health, 86*(7), 956-965.

81. Klepp, K.-I., Kelder, S. H., & Perry, C. L. (1995). Alcohol and marijuana use among adolescents: Long-term outcomes of the Class of 1989 Study. *Annals of Behavioral Medicine, 17*(1), 19-24.

82. Perry, C. L., Williams, C. L., Komro, K. A., Veblen-Mortenson, S., Stigler, M. H., Munson, K. A., . . . Forster, J. L. (2002). Project Northland: Long-term outcomes of community action to reduce adolescent alcohol use. *Health Education Research, 17*(1), 117-132.

83. Pentz, M. A., Dwyer, J. H., MacKinnon, D. P., Flay, B. R., Hansen, W. B., Wang, E. Y. I., & Johnson, C. A. (1989). A multicommunity trial for primary prevention of adolescent drug abuse: Effects on drug use prevalence. *JAMA, 261*(22), 3259-3266.

84. Pentz, M. A., & Valente, T. (1993). Project STAR: A substance abuse prevention campaign in Kansas City. In T. E. Backer & E. M. Rogers (Eds.), *Organizational aspects of health communication campaigns: What works?* (pp. 37-60). Thousand Oaks, CA: Sage.

85. Pentz, M. A., Trebow, E. A., Hansen, W. B., MacKinnon, D. P., Dwyer, J. H., Johnson, C. A., . . . Cormack, C. (1990). Effects of program implementation on adolescent drug use behavior: The Midwestern Prevention Project (MPP). *Evaluation Review, 14*(3), 264-289.

86. Chou, C.-P., Montgomery, S., Pentz, M. A., Rohrbach, L. A., Johnson, C. A., Flay, B. R., & MacKinnon, D. P. (1998). Effects of a community-based prevention program on decreasing drug use in high-risk adolescents. *American Journal of Public Health, 88*(6), 944-948.

87. Riggs, N. R., Chou, C. P., & Pentz, M. A. (2009). Preventing growth in amphetamine use: Long-term effects of the Midwestern Prevention Project (MPP) from early adolescence to early adulthood. *Addiction, 104*(10), 1691-1699.

88. Wagenaar, A. C., Erickson, D. J., Harwood, E. M., & O'Malley, P. M. (2006). Effects of state coalitions to reduce underage drinking: A national evaluation. *American Journal of Preventive Medicine, 31*(4), 307-315.

89. Saltz, R. F., Paschall, M. J., McGaffigan, R. P., & Nygaard, P. M. O. (2010). Alcohol risk management in college settings: The Safer California Universities randomized trial. *American Journal of Preventive Medicine, 39*(6), 491-499.

90. Hingson, R., McGovern, T., Howland, J., Heeren, T., Winter, M., & Zakocs, R. C. (1996). Reducing alcohol-impaired driving in Massachusetts: The Saving Lives program. *American Journal of Public Health, 86*(6), 791-797.

91. Wagenaar, A. C., Murray, D. M., Gehan, J. P., Wolfson, M., Forster, J. L., Toomey, T. L., . . . Jones-Webb, R. (2000). Communities Mobilizing For Change on Alcohol: Outcomes from a randomized community trial. *Journal of Studies on Alcohol, 61*(1), 85-94.

92. Wagenaar, A. C., Murray, D. M., & Toomey, T. L. (2000). Communities Mobilizing for Change on Alcohol (CMCA): Effects of a randomized trial on arrests and traffic crashes. *Addiction, 95*(2), 209-217.

93. Wolfson, M., Champion, H., McCoy, T. P., Rhodes, S. D., Ip, E. H., Blocker, J. N., . . . Durant, R. H. (2012). Impact of a randomized campus/community trial to prevent high-risk drinking among college students. *Alcoholism: Clinical and Experimental Research, 36*(10), 1767-1778.

94. Treno, A. J., Gruenewald, P. J., Lee, J. P., & Remer, L. G. (2007). The Sacramento Neighborhood Alcohol Prevention Project: Outcomes from a community prevention trial. *Journal of Studies on Alcohol and Drugs, 68*(2), 197-207.

95. Community Preventive Services Task Force. (2016). Preventing excessive alcohol consumption. *The guide to community preventive services: The community guide.* Retrieved from http://www.thecommunityguide.org/alcohol/index.html. Accessed on April 11, 2016.

APPENDIX C.
RESOURCE GUIDE

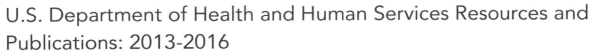

U.S. Department of Health and Human Services Resources and Publications: 2013-2016

Topic	Title	Description	Target Audience
ADHD and Substance Use Disorders	SAMHSA Advisory: Adults With Attention Deficit Hyperactivity Disorder and Substance Use Disorders	This *Advisory* defines ADHD in adults. It discusses the interaction and relationship between ADHD and substance use disorders and provides information on screening for ADHD in adults, treatment of co-occurring ADHD and substance use disorders, and prevention of stimulant abuse in clients with ADHD.	Primary Care Doctors, Nurses, Drug and Alcohol Counselors, Mental Health Clinicians
Complementary Health Approaches	SAMHSA Advisory: Complementary Health Approaches: Advising Clients About Evidence and Risks	This *Advisory* provides behavioral health practitioners a brief overview of complementary health approaches, gives examples of the types of practices and products considered complementary, and discusses how practitioners can offer guidance to clients regarding the benefits and risks of adopting such approaches.	Prevention Professionals, Public Health Professionals, People with Substance Use or Misuse Problems, People with Alcohol Use or Misuse Problems, People with Mental Health Problems, Patients

Topic	Title	Description	Target Audience
Cultural Competence	TIP 59: Improving Cultural Competence	This *Treatment Improvement Protocol (TIP)* uses a multidimensional model for developing cultural competence. Adapted to address cultural competence across behavioral health settings, this model serves as a framework for targeting three organizational levels of treatment: individual counselor and staff, clinical and programmatic, and organizational and administrative. The chapters target specific racial, ethnic, and cultural considerations along with the core elements of cultural competence highlighted in the model. These core elements include cultural awareness, general cultural knowledge, cultural knowledge of behavioral health, and cultural skill development.	Professional Care Providers, Program Planners, Administrators, Project Managers
Disaster Planning	TAP 34: Disaster Planning Handbook for Behavioral Health Treatment Programs	This *Technical Assistance Publication (TAP)* offers guidance in creating a disaster preparedness and recovery plan for programs that provide treatment for mental illness and substance use disorders. It also covers the planning process, preparing for disaster, roles and responsibilities, training, and testing.	Professional Care Providers, Disaster Response Workers, Program Planners, Administrators, Project Managers
Gambling	SAMHSA Advisory: Gambling Problems: An Introduction for Behavioral Health Services Providers	This *Advisory* provides an introduction to pathological gambling, gambling disorder, and problem gambling; it also explores their links with substance use disorders. It describes tools available for screening and diagnosis of gambling disorder as well as strategies for treating people with gambling problems.	Drug and Alcohol Counselors, Mental Health Clinicians, Peer Counselors
Homelessness	TIP 55: Behavioral Health Services for People Who Are Homeless	This *TIP* is for behavioral health service providers and program administrators who want to work more effectively with people who are homeless or at risk of homelessness and who need, or are currently in, substance use disorder or mental health treatment. The TIP addresses treatment and prevention issues. The approach advocated by the TIP is integrated and is aimed at providing services to the whole person to improve quality of life in all relevant domains.	Public Officials, Public Health Professionals, Program Planners, Administrators, Project Managers, Professional Care Providers, Non-Profits & Faith-Based Organizations, Community Coalitions

Topic	Title	Description	Target Audience
Medication-Assisted Treatment	CMCS Informational Bulletin: Medication Assisted Treatment for Substance Use Disorders	This *Bulletin* highlights the use of FDA-approved medications in combination with evidence-based behavioral therapies, commonly referred to as "Medication Assisted Treatment" (MAT), to help persons with substance use disorders (SUD) recover in a safe and cost-effective manner. Specifically, the Bulletin provides background information about MAT, examples of state-based initiatives, and useful resources to help ensure proper delivery of these services.	People with Substance Use or Misuse Problems, People in Recovery, People in Treatment
Medication-Assisted Treatment	DrugFacts: Treatment Approaches for Drug Addiction	This website describes research findings on effective medication and behavioral treatment approaches for drug addiction and discusses special considerations for the criminal justice setting.	General public
Medication-Assisted Treatment	In Brief: Adult Drug Courts and Medication-Assisted Treatment for Opioid Dependence	This *In Brief* highlights the use of MAT for opioid dependence in drug courts. It reviews effective medications, including methadone, buprenorphine, and naltrexone and provides strategies to increase the use of MAT in drug court programs.	Public Health Professionals, Program Planners, Administrators, Project Managers, Policymakers, Public Officials
Medication-Assisted Treatment	MATx Mobile App	This mobile app supports the practice of health care practitioners who provide MAT. MATx features include resources to support ongoing MAT practices, guidance on attaining a Drug Addiction Treatment Act of 2000 (DATA) waiver for treatment with buprenorphine, and tips for conducting effective patient assessments.	Physicians
Medication-Assisted Treatment	Medication-Assisted Treatment of Opioid Use Disorder Pocket Guide	This pocket guide offers guidelines for physicians using MAT for patients with opioid use disorder. It includes a checklist for prescribing medication, approved medications in the treatment of opioid use disorder, screening and assessment tools, and best practices for patient care.	Physicians
Medication-Assisted Treatment	Medication for the Treatment of Alcohol Use Disorder: A Brief Guide	This guide provides evidence on the effectiveness of available medications for the treatment of alcohol use disorder and guidance for the use of medications in clinical practice.	Physicians

Topic	Title	Description	Target Audience
Opioid Prevention	CMCS Informational Bulletin: Best Practices for Addressing Prescription Opioid Overdoses, Misuse and Addiction	This *Bulletin* highlights emerging Medicaid strategies for preventing opioid-related harms and provides background information on overdose deaths involving prescription opioids, describes several Medicaid pharmacy benefit management strategies for mitigating prescription drug abuse and discusses strategies to increase the provision of naloxone to reverse opioid overdose, thereby reducing opioid-related overdose deaths. Wherever possible, the *Bulletin* provides examples of methods states can use to target the prescribing of methadone for pain relief, given the disproportionate share of opioid-related overdose deaths associated with methadone when used as a pain reliever.	People with Substance Use or Misuse Problems, People in Recovery, People in Treatment
Opioid Prevention	Opioid Overdose Prevention Toolkit (updated 2016)	This toolkit provides guidance to develop practices and policies to help prevent opioid-related overdoses and deaths.	Health Care Professionals, First Responders, Treatment Providers, Local Governments, Communities, Those Recovering from Opioid Overdose
Opioid Prevention	Opioid and Pain Management CMEs/CEs: Safe Prescribing for Pain and Managing Pain Patients Who Abuse Rx Drugs	These CME courses developed by NIDA and Medscape Education, with funding from the White House Office of National Drug Control Policy provide practical guidance for physicians and other clinicians in screening pain patients for substance use disorder risk factors before prescribing, and in identifying when patients are abusing their medications.	Health Care Professionals
Recovery	Motivation for Change: John's Story—Consequences of His Heavy Drinking and His Recovery	This comic book/fotonovela uses photographs with captions to help the reader recognize the dangers people face when they have a substance use disorder. It tells the troubles of a family as the son, John, faces his substance use problem, enters treatment, and moves into recovery.	People with Alcohol Use or Misuse Problems, People With Substance Use or Misuse Problems

Topic	Title	Description	Target Audience
Recovery	You Can Manage Your Chronic Pain To Live a Good Life: A Guide for People in Recovery from Mental Illness or Addiction	This consumer brochure equips people who have chronic pain and mental illness or addiction with tips for working with their health care professional to decrease their pain without jeopardizing their recovery. It also explores counseling, exercise, and alternative therapy, as well as medications.	People in Recovery, People in Treatment
Screening and Brief Intervention	Alcohol Screening and Brief Intervention for Youth: A Practitioner's Guide	This Guide helps health care professionals who manage the health and well-being of children and adolescents conduct fast, effective alcohol screens and interventions with patients ages 9-18.	Health Care Professionals
Screening and Referral to Treatment	SAMHSA Advisory: Hepatitis C Screening in the Behavioral Healthcare Setting	This Advisory explains why behavioral health services programs should consider screening clients for Hepatitis C if clients have known risk factors for Hepatitis C viral infection or if they have signs and symptoms of liver disease. The Advisory explains how onsite screening, or referral to screening, can be incorporated into existing intake and monitoring procedures. It also offers guidance on providing clients with viral hepatitis prevention education, counseling, and referral to follow-up evaluation and medical treatment as needed.	Public Health Professionals, Program Planners, Administrators, Project Managers, Health Care Professionals
Screening and Referral to Treatment	NIDA Drug Use Screening Tool	This tool features a one-question Quick Screen as well as the full NIDA-Modified Alcohol, Smoking and Substance Involvement Screening Test.	Health Care Professionals
Screening, Brief Intervention, and Referral to Treatment	TAP 33: Systems-Level Implementation of Screening, Brief Intervention, and Referral to Treatment (SBIRT)	This TAP describes core elements of SBIRT programs for people with or at risk for substance use disorders and also describes SBIRT services implementation, covering challenges, barriers, cost, and sustainability.	Public Health Professionals, Program Planners, Administrators, Project Managers, Professional Care Providers, Grant Seekers and Grantees, Public Officials
Substance Misuse and Mental Health	In Brief: An Introduction to Co-Occurring Borderline Personality Disorder and Substance Use Disorders	This In Brief Introduces professional care providers to borderline personality disorder. It covers signs and symptoms, with or without co-occurring substance use disorder; monitoring clients for self-harm and suicide; and referrals to treatment.	Professional Care Providers, Public Health Professionals

Topic	Title	Description	Target Audience
Substance Misuse and Mental Health	National Prevention Week	National Prevention Week is an annual health observance dedicated to increasing public awareness of, and action around, substance use and mental health issues.	Businesses, Communities, Educators, Health Care Professionals, Law Enforcement, Parents and Caregivers, Prevention Specialists, Youth
Substance Misuse and Mental Health	No Longer Alone (A Story About Alcohol, Drugs, Depression, and Trauma): Addressing the Specific Needs of Women	This comic book tells the stories of three women with substance misuse and mental health problems who have received treatment and improved their quality of life. Featuring flashbacks, the fotonovela is culturally relevant and dispels myths around behavioral health disorders.	Adolescents, Young Adults, Mature Adults
Substance Misuse Prevention	Alcohol Overdose: The Dangers of Drinking Too Much	This fact sheet provides information about the signs and symptoms of alcohol overdose.	Individuals
Substance Misuse Prevention	Center for the Application of Prevention Technologies (CAPT)	SAMHSA's CAPT is a national training and technical assistance (T/TA) system committed to strengthening prevention systems and building the nation's behavioral health workforce.	SAMHSA Substance Use Prevention Grantees and Prevention Professionals
Substance Misuse Prevention	CMCS Informational Bulletin: Prevention and Early Identification of Mental Health and Substance Use Conditions	This Bulletin helps inform states about resources available to help them meet the needs of children under Early and Periodic Screening, Diagnostic, and Treatment (EPSDT), specifically with respect to mental health and substance use disorder services.	Public Officials
Substance Misuse Prevention	Harmful Interactions	This resource provides information about medications that can cause harm when taken with alcohol and describes the effects that can result.	Adolescents, Young Adults, Mature Adults, Health Care Professionals
Substance Misuse Prevention	Health Education Curriculum Analysis Tool (HECAT) and HECAT Module AOD	This tool can help school districts, schools, and others conduct a clear, complete, and consistent analysis of health education curricula based on the National Health Education Standards and CDC's Characteristics of an Effective Health Education Curriculum. Results of the HECAT can help schools select or develop appropriate and effective health education curricula and improve the delivery of health education. The HECAT can be customized to meet local community needs and conform to the curriculum requirements of the state or school district.	Educators

Topic	Title	Description	Target Audience
Substance Misuse Prevention	Marijuana Facts for Teens and Marijuana Facts Parents Need to Know	The teen booklet is presented in question-and-answer format and provides facts about marijuana and its potential harmful effects. The parent booklet provides important facts about marijuana and offers tips for talking with children about the drug and its potential harmful effects.	Teens, parents, caregivers, general public
Substance Misuse Prevention	National Drug & Alcohol Facts Week	This online guide gives organizers everything they need to plan, promote, and host their own National Drug & Alcohol Facts Week (NDAFW) event. NDAFW is a national health observance for teens to promote local events that use NIDA science to SHATTER THE MYTHS about drugs.	Teens, parents, educators, general public
Substance Misuse Prevention	Principles of Substance Abuse Prevention for Early Childhood	This guide begins with a list of 7 principles addressing the specific ways in which early interventions can have positive effects on development; these principles reflect findings on the influence of intervening early with vulnerable populations, on the course of child development, and on common elements of early childhood programs.	Parents, health care providers, and policymakers
Substance Misuse Prevention	Rethinking Drinking	This website is a tool for individuals who want to assess and/or change their drinking habits.	Individuals, Family Members
Substance Use Disorder Services	CMCS Informational Bulletin: Coverage of Behavioral Health Services for Youth with Substance Use Disorders	This *Bulletin*, based on evidence from scientific research and the results of a Substance Abuse and Mental Health Services Administration (SAMHSA)-supported technical expert panel consensus process, is intended to assist states to design a benefit that will meet the needs of youth with substance use disorders (SUD) and their families and help states comply with their obligations under Medicaid's Early and Periodic Screening, Diagnostic, and Treatment (EPSDT) requirements. The services described in this document are designed to enable youth to address their substance use disorders, to receive treatment and continuing care and to participate in recovery services and supports. This *Bulletin* also identifies resources that are available to states to facilitate their work in designing and implementing a benefit package for these youth and their families.	Public Officials

Topic	Title	Description	Target Audience
Substance Use Disorder Services	New Service Delivery Opportunities for Individuals with a Substance Use Disorder	This State Medicaid Director Letter informs states of opportunities to design service delivery systems for individuals with substance use disorder (SUD), including a new opportunity for demonstration projects approved under section 1115 of the Social Security Act (Act) to ensure that a continuum of care is available to individuals with SUD.	Public Officials
Substance Use Disorder Treatment	In Brief: Treating Sleep Problems of People in Recovery From Substance Use Disorders	This In Brief discusses the relationship between sleep disturbances and substance use disorders and provides guidance on how to assess for and treat sleep problems for people in recovery. It also reviews nonpharmacological as well as over-the-counter and prescription medications.	Professional Care Providers
Substance Use Disorder Treatment	Principles of Adolescent Substance Use Disorder Treatment: A Research-Based Guide	This guide presents research-based principles of adolescent substance use disorder treatment; covers treatment for a variety of drugs including, illicit and prescription drugs, alcohol, and tobacco; presents settings and evidence-based approaches unique to treating adolescents.	Professional Care Providers, Administrators, Public Health Professionals, individuals and families
Substance Use Disorder Treatment	Principles of Drug Abuse Treatment for Criminal Justice Populations - A Research-Based Guide	This guide presents research-based principles of addiction treatment that can inform drug treatment programs and services in the criminal justice setting.	Professional Care Providers, Administrators, Public Health Professionals, individuals and families
Substance Use Disorder Treatment	SAMHSA Advisory: Diabetes Care for Clients in Behavioral Health Treatment	This Advisory reviews diabetes and its link with mental illness, stress, and substance use disorders, and it discusses ways to integrate diabetes care into behavioral health treatment, such as screening and intake, staff education, integrated care, and counseling support.	Professional Care Providers, Program Planners, Administrators, Project Managers, Public Health Professionals
Substance Use Disorder Treatment	SAMHSA Advisory: Spice, Bath Salts, and Behavioral Health	This Advisory equips professional health providers with an introduction to spice and bath salts in the context of treating people with substance use disorders and mental illness. It discusses adverse effects of use, patient assessment, and abstinence monitoring, among other issues.	Prevention Professionals, Professional Care Providers, Public Health Professionals, Public Officials

Topic	Title	Description	Target Audience
Substance Use Disorder Treatment	SAMHSA Advisory: Sublingual and Transmucosal Buprenorphine for Opioid Use Disorder: Review and Update	This *Advisory* provides an overview of data on the use of sublingual (medicine that dissolves under the tongues) and transmucosal (medicine that dissolves between the cheeks and gums) buprenorphine to treat opioid use disorder and discusses the implications of using MAT as a recovery support.	Primary Care Doctors and Nurses, Drug and Alcohol Counselors
Substance Use Disorder Treatment	Seeking Drug Abuse Treatment: Know What To Ask	This guide offers guidance in seeking drug abuse treatment and lists five questions to ask when searching for a treatment program.	General Public
Substance Use Disorder Treatment	TIP 56: Addressing the Specific Behavioral Health Needs of Men	This *TIP* is a companion to TIP 51, *Substance Abuse Treatment: Addressing the Specific Needs of Women*. It examines how gender-specific treatment strategies can improve outcomes for men. It also covers differences between men and women in the effects of substance use and misuse and the implications these differences have in behavioral health services. It provides practical information based on available evidence and clinical experience that can help counselors more effectively treat men with substance use disorders.	Public Health Professionals, Program Planners, Administrators, Project Managers, Professional Care Providers, Prevention Professionals, Researchers
Substance Use Disorder Treatment	TIP 51: *Substance Abuse Treatment: Addressing the Specific Needs of Women*	This *TIP* assists treatment providers in offering treatment to adult women with substance use disorders. It reviews gender-specific research and best practices, such as common patterns of initiation of substance use among women and specific treatment issues and strategies.	Public Health Professionals, Program Planners, Administrators, Project Managers, Professional Care Providers, Prevention Professionals, Researchers
Substance Use Disorder Treatment	Treatment for Alcohol Problems: Finding and Getting Help	This guide is written for individuals, and their family and friends who are looking for options to address to address alcohol problems.	Individuals, Families, Friends
Suicide Prevention	In Brief: Substance Use and Suicide: A Nexus Requiring a Public Health Approach	This *In Brief* summarizes the relationship between substance use and suicide and provides state and tribal prevention professionals with information on the scope of the problem, an understanding of traditional barriers to collaboration and current programming, and ways to work together on substance use and suicide prevention strategies.	State and Tribal Prevention Professionals working in the fields of substance use and suicide prevention

Topic	Title	Description	Target Audience
Suicide Prevention	Suicide Prevention Resource Center (SPRC)	SAMHSA's SPRC provides technical assistance, training, and materials to increase the knowledge and expertise of suicide prevention practitioners and other professionals serving people at risk for suicide. While multiple factors influence suicidal behaviors, substance use—especially alcohol use—is a significant factor that is linked to a substantial number of suicides and suicide attempts.	Professionals in a variety of settings (e.g., tribal communities, schools, colleges and universities, primary care, emergency departments, behavioral health care, workplace, and faith communities)
Technology-Assisted Care	TIP 60: Using Technology-Based Therapeutic Tools in Behavioral Health Services	This *TIP* provides an overview of current technology-based behavioral health assessments and interventions, and it summarizes the evidence base supporting the effectiveness of such interventions. It also examines opportunities for technology-assisted care (TAC) in the behavioral health arena. It emphasizes use of TAC with clients who might not otherwise receive treatment or whose treatment might be impeded by physical disabilities, rural or remote geographic locations, lack of transportation, employment constraints, or symptoms of mental illness. The TIP covers programmatic, technological, budgeting, vendor selection, data management, privacy and confidentiality, and regulatory considerations likely to arise during adoption of technology-based interventions.	Program Planners, Administrators, Project Managers, Prevention Professionals, Professional Care Providers
Trauma-Informed Care	TIP 57: Trauma-Informed Care in Behavioral Health Services	This *TIP* presents fundamental concepts that behavioral health service providers and program administrators can use to initiate trauma-related screening and assessment, implement collaborative strengths-based interventions, learn the core principles and practices that reflect trauma-informed care, decrease inadvertent retraumatization, and evaluate and build a trauma-informed organization and workforce.	Professional Care Providers, Program Planners, Administrators, Project Managers
Underage Drinking	College Alcohol Intervention Matrix (CollegeAIM)	This matrix is a resource to help colleges and universities address harmful and underage student drinking. Developed with leading college alcohol researchers and staff, it is an easy-to-use and comprehensive tool to identify effective alcohol interventions.	Higher Education Officials, particularly alcohol and other drug program and student life staff

Topic	Title	Description	Target Audience
Underage Drinking	Stop Underage Drinking website	This interagency Web portal provides key federal resources targeting the prevention of underage alcohol use.	Businesses, Communities, Educators, Health Care Professionals, Law Enforcement, Parents and Caregivers, Prevention Specialists, Youth
Underage Drinking	Talk. They Hear You. - Underage Drinking Prevention	This underage drinking prevention campaign sponsored by SAMHSA provides parents and caregivers with information and resources they need to start addressing the dangers of alcohol with their children, 9 to 15 years old.	Parents and Other Caregivers of Youth 9 to 15 years old

APPENDIX D.
IMPORTANT FACTS ABOUT ALCOHOL AND DRUGS

Appendix D outlines important facts about the following substances:

- Alcohol
- Cocaine
- GHB (gamma-hydroxybutyric acid)
- Heroin
- Inhalants
- Ketamine
- LSD (lysergic acid diethylamide)
- Marijuana (Cannabis)
- MDMA (Ecstasy)
- Mescaline (Peyote)
- Methamphetamine
- Over-the-counter Cough/Cold Medicines (Dextromethorphan or DXM)
- PCP (Phencyclidine)
- Prescription Opioids
- Prescription Sedatives (Tranquilizers, Depressants)
- Prescription Stimulants
- Psilocybin
- Rohypnol® (Flunitrazepam)
- Salvia
- Steroids (Anabolic)
- Synthetic Cannabinoids ("K2"/"Spice")
- Synthetic Cathinones ("Bath Salts")

Sources cited in this Appendix are:

- Drug Enforcement Administration's *Drug Facts Sheets*[1]
- Inhalant Addiction Treatment's *Dangers of Mixing Inhalants with Alcohol and Other Drugs*[2]
- National Institute on Alcohol Abuse and Alcoholism's (NIAAA's) *Alcohol's Effects on the Body*[3]
- National Institute on Drug Abuse's (NIDA's) *Commonly Abused Drugs*[4]
- NIDA's *Treatment for Alcohol Problems: Finding and Getting Help*[5]
- National Institutes of Health (NIH) National Library of Medicine's *Alcohol Withdrawal*[6]
- Rohypnol® *Abuse Treatment FAQs*[7]
- Substance Abuse and Mental Health Services Administration's (SAMHSA's) *Keeping Youth Drug Free*[8]
- SAMHSA's Center for Behavioral Health Statistics and Quality's (CBHSQ's) *Results from the 2015 National Survey on Drug Use and Health: Detailed Tables*[9]

The substances that are considered controlled substances under the Controlled Substances Act (CSA) are divided into five schedules. An updated and complete list of the schedules is published annually in Title 21 Code of Federal Regulations (C.F.R.) §§ 1308.11 through 1308.15.[10] Substances are placed in their respective schedules based on whether they have a currently accepted medical use in treatment in the United States, their relative abuse potential, and likelihood of causing dependence when abused. A description of each schedule is listed below.

- **Schedule I (1):** Substances in this schedule have no currently accepted medical use in the United States, a lack of accepted safety for use under medical supervision, and a high potential for abuse.
- **Schedule II/IIN (2/2N):** Substances in this schedule have a high potential for abuse which may lead to severe psychological or physical dependence.
- **Schedule III/IIIN (3/3N):** Substances in this schedule have a potential for abuse less than substances in Schedules I or II and abuse may lead to moderate or low physical dependence or high psychological dependence.
- **Schedule IV (4):** Substances in this schedule have a low potential for abuse relative to substances in Schedule III.
- **Schedule V (5):** Substances in this schedule have a low potential for abuse relative to substances listed in Schedule IV and consist primarily of preparations containing limited quantities of certain narcotics.

Alcohol

Ethyl alcohol, or ethanol, is an intoxicating ingredient found in beer, wine, and liquor. Alcohol is produced by the fermentation of yeast, sugars, and starches.[i]

Common Commercial Names	Street Names	Common Forms	Common Ways Taken	DEA Schedule / Legal Status
Various	Booze, Juice, Sauce, Brew	Beer, Wine, Liquor/Spirits/Malt Beverages	Ingested by drinking	Not scheduled / Illegal for purchase or use by those under age 21[ii]

Uses & Possible Health Effects[iii]

Short-term Symptoms of Use	Injuries and risky behavior, memory and concentration problems, coma, breathing problems, slurred speech, confusion, impaired judgment and motor skills, drowsiness, nausea and vomiting, emotional volatility, loss of coordination, visual distortions, impaired memory, changes in mood and behavior, and depression. Impaired judgment can result in inappropriate sexual behavior, sexually transmitted infections, and reduced inhibitions.
Long-term Consequences of Use and Health Effects	Some studies have found benefits associated with moderate alcohol consumption,[iv,v] while other studies do not support a role for moderate alcohol consumption in providing health benefits.[vi,vii] Studies have shown alcohol misuse use can lead to: an inability to control drinking; a high tolerance level; changes in mood and behavior; difficulty thinking clearly; impaired coordination; cardiovascular problems including heart muscle injury, irregular heartbeat, stroke, and high blood pressure; liver problems including steatosis (fatty liver), alcoholic hepatitis, fibrosis, and cirrhosis; pancreatitis; increased risk of various cancers (including of the mouth, esophagus, larynx, pharynx, liver, colon, and rectum); weakened immune system; depression; interference with personal relationships; coma, and death due to alcohol overdose. For breast cancer, even moderate drinking may increase the risk.
Other Health-related Issues	Pregnancy-related: sudden infant death syndrome (SIDS), fetal alcohol spectrum disorders (FASD).
In Combination with Alcohol	N/A
Withdrawal Symptoms	Alcohol withdrawal symptoms usually occur within 8 hours after the last drink, but can occur days later. Symptoms usually peak by 24 to 72 hours, but may go on for weeks. Common symptoms include: anxiety or nervousness, depression, fatigue, irritability, jumpiness or shakiness, mood swings, nightmares, and not thinking clearly. Other symptoms may include: clammy skin, enlarged (dilated) pupils, headache, insomnia, loss of appetite, nausea and vomiting, pallor, rapid heart rate, sweating, and tremor of the hands or other body parts. A severe form of alcohol withdrawal called delirium tremens can cause: agitation, fever, hallucinations, seizures, and severe confusion.

i. Source: NIDA, (2016).
ii. Most states prohibit possession and consumption of alcoholic beverages by those under age 21, though some make exceptions for possession or consumption in the presence, or with the consent, of family or on private property.
iii. Sources: NIDA, (2016) & NIAAA, (n.d.). The uses and possible health effects that are listed are illustrative examples and not exhaustive.
iv. Source: Gepner, et al. (2015).[12]
v. Source: Howard, et al. (2004).[13]
vi. Source: Stockwell, et al. (2016).[14]
vii. Source: Fillmore, et al. (2006).[15]

APPENDICES

Alcohol	
Treatment Options[viii]	
Medications	The U.S. Food and Drug Administration (FDA) has approved three medications for treating alcohol dependence, and others are being tested to determine if they are effective. • Naltrexone can help people reduce heavy drinking. • Acamprosate makes it easier to maintain abstinence. • Disulfiram blocks the breakdown (metabolism) of alcohol by the body, causing unpleasant symptoms such as nausea and flushing of the skin. Those unpleasant effects can help some people avoid drinking while taking disulfiram.
Behavioral Therapies	Also known as alcohol counseling, behavioral treatments involve working with a health professional to identify and help change the behaviors that lead to heavy drinking. Behavioral treatments share certain features, which can include: • Developing the skills needed to stop or reduce drinking • Helping to build a strong social support system • Working to set reachable goals • Coping with or avoiding the triggers that might cause relapse
Statistics as of 2015[ix]	
Prevalence	*Lifetime:* 217 million persons (81.0%) aged 12 or older have used alcohol in their lifetime. *Past Year:* 176 million persons (65.7%) aged 12 or older have used alcohol in the past year.
Average Age of Initiation[x]	17.6

viii. Source: NIDA, (2016).
ix. Source: CBHSQ, (2016).
x. Average age of initiation (for all substances) is based on respondents aged 12 to 49 years old.

Cocaine				
A powerfully addictive stimulant drug made from the leaves of the coca plant native to South America.[i]				
Common Commercial Names	Street Names	Common Forms	Common Ways Taken	DEA Schedule / Legal Status
Cocaine hydrochloride topical solution (anesthetic rarely used in medical procedures)	*Cocaine:* Blow, Bump, C, Candy, Charlie, Coke, Crack, Flake, Rock, Snow, Toot, Dust *Crack cocaine:* Crack, Rock, Base, Sugar Block, Rox/Roxanne	White powder, whitish rock crystal	Snorted, smoked, injected, orally, topically	Schedule II / Illegal, except for use in hospital settings (however it's rarely used)
Uses & Possible Health Effects[ii]				
Short-term Symptoms of Use	Narrowed blood vessels; enlarged pupils; increased body temperature, heart rate, and blood pressure; headache; abdominal pain and nausea; euphoria; increased energy, alertness; insomnia; restlessness, irritability, anxiety; erratic and violent behavior, panic attacks, paranoia, psychosis; heart rhythm problems, heart attack; stroke, seizure, coma; and death from cardiac arrest, respiratory arrest, or suicide.			
Long-term Consequences of Use and Health Effects	Loss of sense of smell, nosebleeds, nasal damage and trouble swallowing from snorting; infection and death of bowel tissue from decreased blood flow; poor nutrition and weight loss from decreased appetite; and severe depression.			
Other Health-related Issues	Risk of HIV, hepatitis, and other infectious diseases from shared needles. Pregnancy-related: premature delivery, low birth weight, neonatal abstinence syndrome.[iii]			
In Combination with Alcohol	Greater risk of overdose and sudden death than from alcohol or cocaine alone.			
Withdrawal Symptoms	Depression, tiredness, increased appetite, insomnia, vivid unpleasant dreams, slowed thinking and movement, restlessness.			
Medical Use	Cocaine hydrochloride topical solution is indicated for the introduction of local (topical) anesthesia of accessible mucous membranes of the oral, laryngeal and nasal cavities.			
Treatment Options[iv]				
Medications	There are no FDA-approved medications to treat cocaine addiction.			
Behavioral Therapies	• Cognitive-behavioral therapy (CBT) • Community reinforcement approach plus vouchers • Contingency management, or motivational incentives • The Matrix Model • 12-Step facilitation therapy			

i. Source: NIDA, (2016).
ii. Sources: NIDA, (2016) and DEA, (2015).
iii. Neonatal abstinence syndrome is a group of problems that occur in a newborn who was exposed to addictive opioid drugs while in the mother's womb. At birth, the baby is still dependent on the drug. Because the baby is no longer getting the drug after birth, symptoms of withdrawal may occur.[11]
iv. Source: NIDA, (2016).

	Cocaine
	Statistics as of 2015[v]
Prevalence	*Lifetime:* - Cocaine: 38.7 million persons (14.5%) aged 12 or older have used cocaine in their lifetime. - Crack: 9.0 million persons (3.4%) aged 12 or older have used crack cocaine in their lifetime. *Past Year:* - Cocaine: 4.8 million persons (1.8%) aged 12 or older have used cocaine in the past year. - Crack: 833,000 persons (0.3%) aged 12 or older have used crack cocaine in the past year.
Average Age of Initiation	Cocaine: 21.5
	Crack: 21.3

v. Source: CBHSQ, (2016).

GHB (gamma-hydroxybutyric acid)

A depressant approved for use in the treatment of narcolepsy, a disorder that causes daytime "sleep attacks".[i]

Common Commercial Names	Street Names	Common Forms	Common Ways Taken	DEA Schedule / Legal Status
Gamma-hydroxybutyrate or sodium oxybate (Xyrem®)	G, Georgia Home Boy, Goop, Grievous Bodily Harm, Liquid Ecstasy, Liquid X, Soap, Scoop	Colorless liquid, white powder	Ingested (often combined with alcohol or other beverages)	Schedule I / Illegal; GHB products such as Xyrem®, are Schedule III substances

Uses & Possible Health Effects[ii]

Short-term Symptoms of Use	Euphoria, drowsiness, decreased anxiety, confusion, memory loss, hallucinations, excited and aggressive behavior, nausea, vomiting, unconsciousness, seizures, slowed heart rate and breathing, lower body temperature, coma, and death.
Long term Consequences of Use and Health Effects	Unknown.
Other Health-related Issues	Sometimes used as a date rape drug.
In Combination with Alcohol	Nausea, problems with breathing, greatly increased depressant effects.
Withdrawal Symptoms	Insomnia, anxiety, tremors, sweating, increased heart rate and blood pressure, and psychosis.
Medical Use	Sodium Osybate (Xyrem®) is approved for use in the treatment of narcolepsy, a disorder that causes daytime "sleep attacks."

Treatment Options[iii]

Medications	Benzodiazepines
Behavioral Therapies	More research is needed to determine if behavioral therapies can be used to treat GHB addiction.

Statistics as of 2015[iv]

Prevalence	*Lifetime:* 1.2 million persons (0.4%) aged 12 or older have used GHB in their lifetime. *Past Year:* 136,000 persons (0.1%) aged 12 or older have used GHB in the past year.
Average Age of Initiation	Sedatives in general: 28.3

i. Source: NIDA, (2016).
ii. Sources: NIDA, (2016) & DEA, (2015).
iii. Sources: NIDA, (2016).
iv. Source: CBHSQ, (2016).

Heroin				
An opioid drug made from morphine, a natural substance extracted from the seed pod of the Asian opium poppy plant.[i]				
Common Commercial Names	Street Names	Common Forms	Common Ways Taken	DEA Schedule / Legal Status
No commercial uses	Brown sugar, China White, Dope, H, Horse, Junk, Skag, Skunk, Smack, White Horse With OTC cold medicine and antihistamine: Cheese	White or brownish powder, or black sticky substance known as "black tar heroin"	Injected, smoked, snorted	Schedule I / Illegal
Uses & Possible Health Effects[ii]				
Short-term Symptoms of Use	Euphoria; warm flushing of skin; dry mouth; heavy feeling in the hands and feet; clouded thinking, impaired coordination; alternate wakeful and drowsy states; itching; nausea; vomiting; slowed breathing and heart rate; and fatal overdose.			
Long-term Consequences of Use and Health Effects	Collapsed veins; abscesses (swollen tissue with pus); infection of the lining and valves in the heart (endocarditis); constipation and stomach cramps; liver or kidney disease; and pneumonia.			
Other Health-related Issues	Pregnancy-related: miscarriage, low birth weight, neonatal abstinence syndrome. Risk of HIV, hepatitis, and other infectious diseases from shared needles.			
In Combination with Alcohol	Dangerous slowdown of heart rate and breathing, coma, and death.			
Withdrawal Symptoms	Restlessness, muscle and bone pain, insomnia, diarrhea, vomiting, and cold flashes with goose bumps.			
Treatment Options[iii]				
Medications	Methadone, Buprenorphine, and Naltrexone.			
Behavioral Therapies	Contingency management, or motivational incentives 12-Step facilitation therapy			
Statistics as of 2015[23]				
Prevalence	*Lifetime:* 5.1 million persons (1.9%) aged 12 or older have used heroin in their lifetime. • Heroin needle use: 2.2 million persons (0.8%) • Smoked heroin: 2.0 million persons (0.7%) • Sniffed or snorted heroin: 3.3 million persons (1.2%) *Past Year:* 828,000 persons (0.3%) aged 12 or older have used heroin in the past year.			
Average Age of Initiation	25.4			

i. Source: NIDA, (2016).
ii. Sources: NIDA, (2016) & DEA, (2015).
iii. Sources: NIDA, (2016).

Inhalants				
Solvents, aerosols, and gases found in household products such as spray paints, markers, glues, and cleaning fluids; also nitrites (e.g., amyl nitrite), which are prescription medications for chest pain. Precise categorization of inhalants is difficult, however one classification system lists four general categories of inhalants — volatile solvents, aerosols, gases, and nitrites — based on the forms in which they are often found in household, industrial, and medical products.[i]				
Common Commercial Names	Street Names	Common Forms	Common Ways Taken	DEA Schedule / Legal Status
Solvents (paint thinners, gasoline, glues, organic solvents, nail polish remover); gases (butane, propane, aerosol propellants), nitrous oxide, hair spray; and nitrites (isoamyl, isobutyl, and cyclohexyl)	Poppers, snappers, whippets, laughing gas	Paint thinners or removers, degreasers, dry-cleaning fluids, gasoline, lighter fluids, correction fluids, permanent markers, electronics cleaners and freeze sprays, glue, spray paint, hair or deodorant sprays, fabric protector sprays, aerosol computer cleaning products, vegetable oil sprays, butane lighters, propane tanks, whipped cream aerosol containers, refrigerant gases, ether, chloroform, halothane, nitrous oxide	Inhaled through the nose or mouth	N/A
Uses & Possible Health Effects[ii]				
Short-term Symptoms of Use	While symptoms vary by chemical, potential symptoms include: confusion; nausea or vomiting; slurred speech; loss of coordination; euphoria; dizziness; drowsiness; loss of inhibition, lightheadedness, hallucinations/delusions; headaches; sudden sniffing death due to heart failure (from butane, propane, and other chemicals in aerosols); death from asphyxiation, suffocation, convulsions or seizures, coma, or choking. *Nitrites:* Enlarged blood vessels, enhanced sexual pleasure, increased heart rate, brief sensation of heat and excitement, dizziness, and headache.			
Long-term Consequences of Use and Health Effects	Liver and kidney damage; damage to cardiovascular and nervous systems; bone marrow damage; nerve damage; and brain damage from lack of oxygen that can cause problems with thinking, movement, vision, and hearing. *Nitrites:* Increased risk of pneumonia.			
Other Health-related Issues	Pregnancy-related: low birth weight, bone problems, delayed behavioral development due to brain problems, altered metabolism and body composition.			
In Combination with Alcohol[iii]	Intensifies the toxic effects of inhalants; serious mental impairment can result, leading the user to engage in deadly behavior; and may lead to coma or death. Nitrites: dangerously low blood pressure.			
Withdrawal Symptoms	Nausea, loss of appetite, sweating, tics, problems sleeping, and mood changes.			
Medical Use[iv]	Nitrous oxide only, for anesthesia: amyl nitrate indicated for rapid relief of angina pectoris.			
Treatment Options[v]				
Medications	There are no FDA-approved medications to treat inhalant addiction.			

i. Source: NIDA, (2016).
ii. Sources: NIDA, (2016).
iii. Source: Inhalant Addiction Treatment, (n.d.).
iv. Source: SAMHSA, (2004).
v. Source: NIDA, (2016).

	Inhalants
Behavioral Therapies	More research is needed to determine if behavioral therapies can be used to treat inhalant addiction.
Statistics as of 2015[vi]	
Prevalence	*Lifetime:* 25.8 million persons (9.6%) aged 12 or older have used inhalants in their lifetime. • Amyl Nitrite, Poppers, Locker Room Odorizers, or Rush: 7.4 million persons (2.8%) • Computer Cleaner/Air Duster: 3.0 million persons (1.1 %) • Correction Fluid, Degreaser, or Cleaning Fluid: 1.6 million persons (0.6%) • Felt-Tip Pens, Felt-Tip Markers, or Magic Markers: 6.8 million persons (2.5 %) • Gasoline or Lighter Fluid: 3.2 million persons (1.2%) • Glue, Shoe Polish, or Toluene: 3.2 million persons (1.2%) • Halothane, Ether, or Other Anesthetics: 809,000 persons (0.3%) • Lacquer Thinner or Other Paint Solvents: 1.5 million persons (0.6%) • Lighter Gases (Butane, Propane): 767,000 persons (0.3%) • Nitrous Oxide or Whippits: 12.4 million persons (4.6%) • Spray Paints: 1.9 million persons (0.7%) • Other Aerosol Sprays: 1.5 million persons (0.6%) *Past Year:* 1.8 million persons (0.7%) aged 12 or older have used inhalants in the past year.
Average Age of Initiation	17.4

vi. Source: CBHSQ, (2016).

Ketamine

A dissociative drug, hallucinogen, which causes the user to feel detached from reality.[i]

Common Commercial Names	Street Names	Common Forms	Common Ways Taken	DEA Schedule / Legal Status
Ketalar	Cat Valium, K, Special K, Vitamin K	Liquid, white powder	Injected, snorted, smoked (powder added to tobacco or marijuana cigarettes), ingested	Schedule III / Legal by prescription only

Uses & Possible Health Effects[ii]

Short-term Symptoms of Use	Problems with attention, learning, and memory; dreamlike states, hallucinations; sedation; confusion and problems speaking; memory loss; stiffening of the muscles and numbness; problems moving, to the point of being immobile; increased blood pressure; nausea; unconsciousness; slowed breathing (respiratory depression) that can lead to death.
Long-term Consequences of Use and Health Effects	Ulcers and pain in the bladder; kidney problems; stomach pain; depression; flashbacks; and poor memory.
Other Health-related Issues	Sometimes used as a date rape drug. Risk of HIV, hepatitis, and other infectious diseases from shared needles.
In Combination with Alcohol	Increased risk of adverse effects.
Withdrawal Symptoms	Unknown.
Medical Use	Used as an anesthetic agent.

Treatment Options[iii]

Medications	There are no FDA-approved medications to treat addiction to ketamine or other dissociative drugs.
Behavioral Therapies	More research is needed to determine if behavioral therapies can be used to treat addiction to dissociative drugs.

Statistics as of 2015[iv]

Prevalence	*Lifetime:* 3.0 million persons (1.1%) aged 12 or older have used ketamine in their lifetime. *Past Year:* Data not collected.
Average Age of Initiation	Hallucinogens in general: 19.6

---

i. Source: NIDA, (2016).
ii. Sources: NIDA, (2016) & DEA, (2015).
iii. Source: NIDA, (2016).
iv. Source: CBHSQ, (2016).

LSD (lysergic acid diethylamide)

A hallucinogen manufactured from lysergic acid, which is found in ergot, a fungus that grows on rye and other grains. LSD is an abbreviation of the scientific name lysergic acid diethylamide.[i]

Common Commercial Names	Street Names	Common Forms	Common Ways Taken	DEA Schedule / Legal Status
No commercial uses	Acid, Blotter, Blue Heaven, Cubes, Microdot, Yellow Sunshine, A, Windowpane	Tablet; capsule; clear liquid; small, decorated squares of absorbent paper that liquid has been added to	Ingested, absorbed through mouth tissues (paper squares)	Schedule I / Illegal

Uses & Possible Health Effects[ii]

Short-term Symptoms of Use	Rapid mood swings; distortion of a person's ability to recognize reality, think rationally, or communicate with others; raised blood pressure, heart rate, body temperature; dizziness and insomnia; loss of appetite; dry mouth; sweating; numbness; weakness; tremors; enlarged pupils; and impulsive behavior.
Long-term Consequences of Use and Health Effects	Frightening flashbacks (called Hallucinogen Persisting Perception Disorder [HPPD]); ongoing visual disturbances, disorganized thinking, paranoia, mood swings; and prolonged depression.
Other Health-related Issues	Unknown.
In Combination with Alcohol	May decrease the perceived effects of alcohol.
Withdrawal Symptoms	Unknown.

Treatment Options[iii]

Medications	There are no FDA-approved medications to treat addiction to LSD or other hallucinogens.
Behavioral Therapies	More research is needed to determine if behavioral therapies can be used to treat addiction to hallucinogens.

Statistics as of 2015[iv]

Prevalence	*Lifetime:* 25.3 million persons (9.5%) aged 12 or older have used LSD in their lifetime. *Past Year:* 1.5 million persons (0.6%) aged 12 or older have used LSD in the past year.
Average Age of Initiation	19.6

i. Source: NIDA, (2016).
ii. Sources: NIDA, (2016) & DEA, (2015).
iii. Source: NIDA, (2016).
iv. Source: CBHSQ, (2016).

Marijuana (Cannabis)

Marijuana is Cannabis sativa, a plant with psychoactive properties. The main psychoactive (mind-altering) chemical in marijuana is delta-9-tetrahydrocannabinol, or THC.[i]

Common Commercial Names	Street Names	Common Forms	Common Ways Taken	DEA Schedule / Legal Status
Various brand names in states where the sale of marijuana is legal	Marijuana: Blunt, Bud, Dope, Ganja, Grass, Green, Herb, Joint, Mary Jane, Pot, Reefer, Sinsemilla, Skunk, Smoke, Trees, Weed Hashish: Boom, Gangster, Hash, Hemp, THC	Greenish-gray mixture of dried, shredded leaves, stems, seeds, and/or flowers; resin (hashish) or sticky, black liquid (hash oil)	Smoked, ingested (mixed in food or brewed as tea)	Schedule I/ Illegal[ii] for both marijuana and THC, the active ingredient in marijuana, which is listed separately from marijuana. Marinol®, containing THC as synthetically-derived dronabinol, is an FDA-approved drug product, controlled in Schedule III / Legal by prescription only

Uses & Possible Health Effects[iii]

Short-term Symptoms of Use	Enhanced sensory perception and euphoria followed by drowsiness/relaxation; disinhibition, increased sociability; dry mouth; slowed reaction time; time distortion; impaired balance and coordination; increased heart rate and appetite; decreased blood pressure; problems with learning and memory; heightened imagination, hallucinations and delusions; anxiety; panic attacks; and psychosis.
Long-term Consequences of Use and Health Effects	Mental health problems, chronic cough, frequent respiratory infections, increased risk for cancer, and suppression of the immune system.
Other Health-related Issues	Breathing problems and increased risk of cancer of the head, neck, lungs, and respiratory tract. *Youth:* Possible loss of IQ points when repeated use begins in adolescence. *Pregnancy-related:* Babies born with problems with attention, memory, and problem solving.
In Combination with Alcohol	Increased heart rate, blood pressure; further slowing of mental processing and reaction time.
Withdrawal Symptoms	Irritability, trouble sleeping, decreased appetite, anxiety.
Medical Uses	Marino® is indicated for the treatment of: • Anorexia associated with weight loss in patients with AIDS; and • Nausea and vomiting associated with cancer chemotherapy in patients who have failed to respond adequately to conventional antiemetic treatments.

Treatment Options[iv]

Medications	There are no FDA-approved medications to treat marijuana addiction.
Behavioral Therapies	• Behavioral treatments tested with adolescents • Cognitive-behavioral therapy (CBT) • Contingency management, or motivational incentives • Motivational Enhancement Therapy (MET)

Marijuana (Cannabis)	
Statistics as of 2015[v]	
Prevalence	*Lifetime:* 117.9 million persons (44.0%) aged 12 or older have used marijuana in their lifetime.
	Past Year: 36.0 million persons (13.5%) aged 12 or older have used marijuana in the past year.
Average Age of Initiation	19.0

i. Source: NIDA, (2016).
ii. As of this writing, 25 states and the District of Columbia have legalized medical marijuana use, four states have legalized retail marijuana sales, and the District of Columbia has legalized personal use and home cultivation (both medical and recreational). See Chapter 3 - Prevention Programs and Policies for more detail on this issue.
iii. Sources: NIDA, (2016) & DEA, (2015).
iv. Source: NIDA, (2016).
v. Source: CBHSQ, (2016).

MDMA (Ecstasy)

A synthetic, psychoactive drug that has similarities to both the stimulant amphetamine and the hallucinogen mescaline. MDMA is an abbreviation of the scientific name 3,4-methylenedioxy-methamphetamine.[i]

Common Commercial Names	Street Names	Common Forms	Common Ways Taken	DEA Schedule / Legal Status
No commercial uses	Adam, Clarity, Eve, Lover's Speed, Peace, Uppers, E, X, XTC, Molly	Colorful tablets with imprinted logos, capsules, powder, liquid	Ingested, snorted	Schedule I / Illegal

Uses & Possible Health Effects[ii]

Short-term Symptoms of Use	Lowered inhibition and coordination; sleep disturbances; enhanced sensory perception; confusion; depression; sleep problems; anxiety; increased heart rate and blood pressure; muscle tension; teeth clenching; increased motor activity, alertness; nausea; blurred vision; faintness; chills or sweating; sharp rise in body temperature leading to liver, kidney, or heart failure and death.
Long-term Consequences of Use and Health Effects	Long lasting confusion; depression; damage to the serotonin system; problems with attention, memory, and sleep; increased anxiety, impulsiveness, and aggression; loss of appetite; and less interest in sex.
Other Health-related Issues	Unknown.
In Combination with Alcohol	May increase the risk of cell and organ damage.
Withdrawal Symptoms	Fatigue, loss of appetite, depression, and trouble concentrating.

Treatment Options[iii]

Medications	There is conflicting evidence about whether MDMA is addictive. There are no FDA-approved medications to treat MDMA addiction.
Behavioral Therapies	More research is needed to determine if behavioral therapies can be used to treat potential MDMA addiction.

Statistics as of 2015[iv]

Prevalence	*Lifetime:* 18.3 million persons (6.8%) aged 12 or older have used ecstasy in their lifetime. *Past Year:* 2.6 million persons (1.0%) aged 12 or older have used ecstasy in the past year.
Average Age of Initiation	20.7

i. Source: NIDA, (2016).
ii. Sources: NIDA, (2016) & DEA, (2015).
iii. Source: NIDA, (2016).
iv. Source: CBHSQ, (2016).

Mescaline (Peyote)				
A hallucinogen found in disk-shaped "buttons" in the crown of several cacti, including peyote, and can also be created synthetically.[i]				
Common Commercial Names	Street Names	Common Forms	Common Ways Taken	DEA Schedule / Legal Status
No commercial uses	Buttons, Cactus, Mesc, Peyote	Fresh or dried buttons, capsule	Ingested (chewed or soaked in water and drunk) or smoked	Schedule I / Illegal
Uses & Possible Health Effects[ii]				
Short-term Symptoms of Use	Enhanced perception and feeling; hallucinations; euphoria; anxiety; increased body temperature, heart rate, blood pressure; sweating; headaches; and impaired motor coordination.			
Long-term Consequences of Use and Health Effects	Unknown.			
Other Health-related Issues	Unknown.			
In Combination with Alcohol	Unknown.			
Withdrawal Symptoms	Unknown.			
Treatment Options[iii]				
Medications	There are no FDA-approved medications to treat addiction to mescaline or other hallucinogens.			
Behavioral Therapies	More research is needed to determine if behavioral therapies can be used to treat addiction to hallucinogens.			
Statistics as of 2015[iv]				
Prevalence	*Lifetime:* • Mescaline: 8.0 million persons (3.0%) aged 12 or older have used mescaline in their lifetime. • Peyote: 5.5 million persons (2.0%) aged 12 or older have used peyote in their lifetime. *Past Year:* 4.7 million persons (1.8%) aged 12 or older have used hallucinogens in the past year.			
Average Age of Initiation	Hallucinogens in general: 19.6			

i. Source: NIDA, (2016).
ii. Sources: NIDA, (2016) & DEA, (2015).
iii. Source: NIDA, (2016).
iv. Source: CBHSQ, (2016).

Methamphetamine

An extremely addictive stimulant amphetamine drug.[i]

Common Commercial Names	Street Names	Common Forms	Common Ways Taken	DEA Schedule / Legal Status
Desoxyn®	Crank, Chalk, Crystal, Fire, Glass, Go Fast, Ice, Meth, Speed	White powder or pill; crystal meth looks like pieces of glass or shiny blue-white "rocks" of different sizes	Ingested, snorted, smoked, injected	Schedule II / Illegal (except for Desoxyn® by prescription only)

Uses & Possible Health Effects[ii]

Short-term Symptoms of Use	Increased wakefulness and physical activity; decreased appetite; hyperthermia; increased breathing, heart rate, blood pressure, temperature; irregular heartbeat; and death from cardiac arrest, stroke, or suicide.
Long-term Consequences of Use and Health Effects	Anxiety, confusion, insomnia, mood problems, violent behavior, paranoia, hallucinations, delusions, weight loss, severe dental problems ("meth mouth"), memory loss, intense itching leading to skin sores from scratching and high-risk for addiction.
Other Health-related Issues	Sharing needles increases the risk of contracting infectious diseases like HIV and Hepatitis B and C. Pregnancy-related: premature delivery; separation of the placenta from the uterus; low birth weight; lethargy; heart and brain problems.
In Combination with Alcohol	Masks the depressant effect of alcohol, increasing risk of alcohol overdose; may increase blood pressure and jitters.
Withdrawal Symptoms	Depression, anxiety, tiredness.
Medical Uses	Desoxyn® is indicated for the treatment of: • Attention Deficit Disorder with Hyperactivity • Exogenous Obesity

Treatment Options[iii]

Medications	There are no FDA-approved medications to treat methamphetamine addiction.
Behavioral Therapies	• Cognitive-behavioral therapy (CBT) • Contingency management or motivational incentives • The Matrix Model • 12-Step facilitation therapy

Statistics as of 2015[iv]

Prevalence	*Lifetime:* 14.5 million persons (5.4%) aged 12 or older have used methamphetamine in their lifetime. Methamphetamine needle use: 1.9 million persons (0.7%) *Past Year:* 1.7 million persons (0.6%) aged 12 or older have used methamphetamine in the past year.
Average Age of Initiation	25.8

i. Source: NIDA, (2016).
ii. Sources: NIDA, (2016) & DEA, (2015).
iii. Source: NIDA, (2016).
iv. Source: CBHSQ, (2016).

Over-the-counter Cough/Cold Medicines (Dextromethorphan or DXM)				
Psychoactive when taken in higher-than-recommended amounts.[i]				
Common Commercial Names	Street Names	Common Forms	Common Ways Taken	DEA Schedule / Legal Status
Various (many brand names include "DM")	Robotripping, Robo, Triple C	Suspension, capsule	Ingested	Cough medicines with codeine are Schedule V. DXM is not Scheduled and is an over-the-counter medication
Uses & Possible Health Effects[ii]				
Short-term Symptoms of Use	Euphoria; slurred speech; increased heart rate, blood pressure, and body temperature; numbness; dizziness; nausea; vomiting; confusion; hallucinations; paranoia; agitation; altered visual perceptions; loss of coordination, problems with movement; buildup of excess acid in body fluids; liver damage; seizures; and coma.			
Long-term Consequences of Use and Health Effects	Unknown.			
Other Health-related Issues	Breathing problems, seizures, and increased heart rate may occur from other ingredients in cough/cold medicines.			
In Combination with Alcohol	Increased risk of adverse effects.			
Withdrawal Symptoms	Unknown.			
Medical Use[iii]	Used for cough suppression.			
Treatment Options[iv]				
Medications	There are no FDA-approved medications to treat addiction to over-the-counter cough/cold medicines.			
Behavioral Therapies	More research is needed to determine if behavioral therapies can be used to treat addiction to over-the-counter cough/cold medicines.			
Statistics as of 2015[v]				
Prevalence	*Lifetime:* Data not collected. *Past Year:* Data not collected.			
Average Age of Initiation	Stimulants in general: 22.3			

i. Source: NIDA, (2016).
ii. Sources: NIDA, (2016) & DEA, (2015).
iii. Source: SAMHSA, (2004).
iv. Source: NIDA, (2016).
v. Source: CBHSQ, (2016).

PCP (Phencyclidine)

A dissociative drug developed as an intravenous anesthetic that has been discontinued due to serious adverse effects. Dissociative drugs are hallucinogens that cause the user to feel detached from reality.[i]

Common Commercial Names	Street Names	Common Forms	Common Ways Taken	DEA Schedule / Legal Status
No commercial uses	Angel Dust, Boat, Hog, Love Boat, Peace Pill, Angel Mist	White or colored powder, tablet, or capsule; clear liquid	Injected, snorted, ingested, smoked (powder added to mint, parsley, oregano, or marijuana)	Schedule I, II / Illegal

Uses & Possible Health Effects[ii]

Short-term Symptoms of Use	Delusions, hallucinations, paranoia, problems thinking, a sense of distance from one's environment, anxiety. *Low doses:* slight increase in pulse and breathing rate; increased blood pressure and heart rate; shallow breathing; face redness and sweating; numbness of the hands or feet; and loss of coordination. *High doses:* lowered blood pressure, heart rate, and breathing; nausea; vomiting; blurred vision; flicking up and down of the eyes; drooling; loss of balance; dizziness; violence; suicidal thoughts; seizures, coma, and death.
Long-term Consequences of Use and Health Effects	Memory loss, problems with speech and thinking, depression, psychosis, weight loss, anxiety.
Other Health-related Issues	PCP has been linked to self-injury. Risk of HIV, hepatitis, and other infectious diseases from shared needles.
In Combination with Alcohol	Increased risk of coma.
Withdrawal Symptoms	Headaches and sweating.

Treatment Options[iii]

Medications	There are no FDA-approved medications to treat addiction to PCP or other dissociative drugs.
Behavioral Therapies	More research is needed to determine if behavioral therapies can be used to treat addiction to dissociative drugs.

Statistics as of 2015[iv]

Prevalence	*Lifetime:* 6.3 million persons (2.4%) aged 12 or older have used PCP in their lifetime. *Past Year:* 120,000 persons (<0.1%) aged 12 or older have used PCP in the past year.
Average Age of Initiation	15.3

i. Source: NIDA, (2016).
ii. Source: NIDA, (2016).
iii. Source: NIDA, (2016).
iv. Source: CBHSQ, (2016).

Prescription Opioids

Pain relievers with an origin similar to that of heroin. Opioids can cause euphoria and are sometimes used nonmedically, leading to overdose deaths.[i]

Common Commercial Names	Street Names	Common Forms	Common Ways Taken	DEA Schedule / Legal Status
Codeine (various brand names)	Captain Cody, Cody, Lean, Schoolboy, Sizzurp, Purple Drank With glutethimide: Doors & Fours, Loads, Pancakes and Syrup	Tablet, capsule, liquid	Injected, ingested (often mixed with soda and flavorings)	Schedule II, III, V / Legal by prescription only
Fentanyl (Actiq®, Duragesic®, Sublimaze®)	Apache, China Girl, China White, Dance Fever, Friend, Goodfella, Jackpot, Murder 8, Tango and Cash, TNT	Lozenge, sublingual tablet, film, buccal tablet	Injected, smoked, snorted	Schedule II / Legal by prescription only
Hydrocodone or dihydrocodeinone (Vicodin®, Lortab®, Lorcet®, and others)	Vike, Watson-387	Capsule, liquid, tablet	Ingested, snorted, injected	Schedule II / Legal by prescription only
Hydromorphone (Dilaudid®)	D, Dillies, Footballs, Juice, Smack	Liquid, suppository	Injected, rectally inserted	Schedule II / Legal by prescription only
Meperidine (Demerol®)	Demmies, Pain Killer	Tablet, liquid	Ingested, snorted, injected	Schedule II / Legal by prescription only
Methadone (Dolophine®)	Amidone, Fizzies With MDMA: Chocolate Chip Cookies	Tablet	Ingested, injected	Schedule II / Legal by prescription only for pain indication
Morphine, various brand names	M, Miss Emma, Monkey, White Stuff	Tablet, liquid, capsule, suppository	Ingested, injected, smoked	Schedule II, III / Legal by prescription only
Oxycodone (OxyContin®, Percodan®, Percocet®, and others)	O.C., Oxycet, Oxycotton, Oxy, Hillbilly Heroin, Percs	Capsule, liquid, tablet	Ingested, snorted, injected	Schedule II / Legal by prescription only
Oxymorphone (Opana®)	Biscuits, Blue Heaven, Blues, Mrs. O, O Bomb, Octagons, Stop Signs	Tablet	Ingested, snorted, injected	Schedule II / Legal by prescription only

i. Sources: NIDA, (2016) & DEA, (2015).

Prescription Opioids

Uses & Possible Health Effects[ii]

Short-term Symptoms of Use	Pain relief, drowsiness, nausea, constipation, altered judgment and decision making, sedation, euphoria, confusion, clammy skin, muscle weakness, slowed breathing, lowered heart rate and blood pressure, coma, heart failure, and death. For oxycodone specifically: Pain relief, sedation, respiratory depression, constipation, papillary constriction, and cough suppression. For fentanyl specifically: Fentanyl is about 100 times more potent than morphine as an analgesic and results in frequent overdoses.
Long-term Consequences of Use and Health Effects	Heart or respiratory problems. Extended or chronic use of oxycodone containing acetaminophen may cause severe liver damage. Abuse of opioid medications can lead to psychological dependence.
Other Health-related Issues	Pregnancy-related: Miscarriage, low birth weight, neonatal abstinence syndrome. Older adults: higher risk of accidental misuse or abuse because many older adults have multiple prescriptions, increasing the risk of drug-drug interactions, and breakdown of drugs slows with age; also, many older adults are treated with prescription medications for pain. Risk of HIV, hepatitis, and other infectious diseases from shared needles.
In Combination with Alcohol	Dangerous slowing of heart rate and breathing leading to coma or death.
Withdrawal Symptoms	Restlessness, anxiety, muscle and bone pain, insomnia, diarrhea, vomiting, cold flashes with goose bumps, and muscle tremors.
Medical Use[iii]	Used for pain relief. Methadone is also used to treat opioid use disorders.

Treatment Options[iv]

Medications	• Methadone • Buprenorphine • Naltrexone (oral and extended-release injectable)
Behavioral Therapies	Behavioral therapies that have helped treat addiction to heroin may be useful in treating prescription opioid addiction.

Statistics as of 2015[v]

Prevalence	*Lifetime:* 36 million persons (13.6%) aged 12 or older have misused pain relievers in their lifetime. *Past Year:* 12.5 million persons (4.7 %) aged 12 or older have misused pain relievers in the past year. • OxyContin®: 1.7 million persons (0.7%) aged 12 or older have used OxyContin® non-medically in the past year.
Average Age of Initiation	Prescription Opioids: 25.8

---

ii. Sources: NIDA, (2016) & DEA, (2015).
iii. Source: SAMHSA, (2004).
iv. Source: NIDA, (2016).
v. Source: CBHSQ, (2016).

Prescription Sedatives (Tranquilizers, Depressants)				
Medications that slow brain activity, which makes them useful for treating anxiety and sleep problems.[i]				
Common Commercial Names	Street Names	Common Forms	Common Ways Taken	DEA Schedule / Legal Status
Barbiturates: pentobarbital (Nembutal®), phenobarbital (Luminal®)	Barbs, Phennies, Red Birds, Reds, Tooies, Yellow Jackets, Yellows	Pill, capsule, liquid	Ingested, injected	Schedule II, III, IV / Legal by prescription only
Benzodiazepines: alprazolam (Xanax®), chlordiazepoxide (Limbitrol®), diazepam (Valium®), lorazepam (Ativan®), triazolam (Halcion®)	Candy, Downers, Sleeping Pills, Tranks	Pill, capsule, liquid	Ingested, snorted	Schedule IV / Legal by prescription only
Sleep Medications: eszopiclone (Lunesta®), zaleplon (Sonata®), zolpidem (Ambien®)	Forget-me Pill, Mexican Valium, R2, Roche, Roofies, Roofinol, Rope, Rophies	Pill, capsule, liquid	Ingested, snorted	Schedule IV / Legal by prescription only
Uses & Possible Health Effects[ii]				
Short-term Symptoms of Use	Drowsiness, sedation; slurred speech; poor concentration, confusion, dizziness; clammy skin; impaired judgment, coordination and memory; reduced anxiety; lowered blood pressure; slowed breathing and central nervous system; coma, and death.			
Long-term Consequences of Use and Health Effects	Increased risk of respiratory distress.			
Other Health-related Issues	Sleep medications are sometimes used as date rape drugs. Risk of HIV, hepatitis, and other infectious diseases from shared needles.			
In Combination with Alcohol	Dangerous slowdown of heart rate and breathing, coma, and death.			
Withdrawal Symptoms	Must be discussed with a health care professional; barbiturate withdrawal can cause a serious abstinence syndrome that may even include seizures.			
Medical Use[iii]	For tranquilization, sedation, and sleep.			
Treatment Options[iv]				
Medications	There are no FDA-approved medications to treat addiction to prescription sedatives; lowering the dose over time must be done with the help of a health care professional.			
Behavioral Therapies	More research is needed to determine if behavioral therapies can be used to treat addiction to prescription sedatives.			
Statistics as of 2015[v]				
Prevalence	*Lifetime:* Data not collected. *Past Year:* • 1.5 million persons (0.6%) aged 12 or older have misused sedatives in the past year. • 6.1 million persons (2.3%) aged 12 or older have misused tranquilizers in the past year.			
Average Age of Initiation	Sedatives: 28.3 Tranquilizers: 25.9			

i. Source: NIDA, (2016).
ii. Sources: NIDA, (2016) & DEA, (2015).
iii. Source: SAMHSA, (2004).
iv. Source: NIDA, (2016).
v. Source: CBHSQ, (2016).

Prescription Stimulants

Medications that increase alertness, attention, energy, blood pressure, heart rate, and breathing rate.[i]

Common Commercial Names	Street Names	Common Forms	Common Ways Taken	DEA Schedule / Legal Status
Amphetamine (Adderall®, Benzedrine®)	Bennies, Black Beauties, Crosses, Hearts, LA Turnaround, Speed, Truck Drivers, Uppers	Tablet, capsule	Ingested, snorted, smoked, injected	Schedule II / Legal by prescription only
Methylphenidate (Concerta®, Ritalin®)	JIF, MPH, R-ball, Skippy, The Smart Drug, Vitamin R	Liquid, tablet, chewable tablet, capsule	Ingested, snorted, smoked, injected, chewed	Schedule II / Legal by prescription only

Uses & Possible Health Effects[ii]

Short-term Symptoms of Use	Increased alertness, attention, energy; euphoria; insomnia, wakefulness; increased blood pressure and body temperature, metabolism, and heart rate; narrowed blood vessels; increased blood sugar; agitation; opened-up breathing passages; and violent and erratic behavior. High doses: dangerously high body temperature and irregular heartbeat; seizures; and death from heart failure or suicide. For amphetamines specifically: Paranoia, picking at the skin, preoccupation with one's own thoughts, and auditory and visual hallucinations.
Long-term Consequences of Use and Health Effects	Heart problems, psychosis, anger, paranoia, addiction, and chronic sleep problems.
Other Health-related Issues	Risk of HIV, hepatitis, and other infectious diseases from shared needles.
In Combination with Alcohol	Masks the depressant action of alcohol, increasing risk of alcohol overdose; may increase blood pressure and jitters.
Withdrawal Symptoms	Depression, tiredness, and sleep problems.
Medical Use[iii]	For narcolepsy, obesity, and hyperkinesis.

Treatment Options[iv]

Medications	There are no FDA-approved medications to treat stimulant addiction.
Behavioral Therapies	Behavioral therapies that have helped treat addiction to cocaine or methamphetamine may be useful in treating prescription stimulant addiction.

Statistics as of 2015[v]

Prevalence	*Lifetime:* Data not collected. *Past Year:* 5.3 million (2.0%) aged 12 or older have misused stimulants in the past year.
Average Age of Initiation	Stimulants in general: 22.3

---

i. Source: NIDA, (2016).
ii. Sources: NIDA, (2016) & DEA, (2015).
iii. Source: SAMHSA, (2004).
iv. Source: NIDA, (2016).
v. Source: CBHSQ, (2016).

Psilocybin				
A hallucinogen in certain types of mushrooms that grow in parts of South America, Mexico, and the United States.[i]				
Common Commercial Names	Street Names	Common Forms	Common Ways Taken	DEA Schedule / Legal Status
No commercial uses	Little Smoke, Magic Mushrooms, Purple Passion, Shrooms	Fresh or dried mushrooms with long, slender stems topped by caps with dark gills	Ingested (eaten, brewed as tea, or added to other foods)	Schedule I / Illegal
Uses & Possible Health Effects[ii]				
Short-term Symptoms of Use	Hallucinations, altered perception of time, inability to tell fantasy from reality, panic, muscle relaxation or weakness, loss of coordination, enlarged pupils, nausea, vomiting, and drowsiness.			
Long-term Consequences of Use and Health Effects	Risk of flashbacks, psychosis, and memory problems.			
Other Health-related Issues	Risk of poisoning if a poisonous mushroom is accidentally used.			
In Combination with Alcohol	May decrease the perceived effects of alcohol.			
Withdrawal Symptoms	Unknown.			
Treatment Options[iii]				
Medications	It is not known whether psilocybin is addictive. There are no FDA-approved medications to treat addiction to psilocybin or other hallucinogens.			
Behavioral Therapies	More research is needed to determine if psilocybin is addictive and whether behavioral therapies can be used to treat addiction to this or other hallucinogens.			
Statistics as of 2014[iv]				
Prevalence	*Lifetime:* 22.8 million persons (8.5%) aged 12 or older have used psilocybin in their lifetime. *Past Year:* Data not collected.			
Average Age of Initiation	Hallucinogens in general: 19.6			

i. Source: NIDA, (2016).
ii. Sources: NIDA, (2016) & DEA, (2015).
iii. Source: NIDA, (2016).
iv. Source: CBHSQ, (2016).

Rohypnol® (Flunitrazepam)

A benzodiazepine chemically similar to prescription sedatives such as Valium® and Xanax®. Teens and young adults tend to abuse this drug at bars, nightclubs, concerts, and parties. It has been used to commit sexual assaults due to its ability to sedate and incapacitate unsuspecting victims.[1]

Common Commercial Names	Street Names	Common Forms	Common Ways Taken	DEA Schedule / Legal Status
Flunitrazepam, Rohypnol®	Circles, Date Rape Drug, Forget Pill, Forget-Me Pill, La Rocha, Lunch Money, Mexican Valium, Mind Eraser, Pingus, R2, Reynolds, Rib, Roach, Roach 2, Roaches, Roachies, Roapies, Rochas Dos, Roofies, Rope, Rophies, Row-Shay, Ruffies, Trip-and-Fall, Wolfies	Tablet	Ingested (as a pill or as dissolved in a drink), snorted	Schedule IV / Rohypnol® is not approved for medical use in the United States; it is available as a prescription sleep aid in other countries

Uses & Possible Health Effects[ii]

Short-term Symptoms of Use	Drowsiness, sedation, sleep; amnesia, blackout; decreased anxiety; muscle relaxation, impaired reaction time and motor coordination; impaired mental functioning and judgment; confusion; aggression; excitability; slurred speech; headache; slowed breathing and heart rate.
Long-term Consequences of Use and Health Effects[iii]	Physical and psychological dependence; cardiovascular collapse; and death
Other Health-related Issues	Sometimes used as a date rape drug.
In Combination with Alcohol	Exaggerated intoxication, severe sedation, unconsciousness, and slowed heart rate and breathing, which can lead to death.
Withdrawal Symptoms	Headache; muscle pain; extreme anxiety, tension, restlessness, confusion, irritability; numbness and tingling of hands or feet; hallucinations, delirium, convulsions, seizures, or shock.

Treatment Options[iv]

Medications	There are no FDA-approved medications to treat addiction to Rohypnol® or other prescription sedatives.
Behavioral Therapies	More research is needed to determine if behavioral therapies can be used to treat addiction to Rohypnol® or other prescription sedatives.

Statistics as of 2015[v]

Prevalence	*Lifetime:* Data not collected. *Past Year:* Data not collected.
Average Age of Initiation	Sedatives in general: 23.4

i. Source: NIDA, (2016).
ii. Sources: NIDA, (2016) & DEA, (2015).
iii. Source: Rohypnol Abuse Treatment, (n.d.).
iv. Source: NIDA, (2016).
v. Source: CBHSQ, (2016).

Salvia				
A dissociative drug (Salvia divinorum) that is an herb in the mint family native to southern Mexico. Dissociative drugs are hallucinogens that cause the user to feel detached from reality.[i]				
Common Commercial Names	Street Names	Common Forms	Common Ways Taken	DEA Schedule / Legal Status
Sold legally in most states as Salvia divinorum	Magic mint, Maria Pastora, Sally-D, Shepherdess's Herb, Diviner's Sage	Fresh or dried leaves	Smoked, chewed, or brewed as tea	Not scheduled; labeled drug of concern by DEA / Illegal in some states
Uses & Possible Health Effects[ii]				
Short-term Symptoms of Use	Short-lived but intense hallucinations; loss of coordination, dizziness, slurred speech; altered visual perception, mood, body sensations; mood swings, feelings of detachment from one's body; sweating; uncontrollable laughter; and paranoia.			
Long-term Consequences of Use and Health Effects	Unknown.			
Other Health-related Issues	Unknown.			
In Combination with Alcohol	Unknown.			
Withdrawal Symptoms	Unknown.			
Treatment Options[iii]				
Medications	It is not known whether salvia is addictive. There are no FDA-approved medications to treat addiction to salvia or other dissociative drugs.			
Behavioral Therapies	More research is needed to determine if salvia is addictive, but behavioral therapies can be used to treat addiction to dissociative drugs.			
Statistics as of 2015[iv]				
Prevalence	*Lifetime:* 5.1 million persons (1.9%) aged 12 or older have used salvia in their lifetime. *Past Year:* Data not collected.			
Average Age of Initiation	Hallucinogens in general: 19.6			

i. Source: NIDA, (2016).
ii. Sources: NIDA, (2016) & DEA, (2015).
iii. Source: NIDA, (2016).
iv. Source: CBHSQ, (2016).

Steroids (Anabolic)

Man-made substances used to treat conditions caused by low levels of steroid hormones in the body and abused to enhance athletic and sexual performance and physical appearance.[i]

Common Commercial Names	Street Names	Common Forms	Common Ways Taken	DEA Schedule / Legal Status
Nandrolone (Oxandrin®), oxandrolone (Anadrol®), oxymetholone (Winstrol®), stanozolol (Durabolin®), testosterone cypionate (Depo-testosterone®)	Juice, Gym Candy, Pumpers, Roids	Tablet, capsule, liquid drops, gel, cream, patch, injectable solution	Injected, ingested, applied to skin	Schedule III / Legal by prescription only

Uses & Possible Health Effects[ii]

Short-term Symptoms of Use	Headache, acne, fluid retention (especially in the hands and feet), oily skin, yellowing of the skin and whites of the eyes, and infection at the injection site.
Long-term Consequences of Use and Health Effects	Kidney damage or failure; liver damage; high blood pressure, enlarged heart, or changes in cholesterol leading to increased risk of stroke or heart attack, even in young people; hostility and aggression; extreme mood swings; anger ("roid rage"); paranoid jealousy; extreme irritability; delusions; impaired judgment.
Other Health-related Issues	Risk of HIV, hepatitis, and other infectious diseases from shared needles. *Males:* shrunken testicles, lowered sperm count, infertility, baldness, development of breasts, increased risk for prostate cancer. *Females:* facial hair, male-pattern baldness, menstrual cycle changes, enlargement of the clitoris, deepened voice. *Adolescents:* stunted growth.
In Combination with Alcohol	Increased risk of violent behavior.
Withdrawal Symptoms	Mood swings; tiredness; restlessness; loss of appetite; insomnia; lowered sex drive; depression, sometimes leading to suicide attempts.
Medical Use	Used to treat conditions caused by low levels of steroid hormones in the body.

Treatment Options[iii]

Medications	Hormone therapy
Behavioral Therapies	More research is needed to determine if behavioral therapies can be used to treat steroid addiction.

Statistics as of 2015[iv]

Prevalence	Data not collected.
Average Age of Initiation	Data not collected.

i. Source: NIDA, (2016).
ii. Sources: NIDA, (2016) & DEA, (2015).
iii. Source: NIDA, (2016).
iv. Source: CBHSQ, (2016).

Synthetic Cannabinoids ("K2"/"Spice")

A wide variety of herbal mixtures containing man-made cannabinoid chemicals related to THC in marijuana but often much stronger and more dangerous. Sometimes misleadingly called "synthetic marijuana" and marketed as a "natural," "safe," legal alternative to marijuana.[1]

Common Commercial Names	Street Names	Common Forms	Common Ways Taken	DEA Schedule / Legal Status
No commercial uses	K2, Spice, Black Mamba, Bliss, Bombay Blue, Fake Weed, Fire, Genie, Moon Rocks, Skunk, Smacked, Yucatan, Zohai	Dried, shredded plant material that looks like potpourri and is sometimes sold as "incense"	Smoked, ingested (brewed as tea)	Schedule I

Uses & Possible Health Effects[ii]

Short-term Symptoms of Use	Increased heart rate and blood pressure; vomiting; agitation; confusion; hallucinations, anxiety, paranoia; euphoria, relaxation; headache; numbness and tingling; reduced blood supply to the heart; heart attack; and seizures.
Long-term Consequences of Use and Health Effects	Kidney damage and psychosis.
Other Health-related Issues	Use of synthetic cannabinoids has led to an increase in emergency department visits in certain areas.
In Combination with Alcohol	Unknown.
Withdrawal Symptoms	Headaches, anxiety, depression, irritability.

Treatment Options[iii]

Medications	There are no FDA-approved medications to treat K2/Spice addiction.
Behavioral Therapies	More research is needed to determine if behavioral therapies can be used to treat synthetic cannabinoid addiction.

Statistics as of 2015[iv]

Prevalence	Data not collected.
Average Age of Initiation	Data not collected.

i. Source: NIDA, (2016).
ii. Sources: NIDA, (2016) & DEA, (2015).
iii. Source: NIDA, (2016).
iv. Source: CBHSQ, (2016).

Synthetic Cathinones ("Bath Salts")

An emerging family of drugs containing one or more synthetic chemicals related to cathinone, a stimulant found naturally in the khat plant. Examples of such chemicals include mephedrone, methylone, and 3,4-methylenedioxypyrovalerone (MDPV).[i]

Common Commercial Names	Street Names	Common Forms	Common Ways Taken	DEA Schedule / Legal Status
No commercial names for "bath salts"	Bloom, Cloud Nine, Cosmic Blast, Ivory Wave, Lunar Wave, Scarface, Vanilla Sky, White Lightning *MDPV and mephedrone:* Meow meow, MCAT, drone, plant feeder, bubbles, bliss, blue silk, cloud nine, energy-1, ivory wave, lunar wave, ocean burst, pure ivory, purple wave, red dove, snow leopard, stardust, vanilla sky, white dove, white night, and white lightning	White or brown crystalline powder sold in small plastic or foil packages labeled "not for human consumption" and sometimes sold as jewelry cleaner; tablet, capsule, liquid	Ingested, snorted, injected, ingested, smoked	Schedule I

Uses & Possible Health Effects[ii]

Short-term Symptoms of Use	Increased heart rate and blood pressure; euphoria; increased sociability and sex drive; paranoia, agitation, and hallucinations; psychotic and violent behavior; nosebleeds; sweating; headaches; teeth grinding; nausea, vomiting; insomnia; irritability; dizziness; depression; suicidal thoughts; panic attacks; reduced motor control; and cloudy thinking.
Long-term Consequences of Use and Health Effects	Breakdown of skeletal muscle tissue, kidney failure, psychosis, and death.
Other Health-related Issues	Risk of HIV, hepatitis, and other infectious diseases from injecting with shared needles.
In Combination with Alcohol	Unknown.
Withdrawal Symptoms	Depression, anxiety, problems sleeping, tremors, paranoia.

Treatment Options[iii]

Medications	There are no FDA-approved medications to treat addiction to bath salts.
Behavioral Therapies	<ul><li>Behavioral treatments geared to teens</li><li>Cognitive-behavioral therapy (CBT)</li><li>Contingency management, or motivational incentives</li><li>Motivational Enhancement Therapy (MET)</li></ul>

Statistics as of 2015[iv]

Prevalence	Data not collected.
Average Age of Initiation	Data not collected.

i. Source: NIDA, (2016).
ii. Sources: NIDA, (2016) & DEA, (2015).
iii. Source: NIDA, (2016).
iv. Source: CBHSQ, (2016).

References

1. U.S. Department of Justice, Drug Enforcement Administration. (2015). *Drugs of abuse.* Washington, DC: Drug Enforcement Administration.

2. Inhalant Addiction Treatment. (n.d.). Dangers of mixing inhalants with alcohol and other drugs. Retrieved from http://www.inhalantaddictiontreatment.com/dangers-of-mixing-inhalants-with-alcohol-and-other-drugs. Accessed on June 10, 2016.

3. National Institute on Alcohol Abuse and Alcoholism. (n.d.). Alcohol's effects on the body. Retrieved from http://www.niaaa.nih.gov/alcohol-health/alcohols-effects-body. *Accessed* on June 12, 2016.

4. National Institute on Drug Abuse. (2016). *Commonly abused drugs.* Retrieved from https://www.drugabuse.gov/sites/default/files/commonly_abused_drugs_final_04202016.pdf. Accessed on June 10, 2016.

5. National Institute on Alcohol Abuse and Alcoholism. (2014). *Treatment for alcohol problems: Finding and getting help.* (NIH Publication No. 14–7974). Rockville, MD: National Institutes of Health.

6. U.S. National Library of Medicine. (2015). Alcohol withdrawal. Retrieved from https://www.nlm.nih.gov/medlineplus/ency/article/000764.htm. Accessed on June 12, 2016.

7. Rohypnol Abuse Treatment. (n.d.). Does Rohypnol abuse have permanent side effects? Retrieved from http://rohypnolabusetreatment.com/does-rohypnol-abuse-have-permanent-side-effects. Accessed on June 10, 2016.

8. Substance Abuse and Mental Health Services Administration. (2004). *Keeping youth drug free.* (DHHS Publication No. (SMA)-3772). Rockville, MD: Substance Abuse and Mental Health Services Administration, Center for Substance Abuse Prevention.

9. Center for Behavioral Health Statistics and Quality. (2016). *Results from the 2015 National Survey on Drug Use and Health: Detailed tables.* Rockville, MD: Substance Abuse and Mental Health Services Administration.

10. U.S. Department of Justice. (n.d.). Title 21 code of federal regulations: Part 1308 — Schedules of controlled substances. Retrieved from http://www.deadiversion.usdoj.gov/21cfr/cfr/2108cfrt.htm. Accessed on June 27, 2016.

11. U.S. National Library of Medicine. (2015). Neonatal abstinence syndrome. Retrieved from https://www.nlm.nih.gov/medlineplus/ency/article/007313.htm. Accessed on July 5, 2016.

12. Gepner, Y., Golan, R., Harman-Boehm, I., Henkin, Y., Schwarzfuchs, D., Shelef, I., ... Shai, I. (2015). Effects of initiating moderate alcohol intake on cardiometabolic risk in adults with type 2 diabetes: A 2-year randomized, controlled trial. *Annals of Internal Medicine, 163,* 569–579.

13. Howard, A. A., Arnsten, J. H., & Gourevitch, M. N. (2004). Effect of alcohol consumption on diabetes mellitus: a systematic review. *Annals of Internal Medicine, 140*(3), 211-219.

14. Stockwell, T., Zhao, J., Panwar, S., Roemer, A., Naimi, T., & Chikritzhs, T. (2016). Do "moderate" drinkers have reduced mortality risk? A systematic review and meta-analysis of alcohol consumption and all-cause mortality. *Journal of Studies on Alcohol and Drugs, 77*(2), 185-198.

15. Fillmore, K. M., Kerr, W. C., Stockwell, T., Chikritzhs, T., & Bostrom, A. (2006). Moderate alcohol use and reduced mortality risk: Systematic error in prospective studies. *Addiction Research & Theory,* 14(2), 101-132.

Made in the USA
Lexington, KY
23 December 2017